Medicinal Chemistry for Pharmacy Students

Volume 2

Medicinal Chemistry of Drugs Affecting the Nervous System

Edited by

M. O. Faruk Khan

University of Charleston School of Pharmacy
Charleston, WV
USA

&

Ashok E. Philip

Union University College of Pharmacy
Jackson, TN
USA

Medicinal Chemistry for Pharmacy Students

Volume # 2

Medicinal Chemistry of Drugs Affecting the Nervous System

Editors: M. O. Faruk Khan & Ashok E. Philip

ISSN (Online): 2589-6989

ISSN (Print): 2589-6997

ISBN (Online): 978-981-14-5407-3

ISBN (Print): 978-981-14-5405-9

ISBN (Paperback): 978-981-14-5406-6

Published by Bentham Science Publishers Pte. Ltd. Singapore. All Rights Reserved.

need for a court order if at any point you breach any terms of this License Agreement. In no event will any delay or failure by Bentham Science Publishers in enforcing your compliance with this License Agreement constitute a waiver of any of its rights.

3. You acknowledge that you have read this License Agreement, and agree to be bound by its terms and conditions. To the extent that any other terms and conditions presented on any website of Bentham Science Publishers conflict with, or are inconsistent with, the terms and conditions set out in this License Agreement, you acknowledge that the terms and conditions set out in this License Agreement shall prevail.

Bentham Science Publishers Pte. Ltd.
80 Robinson Road #02-00
Singapore 068898
Singapore
Email: subscriptions@benthamscience.net

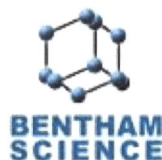

CONTENTS

PREFACE

This is the second volume of the book series, *"Medicinal Chemistry for Pharmacy Students"*. The primary objective of this e-Book series is to educate PharmD students in the area of medicinal chemistry and serve as a reference guide to pharmacists on aspects of chemical basis of drug action. A thorough discussion of key physicochemical parameters of therapeutic agents and how they affect the biochemical, pharmacological, pharmacokinetic processes and clinical use of these agents is the primary focus of the whole book. The rationale for putting together a book of this nature is to equip PharmD students with the scientific basis to competently evaluate, recommend and counsel patients and health care professionals regarding the safe, appropriate, and cost-effective use of medications.

This second volume of the series is comprised of 8 chapters focusing on a comprehensive account of medicinal chemistry of drugs affecting autonomic and central nervous system. It provides the mechanism of drug action, details structure-activity relationships and metabolism as well as clinical significance of drugs affecting the autonomic and central nervous system to give the knowledge base for pharmacist.

Chapter 1 provides a comprehensive account of the medicinal chemistry of "drugs affecting the cholinergic system". This chapter includes s pathophysiologic principles, mechanism of action, structure -activity relationships and metabolism of drugs affecting cholinergic system including cholinergic agonists, antagonists neuromuscular blocking agents and related drugs.

Chapter 2 is a comprehensive account of medicinal chemistry of "drugs affecting the adrenergic system". It details the pathophysiologic principles, mechanism of drug action, structure-activity relationships and metabolism of the adrenergic and related drugs with their clinical significance. This chapter provides a thorough discussion of direct and indirect acting sympathomimetic (adrenergic agonists) and sympatholytic (adrenergic antagonists) drugs.

Chapter 3 focuses on the medicinal chemistry of "phenothiazines and related antipsychotic drugs". This chapter is a comprehensive account of medicinal chemistry of the antipsychotic drugs. It discusses the pathophysiologic principles of schizophrenia and other psychotic disorders and receptor pharmacology, mechanism of action and structure-activity relationships of the first- and second-generation antipsychotics and related drugs. This chapter also delineates the clinical significance of all classes of antipsychotic drugs, their therapeutic indications, side effects and metabolic pathways of selected first- and second-generation antipsychotic agents.

Chapter 4 is a comprehensive account of medicinal chemistry of the "antidepressant drugs" – their pathophysiologic principles, mechanism of action, structure-activity relationships and metabolism. Topics include biogenic amine hypothesis, the roles of dopamine, serotonin and norepinephrine in depression.

Chapter 5 concisely explains the chemical and pharmacological basis of traditional/conventional and newer sedative-hypnotics and anxiolytics that include barbiturates, benzodiazepines and non-benzodiazepine agents. Topics discussed include chemical and pharmacological classes, mechanisms of action, Structure-activity relationships, and key pharmacokinetic (ADMET) characteristics of individual drug molecules.

Chapter 6 is a comprehensive account of the medicinal chemistry of antiepileptic drugs. It discusses the physicochemical principles, mechanism of action, structure-activity relationships and metabolism of the antiepileptic and related drugs, such as barbiturates, hydantoins, oxazolidinediones, succinimides, amides, benzodiazepines, valproic acid and its derivatives, GABA-analogs, and miscellaneous compounds, and their clinical relevance.

Chapter 7 is a comprehensive account of the medicinal chemistry of general and local anesthetic agents. It provides the physicochemical principles, mechanism of drug action, structure-activity relationships, and drug metabolism to build a strong knowledge base for pharmacy students.

Chapter 8 provides a comprehensive account of Parkinson's disease and the medicinal chemistry of antiparkinsonian drugs. It details the mechanism of disease progression, drug action and structure- activity relationships of antiparkinsonian drugs.

The chapters in this volume are designed to guide the reader to review, integrate and apply principles of medicinal chemistry to drug action of therapeutic agents. All concepts are illustrated with diagrams or figures, with the keywords highlighted, bulleted or numbered. Wherever needed, special boxes and case studies are included. In addition, each chapter is reinforced with student's self-study guides and self-assessment questions. Special notations are highlighted using call-out boxes for visual effect. Tables and figures are used to augment the text as needed.

We would like to express our sincere gratitude to the contributing authors for their time and effort in completing this volume. We would also like to thank the Bentham Science Publishers, particularly Ms. Fariya Zulfiqar (Manager Publications) and Mr. Mahmood Alam (Director Publications) for their support. We are confident that this volume of the book series will guide students and educators of pharmacy and related health professions worldwide.

M. O. Faruk Khan
University of Charleston School of Pharmacy
Charleston, WV
USA

&

Ashok E. Philip
Union University College of Pharmacy
Jackson, TN
USA

List of Contributors

Ashok E. Philip   Department of Pharmaceutical Sciences, Union University School of Pharmacy, Jackson, TN 38305, USA

Cory R. Theberge   TechPlace, Brunswick, Maine 04011, USA

Carolyn J. Friel   School of Pharmacy, Massachusetts College of Pharmacy and Health Sciences, Worcester, MA, USA

Donald Sikazwe   Department of Pharmaceutical Sciences, Feik School of Pharmacy, University of the Incarnate Word, San Antonio, TX, USA

George DeMaagd   Department of Pharmaceutical Sciences, Union University School of Pharmacy, Jackson, TN 38305, USA

Horrick Sharma   Department of Pharmaceutical Sciences, College of Pharmacy, Southwestern Oklahoma State University, Weatherford, OK 73096, USA

Kim Lindsey-Goodrich   Department of Pharmacy Practice, Union University School of Pharmacy, Jackson, TN 38305, USA

Les Ramos   College of Pharmacy, Southwestern Oklahoma State University, Weatherford, USA

Michaela Leffler   Department of Pharmacy Practice, University of Charleston School of Pharmacy, Charleston, USA

Mamoon Rashid   Department of Pharmaceutical Sciences, Appalachian College of Pharmacy, Virginia, VA 24631, USA

Mehbuba Rahman   Department of Pharmaceutical Sciences, Appalachian College of Pharmacy, Virginia, VA 24631, USA

M. O. Faruk Khan   Department of Pharmacy, University of Charleston School of Pharmacy, Charleston, WV, USA

Michaela Leffler   Department of Pharmacy Practice, University Charleston School of Pharmacy, Charleston, WV 25304, USA

Tamer E. Fandy   Department of Pharmaceutical and Administrative Sciences, University of Charleston School of Pharmacy, Charleston, USA

CHAPTER 1

Drugs Affecting the Cholinergic System

Cory R. Theberge[1], Kim Lindsey-Goodrich[2] and Ashok E. Philip[3,*]

[1] *TechPlace, Brunswick, Maine 04011, USA*

[2] *Department of Pharmacy Practice, Union University School of Pharmacy, Jackson, TN 38305, USA*

[3] *Department of Pharmaceutical Sciences, Union University School of Pharmacy, Jackson, TN 38305, USA*

Abstract: This chapter is a comprehensive account of the medicinal chemistry of drugs affecting the cholinergic system. It provides the mechanism of drug action and the structure-activity relationship (SAR) of the cholinergic and related drugs. After a study of this chapter, students will be able to:

• Relate principles of acetylcholine (ACh) discovery, biosynthesis, storage, transport, and metabolism.

• Describe the effects of agonism and antagonism of cholinergic receptors and modulation of ACh levels at the synapse.

• Describe cholinergic biochemistry and neurochemical interactions.

• Compare muscarinic and nicotinic receptor subtypes.

• Illustrate the mechanism of action, structure-activity relationship (SAR), metabolites, and clinical considerations of:

▪ muscarinic receptor agonists

▪ muscarinic receptor antagonists (anticholinergics)

▪ acetylcholinesterase (AChE) inhibitors

　o reversible

　o quasi-irreversible

　o antidotes for irreversible inhibitors

▪ neuromuscular blocking agents

* **Corresponding author Ashok E. Philip:** Department of Pharmaceutical Sciences, Union University School of Pharmacy, Jackson, TN 38305, USA; Tel: 731-661-5704; E-mail: aphilip@uu.edu

M. O. Faruk Khan & Ashok E. Philip (Eds.)

Keywords: Acetylcholine, Acetylcholinesterase inhibitors, Anticholinergics, Alzheimer's Disease, Muscarinic agonists, Neuromuscular Blocking Agents, Structure-activity relationship.

HISTORICAL PERSPECTIVES

During the years 1898 - 1906, Reid Hunt of John Hopkins Medical School and Rene Taveau demonstrated the presence of acetyl choline (ACh) in the extracts of the adrenal cortex as a potent hypotensive agent. ACh was later extracted in 1914 from ergot and was shown to be a parasympathomimetic agent by Arthur Ewins and Henry Dale. Dale and Ewins also proposed that physostigmine could prevent the esterase mediated hydrolysis of ACh, which was later demonstrated by Otto Loewi in 1926. In 1921, Loewi also demonstrated that ACh slowed down the heart rate. Dale and Loewi shared the Nobel Prize for physiology or medicine in 1936 for this work. Long before these discoveries, A.W. Gerrard (London) and E. Hardy (France) independently discovered the cholinomimetic alkaloid, pilocarpine, in 1875 from *Pilocarpus jaborandi* and *P. pinnatus*. Its value in ophthalmology for the treatment of glaucoma was discovered by Adolf Weber in 1877. The historical use of deadly nightshade (*Atropa belladonna*) berry juice in the early 1800s by Italian women to enlarge their pupils for a striking appearance gave the name of the plant "belladonna" (means "beautiful lady"). In 1831, German pharmacist Heinrich F. G. Mein isolated it in pure crystalline form, which was identified as atropine. In 1869, Henry Salter described the use of atropine as well as belladonna in the treatment of asthma, and atropine and its derivatives are now widely used for this purpose, in addition to other antimuscarinic uses.

Physostigmine, an AChE inhibitor, was isolated as an amorphous powder from *Physostigma venenosum* (Calabar bean) by Robert Christinson and his coworker, Thomas Fraser. Christinson examined the effects of the plant extracts which showed that it stopped the heart and/or caused atrial fibrillation. In 1875, Ludwig Laquer revealed the value of physostigmine in preventing blindness, and its use in the treatment of glaucoma. This led to the development of all the carbamate type of anticholinesterases. In 1932, Willy Lang and his student at the University of Berlin experienced marked pressure in the larynx followed by breathlessness, clouding of consciousness and blurred vision, effects similar to those produced by nicotine, when they were preparing phosphorus-fluorine compounds. Garhard Schrader of Leverkussen laboratories then prepared >2000 organic phosphate compounds as potential insecticides. Eberhard Gross of the same company showed that these compounds are irreversible inhibitors of AChE, some of which were highly toxic to the laboratory animals causing death. Tabum, discovered by Schrader in 1936, was the first war gas manufactured on large scale in 1942. Sarin, discovered by Schrader in 1938, was far more toxic than tabum. The first safe insecticide, malathion, was introduced by American Cyanamid in 1951, and in 1952, another insecticide metrifonate (a prodrug of dichlorvos) was developed by Schrader and his colleagues at the Bayer laboratories. Today, drugs affecting the cholinergic system are commonly used with many of these ranked in the top 200 drug list and are shown in Fig. (**1**). For additional information, please refer to the *Further Reading* section at the end of the chapter.

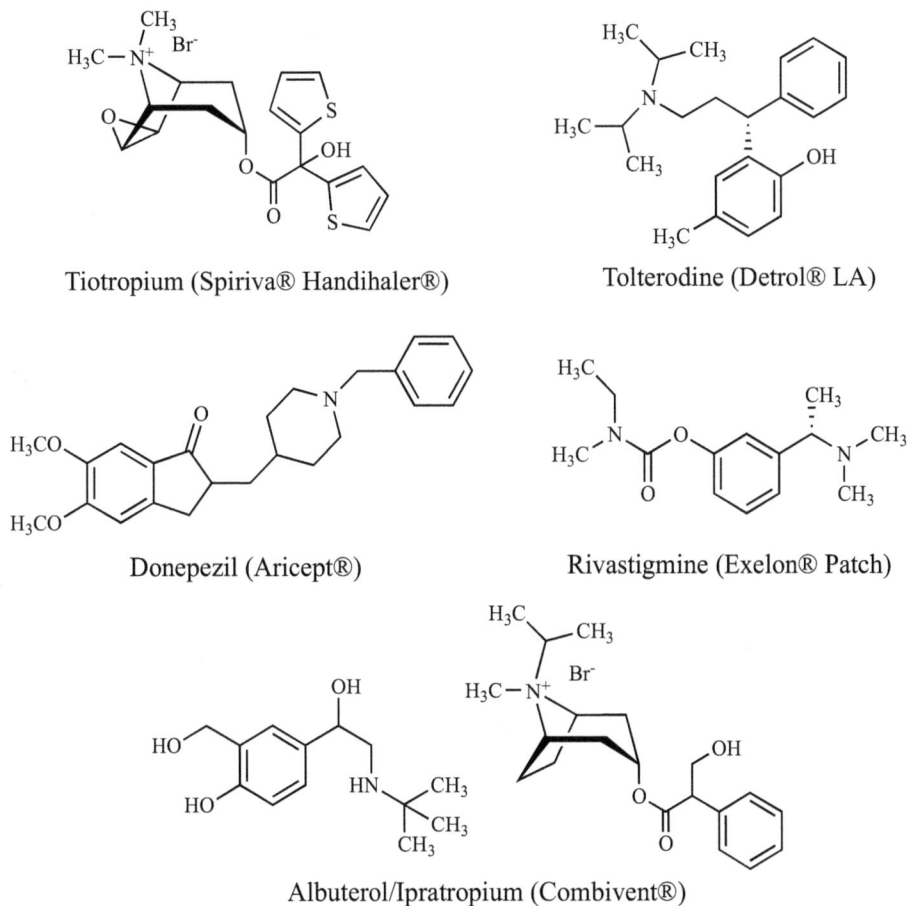

Tiotropium (Spiriva® Handihaler®)

Tolterodine (Detrol® LA)

Donepezil (Aricept®)

Rivastigmine (Exelon® Patch)

Albuterol/Ipratropium (Combivent®)

Fig. (1). Structures of cholinergic drugs frequently ranked in the top 200 drugs list.

INTRODUCTORY CONCEPTS

Choline and Acetylcholine

Circulating levels of molecular choline are essential for human biological homeostasis. Cell membrane structural integrity, lipid transport/metabolism, transmembrane signaling, and cholinergic neurotransmission are all dependent on choline levels that cannot be met by endogenous *de novo* synthesis. Human nutritional needs require the intake of choline-containing foods (*e.g.* eggs, seafood, soy products, broccoli) for proper health and physical performance [1]. Choline requires a carrier-mediated transport system to permeate cell membranes and is taken up by cholinergic neurons via a high-affinity choline transporter (CHT). Choline is a quaternary ammonium cationic molecule necessary for the synthesis and release of the essential chemical neurotransmitter ACh, which contains an acetylated hydroxyl group (Fig. **2**). ACh has a wide range of biochemical activities essential for memory storage, muscle control, and other functions relating to the sympathetic and parasympathetic nervous systems [2 - 4].

Since cholinergic pharmacologic agents usually interact *in vivo* in a manner similar to physiologic ACh, most of the drugs discussed in this chapter contain a nitrogen atom with four substituents that is positively charged, or they contain a nitrogen atom with three substituents that is protonated at physiologic pH. Keep in mind these molecular characteristics when classifying agents that affect cholinergic tone in the patient.

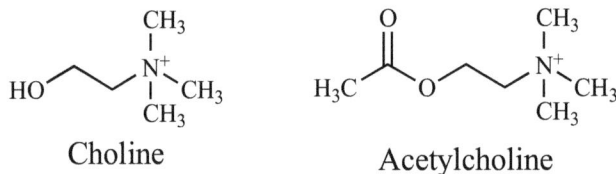

Choline

Acetylcholine

Fig. (2). Choline and acetylcholine structures.

Acetylcholine and Neurotransmission

Pharmacological interest in choline derivatives already existed when ACh was first synthetically produced in 1894 by Nothnagel [5]. It took scientists until 1914 to identify ACh as the component of ergot extract that both inhibited heart muscle and stimulated intestinal muscle [6]. This discovery was effectively made and fully explored by Sir Henry Dale, who also coined the term "cholinergic" to describe the activity of ACh and "adrenergic" to describe the (opposite) activity of adrenaline. The elegant experiments of Otto Loewi later proved the neuromodulatory activity of ACh by demonstrating that it was the essential component of vagus nerve secretions (*"vagusstoff"*) that affected changes in heart muscle activity.

ACh was the first neurotransmitter to be discovered and subsequent experimental work by Dale and others proved that ACh is the neurotransmitter at the terminals of all parasympathetic and some (*e.g.* sweat gland) sympathetic ganglia, as well as at the preganglionic fibers of both parasympathetic and sympathetic nervous systems. Furthermore, ACh was identified at voluntary motor fibers of skeletal muscles and at fibers within the central nervous system (CNS). The combined work of Loewi and Dale led to them being awarded the Nobel Prize in Physiology or Medicine in 1936 "for discoveries relating to the chemical transmission of nerve impulse" [7 - 9].

Cholinergic Neurochemistry: ACh Biosynthesis, Storage, Release, and Metabolism

Acetylcholine has its effect at numerous sites in the body, but let us first consider the biosynthesis, action, and metabolism of ACh near a cholinergic chemical synapse. ACh is formed in the cytosol of a presynaptic cell by the choline acetyltransferase (ChAT) enzyme (Fig. **3**). In this transformation, a molecule of choline receives an acetyl group from mitochondrion-derived acetyl coenzyme A (acetyl-CoA).

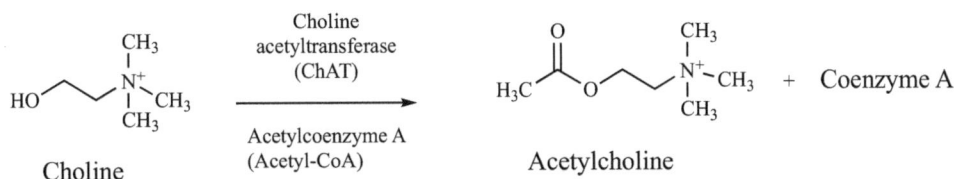

Fig. (3). ACh biosynthesis in the presynaptic nerve cell.

Once formed in the presynaptic environment, much of the ACh is stored in vesicles along with other co-transmitters, where it awaits a release into the synaptic cleft. Vesicular acetylcholine transporter (vAChT) mediates the transport of ACh from the cytoplasm into cholinergic synaptic vesicles. These vesicles contain enzymes and transporters that concentrate and store ACh before neurotransmitter release commences. Estimates of the number of molecules of ACh contained in one vesicle vary between 1000 and 50,000 (defined as one quantum of neurotransmitters), and a single presynaptic cell terminus may contain hundreds of thousands of vesicles. Neurotransmitter release into the synapse is initiated by depolarization of the nerve cell; subsequent calcium ion (Ca^{2+}) influx triggers the fusion of hundreds of vesicles to the presynaptic cell membrane and a release of a quantum of ACh from each vesicle along with co-transmitters into the synaptic cleft. The storage vesicles then reassemble and utilize the same enzymes and transporters to store ACh in the presynaptic area (Fig. **4**).

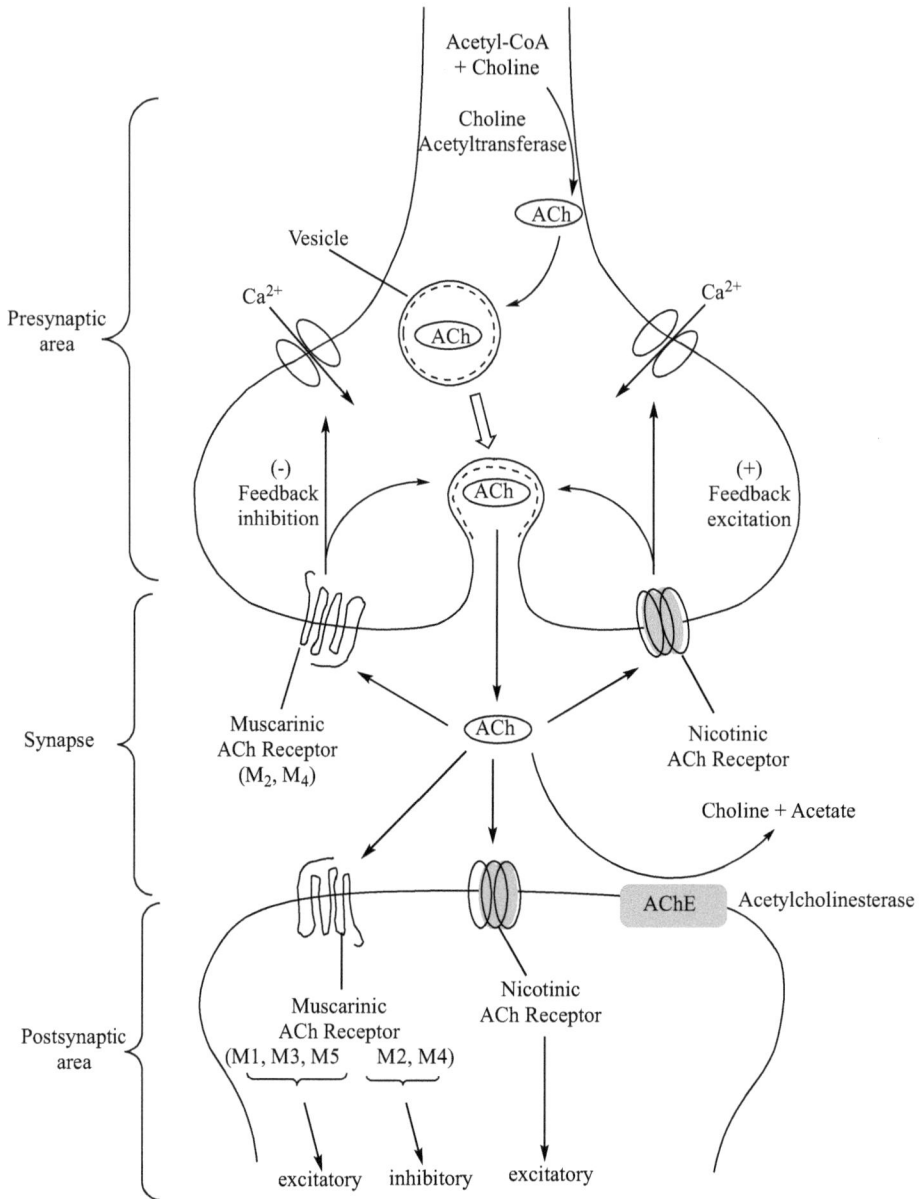

Fig. (4). ACh in the synaptic area.

When vesicles from the presynaptic nerve cell release ACh, stimulation of presynaptic muscarinic receptors (mChR) inhibits the additional release of ACh, whereas stimulated presynaptic nicotinic receptors (nChR) enhance ACh concentrations in the synapse. This feedback modulation of presynaptic receptors is essential for the regulation of synaptic ACh levels.

Once in the synapse, ACh is also susceptible to metabolism into choline and acetyl-CoA via the actions of acetylcholinesterase (AChE) present in local synaptic membranes (Fig. **5**). This metabolic conversion of ACh to choline actively reduces the concentration of ACh in the synapse, and thus modulates the local cholinergic activity

Fig. (5). Breakdown of ACh by the acetylcholinesterase enzyme.

Cholinergic Receptors - Muscarinic and Nicotinic Subtypes

The autonomic nervous system mediates most of the involuntary functions of the body, where essential nerve signals are transmitted to most tissues through two opposing systems, the *sympathetic* and *parasympathetic* (Fig. **6**). The sympathetic and parasympathetic systems innervate many of the same tissues and can be generally considered to have opposite effects. For example, sympathetic stimulation increases heart rate and inhibits digestion, whereas parasympathetic stimulation lowers heart rate and promotes digestion.

Each of the sympathetic and parasympathetic nerves consists of two neurons, a *preganglionic* neuron that originates from the central nervous system and a *postganglionic* neuron that connects to the peripheral effector tissue. These neurons communicate with each other at *ganglia* (clusters of neuronal soma and dendrites) via the release of chemical neurotransmitters into the chemical *synapse*. A chemical synapse is 100-200 angstroms wide and is present wherever nerve cells meet other nerve cells as well as when nerve cells meet gland or muscle cells. Chemical neurotransmitter signaling is therefore intrinsic to normal neurological and physiological functions in human beings.

All preganglionic neurons are cholinergic in both the sympathetic and parasympathetic nervous systems. Postganglionic parasympathetic neurons are cholinergic as well as postganglionic sympathetic neurons that affect the sweat glands, piloerector muscles, and a few blood vessels. All other postganglionic sympathetic neurons are adrenergic [10].

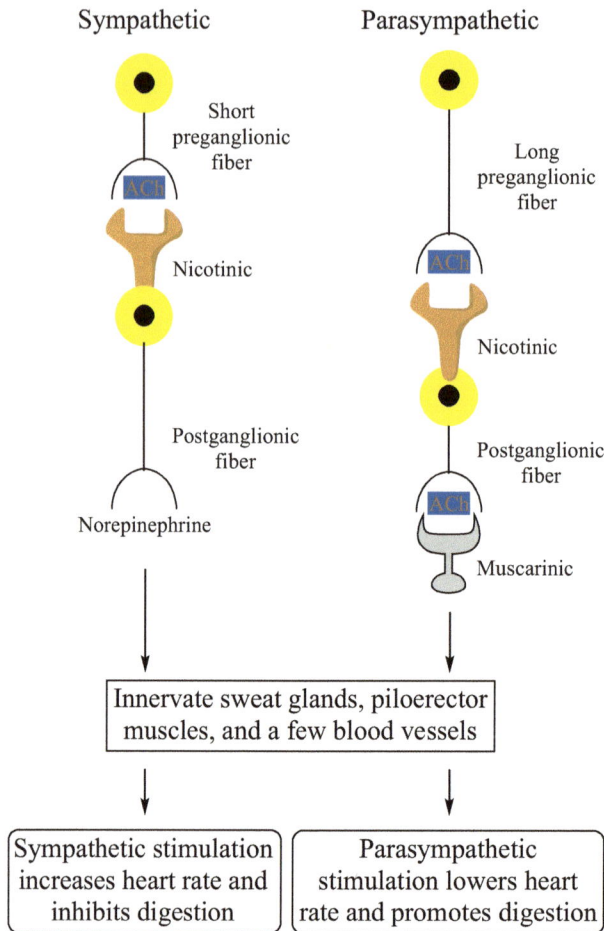

Fig. (6). Peripheral nerve fiber structure and chemical neurotransmitters.

As a neurotransmitter, ACh activates two subtypes of receptors that are classified by their sensitivity to muscarine and nicotine (Fig. **7**). These receptors, as well as the cholinergic drugs that act at these receptors, are termed *muscarinic* and *nicotinic*, respectively. Although nicotine and muscarine are not endogenous to human bodies, these chemical compounds have enabled researchers to identify the location and effect of a number of cholinergic receptors in human tissues.

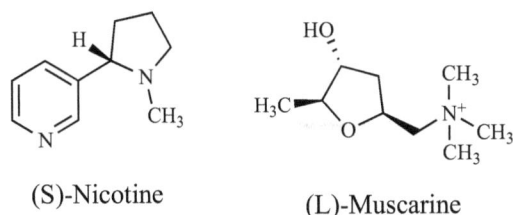

(S)-Nicotine　　　　(L)-Muscarine

Fig. (7). Nicotine and muscarine.

Muscarinic acetylcholine receptors (mAChR) are metabotropic G-protein coupled receptors (GPCRs) that act slowly and may cause excitatory or inhibitory responses (Table **1**).

Table 1. Parasympathetic effects from ACh-mediated stimulation of muscarinic receptors.

Location	Effect of Muscarinic Stimulation
Eyes	Miosis Decreased intra-ocular pressure Near vision adjustment
Digestive Tract	Increased saliva secretion Increased Stomach acid secretion Peristalsis
Other	Decreased heart rate Bronchial constriction Enhanced urination

G-Proteins bind ACh and initiate intracellular signaling through several different pathways. These receptors are expressed at autonomic ganglia and at effector organs. The primary uses of muscarinic agonists and antagonists are to modulate the responses of effector organs. These receptors are numbered by subtype (M_1-M_5) and are found in the CNS, gastric and salivary glands, smooth muscle, and heart (Table **2**). All the muscarinic actions of ACh are *blocked by atropine* (a competitive antagonist). The gene sequences and detailed structural characteristics of muscarinic receptors have been summarized [11 - 13].

Nicotinic acetylcholine receptors (nAChR) are ligand-gated ion channels that cause a rapid increase in the calcium (Ca^{2+}) and sodium (Na^+) ion permeability of the cell, resulting in depolarization and excitation following activation (Table **2**). These ionotropic receptors comprise all of the cholinergic receptors at the neuromuscular junction (N_m), and they predominate at autonomic ganglia (N_n). The primary functions mediated by nAChR are skeletal muscle contraction and autonomic activity. Pharmacologic agents directed at nAChR are applied in neuromuscular blockade through competitive antagonism as well as agonism leading to muscle cell depolarization [11].

Table 2. Anatomical distribution of muscarinic and nicotinic receptors.

Receptor Type	Location
Muscarinic	Nerves
M_1	Heart, nerves, smooth muscle
M_2	Glands, smooth muscle, endothelium
M_3	CNS
M_4	CNS
M_5	
Nicotinic	Skeletal muscle, neuromuscular junction
N_1 (or N_m)	Postganglionic cell body, dendrites
N_2 (or N_n)	

The nicotinic receptor is a pentameric complex assembled from a family of 17 subunits in mammals designated α1-α10, β1-β4, δ, γ, and ε. They are arranged in five wedge-shaped pieces around a central (ion) pore and a single nAChR subunit contains four transmembrane α-helical protein domains designated M_1 through M_4. Since the entire ion channel may be assembled from various subtypes of subunits in various combinations, there is the possibility of a large number of unique nicotinic receptors in the body [12 - 16]. When the subunit composition and subunit stoichiometry is known, the assembled pentamer is indicated by subscript numbers, for example, an $α7_5$ nAChR contains five $α_7$ subunits and an $α1_2β1δγ$ nAChR contains two α1 subunits and one each of the β1, δ, and γ subunits.

Nicotinic receptors contain two agonist sites per receptor and require the binding of two nAChR agonists in order for channel activation to occur. Upon activation, the receptor is stabilized in the open state, allowing an influx of cations such as calcium, sodium, and potassium. The increased permeability of the ion channel to cations affects the release of neurotransmitters and modulates cell sensitivity, potentially influencing the physiological effects of sleep, anxiety, pain, and cognition. Both muscarinic and nicotinic receptors are ubiquitous in the CNS, where ACh plays an essential role in cognition, attention, arousal, and analgesia.

Clinical Use of Acetylcholine

Unmodified ACh (stable in crystalline form as the hydrochloride salt) is not a clinically useful agonist of cholinergic receptors, primarily because the endogenous chemical neurotransmitter lacks specificity for either muscarinic or nicotinic receptor subtypes. It is also highly water-sensitive, especially in the presence of acid or base, and therefore broken down quickly in the gut (Fig. **8**). Parenteral administration is also ineffective because of the metabolic degradation, by cholinesterases, in plasma. Additionally, the quaternary ammonium nitrogen necessary for cholinergic activity renders the molecule highly hydrophilic and therefore incapable of effectively penetrating lipid membranes. Preparations of ACh chloride used to produce miosis during ocular surgery (Miochol-E™) are packaged as two separate ampoules, one containing crystalline ACh chloride and one containing isotonic aqueous solution. These two ampoules must be constituted immediately before topical administration to the eye [17].

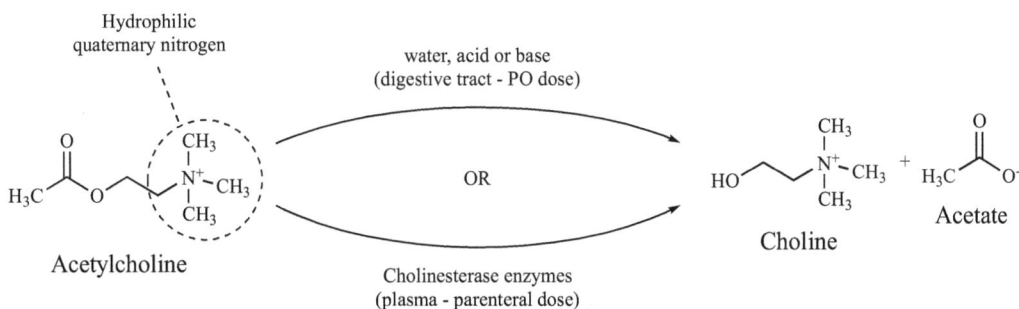

Fig. (8). Liabilities of acetylcholine as a therapeutic agent.

MUSCARINIC RECEPTOR AGONISTS

The mAChR agonists can be divided into two distinct classes: 1) ACh and its synthetic derivatives, and 2) Alkaloids and chemical compounds, including muscarine, that are selective for muscarinic receptors. However, the clinical usefulness of these drugs is limited to only a few compounds.

Exhaustive research has been conducted into the structure-activity relationship (SAR) of simple ACh derivatives for use as muscarinic agonists. There are only a few modifications to ACh that may be made in order to retain the cholinergic activity of the natural neurotransmitter. While there are exceptions to the SAR, the general tenets are (Fig. **9**) [18, 19]:

- The molecule must have a nitrogen atom possessing a positive charge, preferably a quaternary ammonium salt.
- The size of the alkyl groups on this nitrogen may not be larger than a methyl group.
- The molecule must have an oxygen atom analogous to the oxygen in the (acetyl) ester group of ACh.
- There must be no more or less than two carbon atoms linking the

(aforementioned) nitrogen and oxygen atoms.
- Functionality on the carbon atom linker may not exceed the size of methyl groups.
- A β-methyl group on the carbon linker may impart muscarinic receptor selectivity.

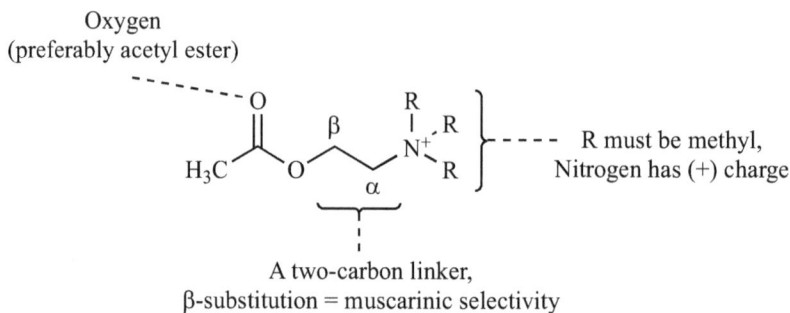

Fig. (9). SAR of acetylcholine-derived cholinergic agonists.

Methacholine is a derivative of ACh that contains a β-methyl substituent (Fig. **10**). While this methyl group imparts significant resistance to metabolism by the AChE enzyme, its therapeutic utility is limited by unpredictable absorption and several cardiovascular side effects (*e.g.* bradycardia, vasodilation). This compound has a specific clinical use in the diagnosis of asthma, where it causes and exaggerates bronchial hyper reactivity response after administration.

Carbachol and bethanechol (Fig. **10**) both contain a carbamoyl group substituted for the acetyl ester of ACh, which has the clinical effect of reducing metabolism by cholinesterase enzymes and extending their duration of action and distribution in tissues. Carbachol has significant nicotinic receptor activity and thus its use is limited to topical administration to the eye to induce miosis and reduce intraocular pressure in glaucoma patients. Bethanechol has very high muscarinic receptor selectivity and is the agent of choice for stimulating urination and gastrointestinal motility, particularly to counteract pre-surgical atropine administered to prevent bowel emptying. Nicotinic symptoms of cholinergic stimulation are usually absent or minimal when ACh derivatives carbachol and bethanechol are orally or subcutaneously administered in therapeutic doses. Muscarinic effects typically occur within minutes of subcutaneous injection, reach a maximum in 15 to 30 minutes, and disappear in 1-2 hours [20, 21].

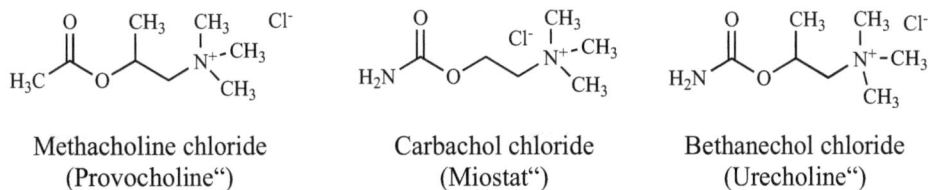

Methacholine chloride   Carbachol chloride   Bethanechol chloride
(Provocholine")   (Miostat")   (Urecholine")

Fig. (10). Carbachol, methacholine, and bethanechol cholinergic agonists.

Muscarine (Fig. **11**) is found in pharmacologically dangerous levels in certain types of mushrooms (*Inocybe* and *Clitocybe*), and it is interesting to note the structural similarities it shares with ACh even though it is not a synthetic derivative of the ACh core structure. Muscarine poisoning (and the effects of muscarinic agonists) may be readily counteracted by atropine (itself an extract of plants from the *Solanaceae* family) since atropine is a competitive muscarinic receptor antagonist.

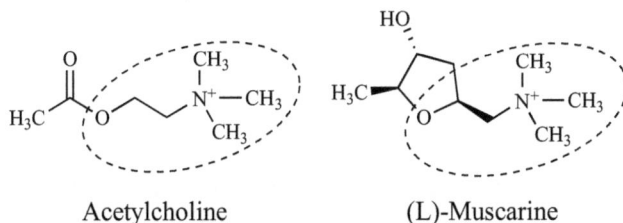

Acetylcholine   (L)-Muscarine

Fig. (11). Structural similarity of ACh and muscarine.

The other clinically relevant muscarinic agonists are pilocarpine and cevimeline (Fig. **12**). Pilocarpine is primarily used to decrease intraocular pressure in glaucoma patients, but both pilocarpine and cevimeline have been specifically labeled for oral administration in the treatment of dry mouth secondary to Sjögren's syndrome (which causes autoimmune degradation of the salivary glands). The sulfur in cevimeline is susceptible to oxidative metabolism and over 40% of the drug is excreted as a mixture of the R and S sulfoxide [22]. Pilocarpine has a significantly shorter half-life than cevimeline (Table **3**) and is associated with a greater incidence of side effects. Studies have shown that patients are more likely to continue cevimeline than pilocarpine for long-term therapy [23].

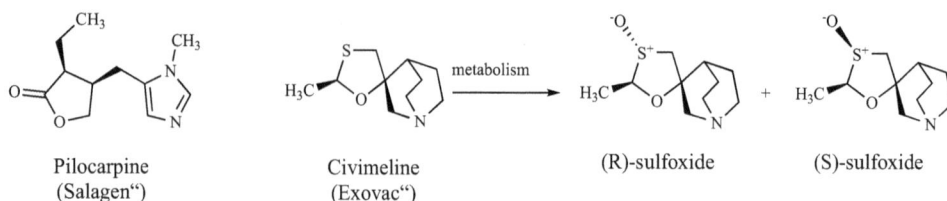

Fig. (12). Pilocarpine and cevimeline plus sulfoxide cevimeline metabolites.

Table 3. PK/PD Summary of pilocarpine and cevimeline.

	Pilocarpine (Salagen·)	Cevimeline (Exovac·)
Dosage Forms	Tablet	Capsule
Initial Dose	5 mg TID	30 mg TID
Max Dose	10 mg TID	30 mg TID
FDA Indication	Dry mouth from radiation therapy or secondary to Sjögren's	Dry mouth secondary to Sjögren's
Mechanism of action (MOA)	mAChR agonist	mAChR agonist
Half-life ($T_{1/2}$)	0.76-1.35h	5 +/-1h
Protein Binding	low	<20%

MUSCARINIC RECEPTOR ANTAGONISTS (ANTICHOLINERGICS)

Antagonists of ACh receptors act by blocking stimulation of ACh receptors by endogenous ACh or exogenous agonists of ACh receptors. These compounds are sometimes called *parasympatholytics* because they stop parasympathetic stimulation and allow sympathetic effects to dominate. These drugs are also sometimes referred to as *antimuscarinics* or, more generally, *anticholinergics* since mAChR dominates the autonomic nervous system.

Atropine saw its first use as a cosmetic agent in the Renaissance era. Italian women would apply or ingest extracts of the nightshade plant (*Atropa belladonna*) to induce dilation of the pupils (mydriasis), which was perceived as an attractive physical feature in that time period. Atropine is still extracted from the plant material and is still used clinically to induce mydriasis before optical examinations. It also has uses to inhibit salivation and mucus secretions as well as to prevent vagal nerve reflex responses during surgical procedures.

The tropine ring in atropine is a 3-endo-hydroxy tropane derivative that is the core structure for many of the alkaloid mAChR antagonists (Fig. **13**). Atropine is a mixture of D- and L-isomers and has very low activity at nicotinic receptors;

effects at the neuromuscular junction are therefore only seen with very high doses.

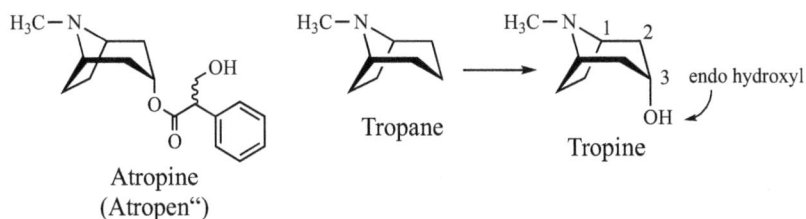

Fig. (13). Atropine and tropine core structure.

Scopolamine (Fig. **14**) is also obtained from plant extracts and differs from atropine in that it has an epoxide on the tropine ring system. It has greater CNS activity than atropine and these effects are often adverse, affecting memory and psychomotor reflexes. Scopolamine is most often administered for nausea associated with motion sickness; a transdermal route of administration minimizes CNS effects and acts to control the rate of delivery. It may be administered intravenously to reduce nausea in chemotherapy if a reduction in mucus secretions is also desired. Scopolamine is administered as a single enantiomer and is rapidly metabolized *in vivo*. The PK/PD profile of scopolamine has not been fully clarified, but it has a long half-life. Scopolamine does not induce or inhibit liver enzymes and the exact enzymes involved in metabolism have not been identified, but scopolamine is extensively metabolized and conjugated with less than 5% of a dose excreted in intact form. Since atropine is extensively used as a rescue agent, its PK profile is age- and sex-specific. In pediatric subjects under 2 years, the $T_{1/2}$ is 6.9 ± 3.3; in adults 16-58 years, it is 3.0 ± 0.9h; in geriatric patients 65-75 years, it is 10.0 ± 7.3. The protein binding of atropine is 14 to 22% in plasma. Gender differences include an $AUC_{(0\text{-inf})}$ and C_{max} that were 15% higher in females than males. The half-life of atropine is slightly shorter (approximately 20 minutes) in females than males [24].

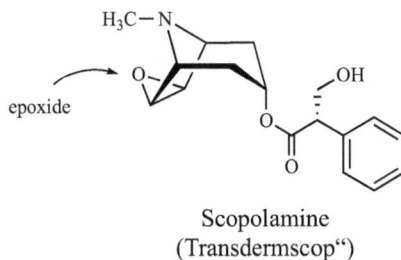

Scopolamine
(Transdermscop")

Fig. (14). Scopolamine.

Methscopolamine and glycopyrrolate (Fig. **15**) are both mAChR antagonists that have a quaternary ammonium nitrogen atom that has the effect of reducing CNS penetration and therefore renders these compounds more effective as peripherally acting drugs. Note that the glycopyrrolate structure lacks the tropine ring system, but retains quaternary nitrogen, hydroxyl, and ester functional groups seen in the tropine analogs. Both drugs are used to reduce the acidity of gastric secretions. Glycopyrrolate is used parenterally as a peripheral mAChR antagonist to counteract the adverse bradycardia seen when neostigmine is used post-surgically to reverse the effects of non-depolarizing muscle relaxants. The reduction of gastric secretions by mAChR antagonists is also useful clinically in the treatment of peptic ulcers, and pirenzepine, specifically for the M_1 and M_4 receptor subtypes, is used for this purpose.

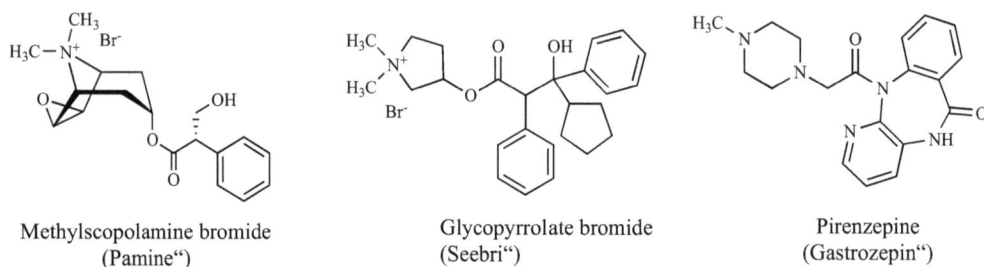

Methylscopolamine bromide (Pamine")	Glycopyrrolate bromide (Seebri")	Pirenzepine (Gastrozepin")

Fig. (15). Methscopolamine, glycopyrrolate, and pirenzepine.

A few mAChR antagonists have widespread clinical use in the treatment of asthma and chronic obstructive pulmonary disease (COPD). Reduction in bronchial secretions is seen with mAChR antagonists when dosed internally, and this effect might be counterproductive in a patient with compromised lung function since natural mucus formation and expulsion is essential to prevent infections and blockages of the lung airways. Ipratropium (Atrovent™) and tiotropium (Spiriva™) administered by inhalation both act to relax smooth muscles in the lungs and therefore result in bronchodilation and alleviation of respiratory distress (Fig. **16**). Tiotropium is more selective for the M_3 receptor subtype and has a lower incidence of adverse effects, and it is labeled for use long-term as a once-daily maintenance treatment for COPD [25, 26]. Both compounds do not reduce mucociliary clearance, so their anticholinergic properties may safely treat the symptoms of asthma and COPD [25]. As observed in excretion and blood level studies, a significant amount of the compound is usually administered orally when the powder is inhaled, but the quaternary ammonium salts are not readily absorbed into the systemic circulation either from the surface of the lung or from the gastrointestinal tract [27, 28]. A majority of administered tiotropium (74%) and ipratropium (50%) is excreted unchanged in the urine, and both drugs contain esters that are susceptible to non-enzymatic hydrolysis. It should be noted that short-acting β-adrenergic agonists are usually the first-line agents for the treatment of asthma.

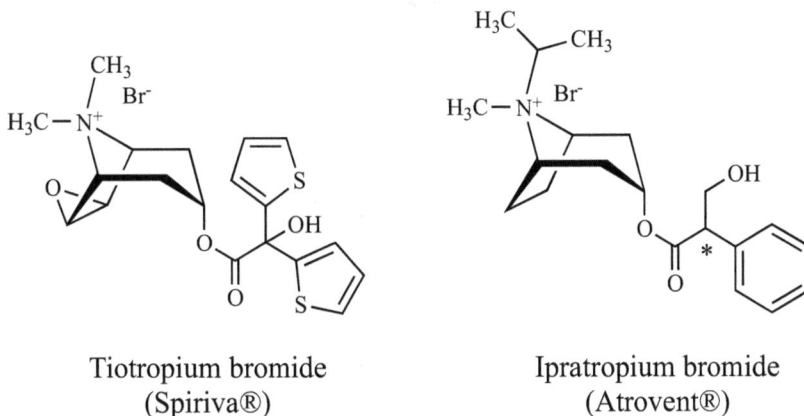

Tiotropium bromide
(Spiriva®)

Ipratropium bromide
(Atrovent®)

Fig. (16). Tiotropium and ipratropium.

Muscarinic receptor antagonists also see a significant amount of use in the treatment of overactive bladder and urinary incontinence. Antimuscarinics have the effect of relaxing the bladder detrusor muscle and tightening the bladder sphincter, and many compounds are approved for use in the treatment of overactive bladder.

Oxybutynin is metabolized primarily by the cytochrome P450 enzyme systems, particularly CYP3A4 found mostly in the liver and gut wall (Fig. **17**). Its metabolic products include inactive phenylcyclohexylglycolic acid and pharmacologically active desethyloxybutynin, which can achieve plasma levels six times that of parent drug after administration of the immediate-release formulation. Extended-release formulations will reduce blood levels of desethyloxybutynin and achieve steadier plasma concentrations of oxybutynin, and transdermal formulations bypass first-pass hepatic metabolism, resulting in significantly lowered plasma levels of the desethyloxybutynin metabolite [29].

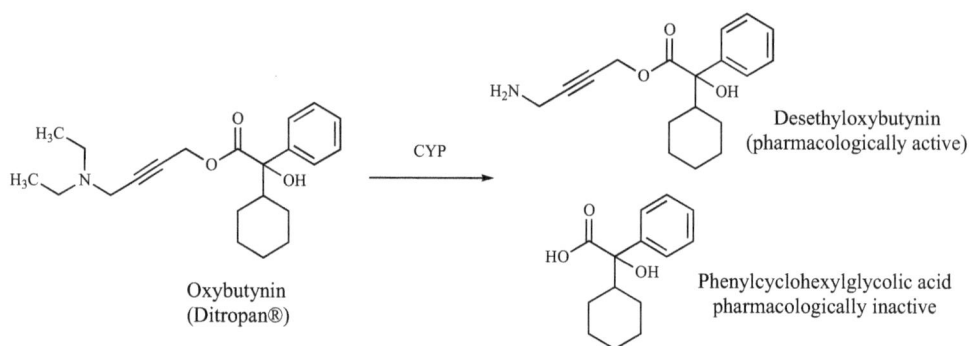

Fig. (17). Oxybutynin metabolism products.

Tolterodine (Detrol™) is one of the most prescribed cholinergic drugs in the US and its 5-hydroxy CYP2D6 liver enzyme metabolite (5-HMT) is equally active at the mAChR (Fig. **18**). The logD value for 5-HMT (0.74) is considerably lower versus tolterodine (1.83). This clinical observation resulted in the development of the prodrug fesoterodine in order to improve the systemic bioavailability of 5-HMT after oral administration. In contrast to the metabolism of tolterodine, 5-HMT is produced from fesoterodine via ubiquitous nonspecific esterases. Consequently, treatment with fesoterodine results in consistent, genotype-independent exposure to a singular active moiety (5-HMT); treatment with tolterodine results in CYP2D6 genotype-dependent exposure to varying proportions of the two active moieties (5-HMT and tolterodine) [30, 31].

While most antimuscarinic drugs for urinary incontinence are not selective for receptor subtypes, darifenacin and solifenacin are more selective for the M_3-subtype of the mAChR and are associated with lowered adverse effects during clinical use (Fig. **19**). The half-life of darifenacin may be longer in individuals who are poor metabolizers (PM) of drugs metabolized by CYP 2D6. Solifenacin has a very large half-life but is not recommended for patients with a history of congenital or acquired QT prolongation [32, 33]. A summary of muscarinic receptor antagonists that are used for the treatment of overactive bladder is provided in Table **4**.

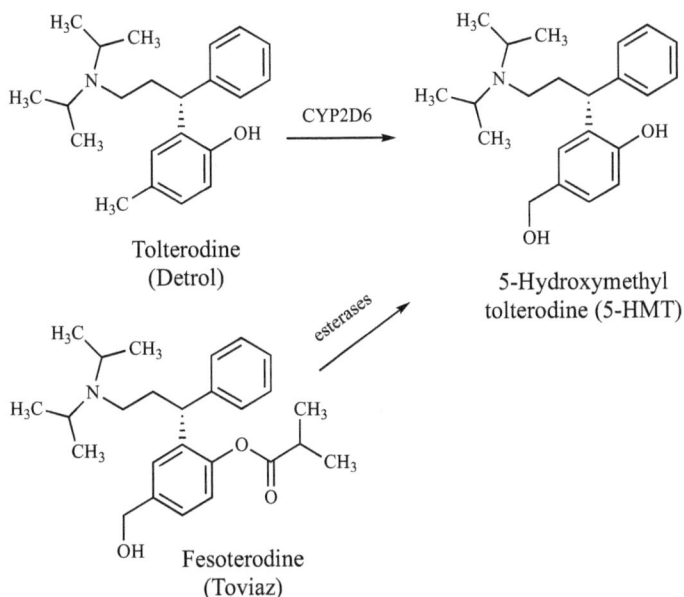

Fig. (18). Tolterodine, 5-HMT metabolite and fesoterodine prodrug.

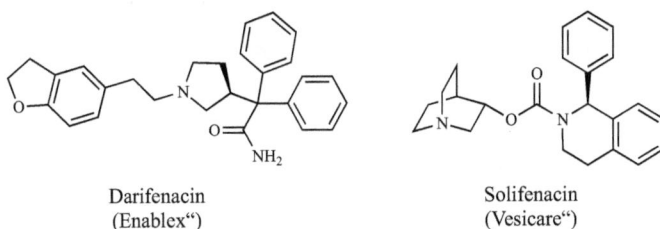

Fig. (19). Darifenacin and solifenacin.

Table 4. PK/PD Summary of muscarinic receptor antagonists for overactive bladder and urinary incontinence

	Oxybutynin (Ditropan XL·)	Tolterodine (Detrol LA·)	Fesoterodine (Toviaz·)	Darifenacin (Enablex·)	Solifenacin (Vesicare·)
Dosage Forms	Tablet, Gel, Syrup, Patch	Capsule	Tablet	Tablet	Tablet
Initial Dose	5-10 mg QD	4 mg QD	4mg QD	7.5 mg QD	5 mg QD
Max Dose	30 mg QD	5 mg QD	8 mg QD	15 mg QD	10 mg QD

(Table 4) cont.....

	Oxybutynin (Ditropan XL·)	Tolterodine (Detrol LA·)	Fesoterodine (Toviaz·)	Darifenacin (Enablex·)	Solifenacin (Vesicare·)
Half-life ($T_{1/2}$)	13h (XL Tab)	8h (LA Tab)	5h	12h (EM) 20h (PM)*	55h
Protein Binding	>97%	>96%	50%	98%	98%
Clearance/ Metabolism	Hepatic CYP 3A4	Hepatic CYP 2D6	Esterases Hepatic CYP 3A4/2D6	Hepatic CYP 3A4/2D6	Hepatic CYP 3A4

* EM = patients who are extensive metabolizers of CYP2D6 susceptible drugs, PM = patients who are poor metabolizers of CYP2D6 susceptible drugs.

The antimuscarinics benztropine and trihexphenidyl (Fig. **20**) were the first types of drugs used to reduce tremors and rigidity associated with idiopathic Parkinson's disease (IPD). Dopamine depletion in Parkinson's patients results in an excess cholinergic activity that is believed to contribute to tremors. Although antimuscarinics may be used in conjunction with L-dopa or other antiparkinson agents, they are contraindicated for use in the elderly and cognitively impaired due to the high incidence of adverse effects [34].

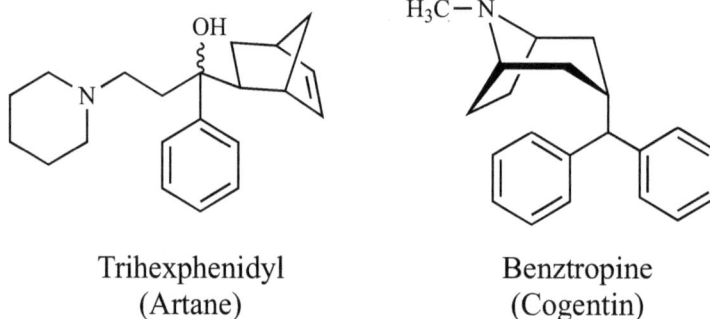

Trihexphenidyl (Artane)

Benztropine (Cogentin)

Fig. (20). Trihexphenidyl and benztropine antiparkinsonian agents.

The peripheral effects of antimuscarinics may be exploited in a variety of clinical applications. Quaternary ammonium antimuscarinics will not effectively cross the blood-brain barrier and thus have fewer CNS effects, yet are more likely to exhibit nicotinic blocking activity (Fig. **21**). Propantheline bromide is a nonselective muscarinic antagonist used for the treatment of mydriasis and IBS that acts as a ganglionic blocker at high doses. Atropine methonitrate has the same effect as atropine with reduced CNS activity. Glycopyrrolate is used preoperatively to inhibit gastrointestinal motility and may be used as a vagal nerve blocker in a parenteral application [35, 36].

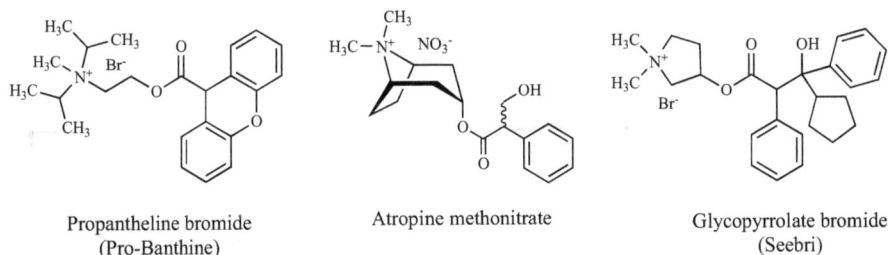

Propantheline bromide
(Pro-Banthine)

Atropine methonitrate

Glycopyrrolate bromide
(Seebri)

Fig. (21). Quaternary antimuscarinics utilized for peripheral effects.

Tropicamide finds utility as a short-acting topical antimuscarinic that induces mydriasis and cycloplegia after application to the eye. The activity of mebeverine is highly localized in the musculature of the gastrointestinal tract and colon and is also used for the treatment of IBS (Fig. **22**).

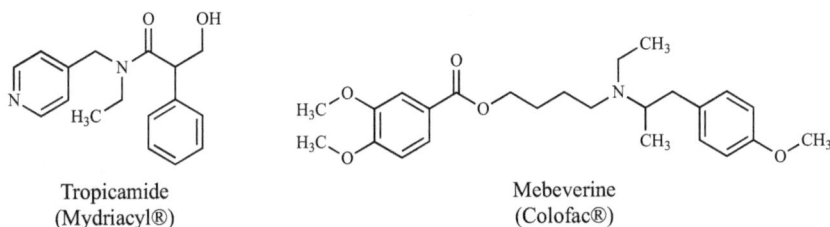

Tropicamide
(Mydriacyl®)

Mebeverine
(Colofac®)

Fig. (22). Non-quaternary antimuscarinics utilized for peripheral effects.

Acetylcholinesterase (AChE) Inhibitors

- Reversible noncovalent inhibitors – Short-acting (~minutes) inhibitors that do not covalently modify the AChE active site serine hydroxyl group.
- Reversible covalent inhibitors – Intermediate-acting (~hours) inhibitors that covalently modify the AChE active site serine hydroxyl group in a reversible manner.
- Irreversible covalent inhibitors – Agents that form stable, persistent covalent bonds with the AChE active site serine hydroxyl group and may permanently deactivate the AChE enzyme.

Cholinergic substances may act directly by imitating the action of ACh at receptors, or indirectly through the increase or decrease of ACh available for neurotransmission at those receptors. Since AChE is the enzyme responsible for the breakdown of free ACh at the synapse, antagonism of this enzyme will cause a local increase in ACh levels (Fig. **23**). These types of drugs may, therefore, be considered *indirectly-acting ACh receptor agonists*.

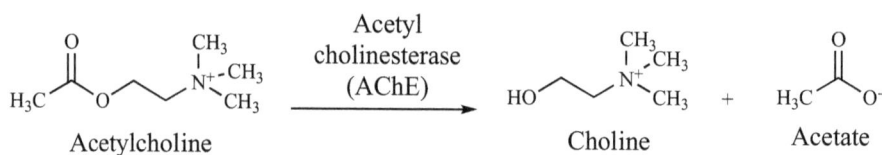

Fig. (**23**). ACh is decomposed by the acetylcholinesterase enzyme into choline and acetate.

The AChE enzyme is a serine protease, so its activity depends on a nucleophilic serine hydroxyl group positioned in the active site that facilitates cleavage of the acetate ester on ACh. The AChE serine hydroxyl covalently attaches to the acetate group and liberates choline from ACh. Aqueous hydrolysis of the acetylated enzyme then takes only milliseconds, regenerating AChE enzyme and acetate anion (acetic acid). This reaction occurs at both pre- and post-synaptic membranes, where AChE is densely localized and has the effect of modulating chemical neurotransmission at the cholinergic synapse (Fig. **24**).

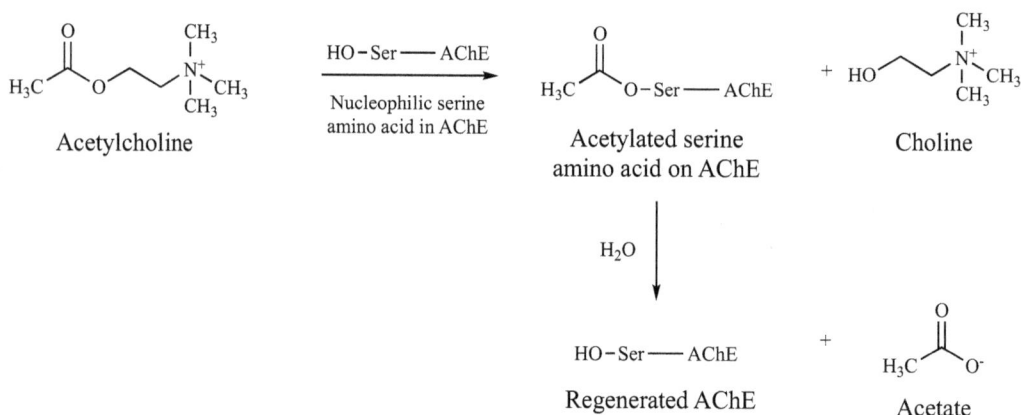

Fig. (**24**). Decomposition of ACh by AChE: The active site serine amino acid hydroxyl in AChE becomes acetylated when extracting the acetyl group of ACh. The acetylated enzyme is then rapidly hydrolyzed, regenerating the enzyme.

Reversible Noncovalent Inhibitors

There are three effective chemical classes of molecules used in controlling the activity of the AChE enzyme. The first are structures that contain quaternary ammonium nitrogen atoms and are selective for the AChE enzyme active site. These inhibitors do not covalently modify the essential serine amino acid in the active site as physiologic ACh does, but they are effective at decreasing enzyme activity and increasing levels of ACh at the synapse. Edrophonium is a rapid-acting drug that is used for acute clinical situations and has effects that last around 10 minutes. Ambenonium is another reversibly binding inhibitor that has a longer duration of action (Fig. **25**).

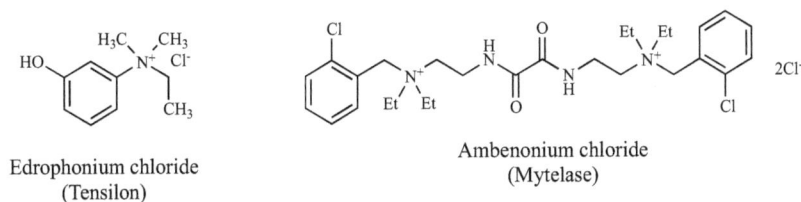

Edrophonium chloride
(Tensilon)

Ambenonium chloride
(Mytelase)

Fig. (25). Reversible noncovalent AChE inhibitors edrophonium and ambenonium.

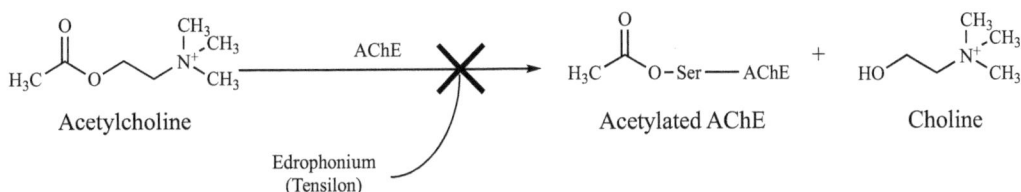

Acetylcholine

Acetylated AChE

Choline

Edrophonium
(Tensilon)

Fig. (26). Reversible noncovalent inhibitor edrophonium. Synaptic ACh is not degraded by the enzyme.

Reversible AChE inhibitors are used in the treatment of myasthenia gravis, where autoimmune production of antibodies directed against cholinergic (N_m) receptors at the neuromuscular junction cause muscle weakness and paralysis. The muscle effects of myasthenia gravis can be minimized by utilizing reversible AChE inhibitors like edrophonium to increase ACh concentrations at the synapse (Fig. **26**). When chronic treatment of myasthenia gravis is indicated, longer-acting inhibitors such as ambenonium, pyridostigmine, and neostigmine may be used.

Reversible Covalent Inhibitors

The second category of AChE inhibitors is comprised of carbamates of simple alcohols that also contain quaternary nitrogen atoms or structural features that ensure interaction with the AChE active site. Physostigmine is an example of a compound with a high affinity for AChE that has a methyl carbamate functional group. The carbamate is positioned in the active site to covalently modify the AChE serine hydroxyl and decrease catalytic activity. While the carbamylated enzyme is deactivated, synaptic ACh levels are not degraded. The carbamylated serine hydroxyl eventually hydrolyzes to regenerate the AChE enzyme, but this hydrolysis takes longer than the hydrolysis of acetylated AChE detailed in Fig.

27. Covalently binding reversible ACh inhibitors drugs have a longer duration of effect (measured in hours) when compared to noncovalently binding inhibitors (measured in minutes). The eseroline metabolite has been shown to be an opioid agonist [37].

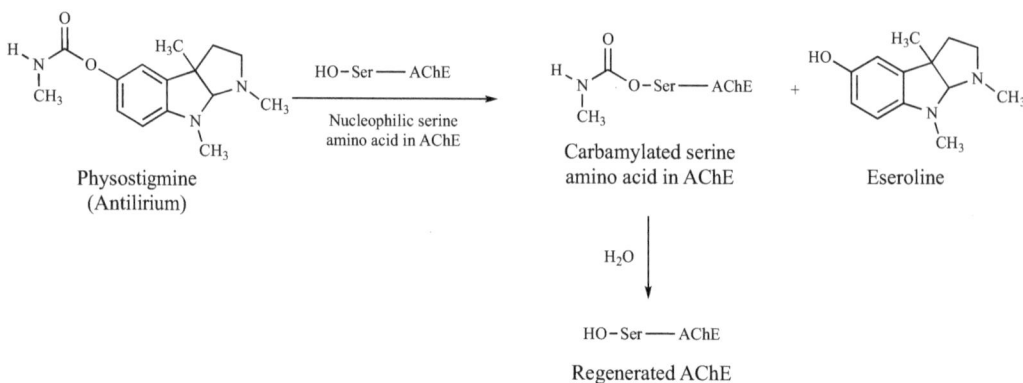

Fig. (27). Carbamylation of serine hydroxyl in ACh by physostigmine results in slower hydrolysis and slower regeneration of ACh.

Physostigmine is a CNS-penetrant tertiary amine and may be used for the reversal of the CNS effects of anticholinergic poisoning. Rivastigmine also penetrates CNS and is used for the treatment of dementia associated with Parkinson's Disease (PD) and Alzheimer's Disease (AD). Many reversible covalent AChE inhibitors have quaternary ammonium nitrogens that prevent CNS penetration and limit their effect to peripheral synaptic ACh levels (Fig. **28**). Pyridostigmine and neostigmine are used as peripherally acting agents for enhancing cholinergic activity for the symptomatic treatment of myasthenia gravis. The efficacy and pharmacokinetics of FDA approved AChE inhibitors for the treatment of Alzheimer's disease (AD) are discussed in detail later in this chapter.

Irreversible Covalent Inhibitors

The third class of AChE inhibitors is highly electrophilic alkoxy derivatives of phosphoric acid. Diisopropyl fluorophosphate and ecothiopate are examples of 2 phosphoric acid ester AChE inhibitors that have limited use as a miotic agent in the treatment of glaucoma. Compounds in this structural series react with the serine hydroxyl in AChE and form very stable phosphate esters. The phosphorylated serine may persist for hours. Additionally, the phosphorylated AChE may undergo a process of "aging", wherein one of the phosphoester alkyl groups is eliminated. This renders the phosphate ester of AChE impervious to hydrolysis and permanently deactivates AChE activity (Fig. **29**). Diisopropyl fluorophosphate and ecothiopate are thus extremely toxic and have very low LD_{50} values (Fig. **30**) [38, 39].

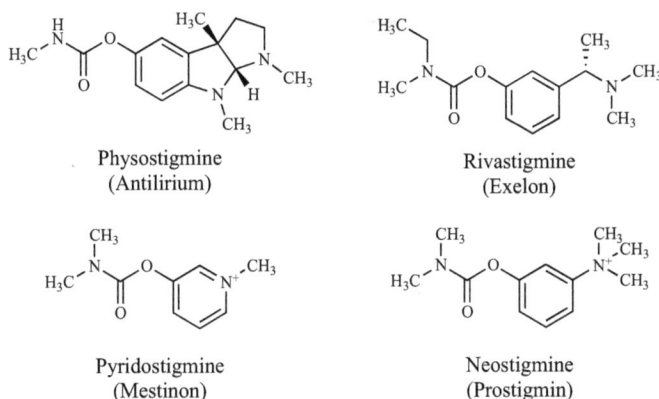

Physostigmine
(Antilirium)

Rivastigmine
(Exelon)

Pyridostigmine
(Mestinon)

Neostigmine
(Prostigmin)

Fig. (28). Reversible covalent AChE inhibitors affecting the CNS (tertiary amines physostigmine and rivastigmine) and peripheral effects (quaternary amines pyridostigmine and neostigmine).

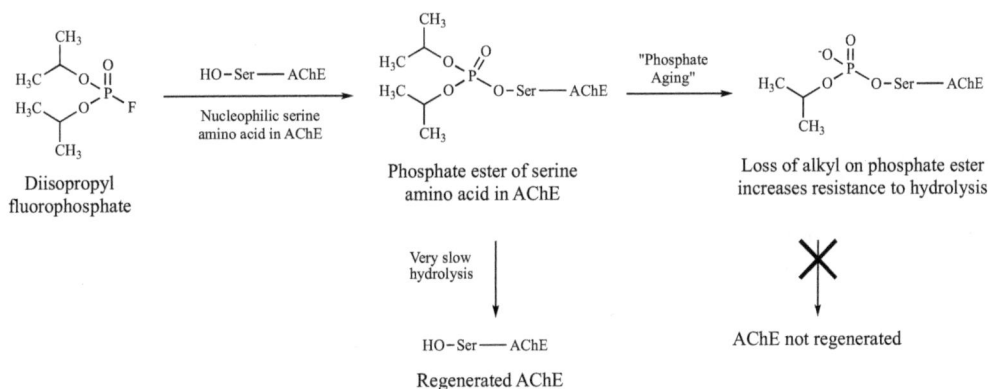

Diisopropyl
fluorophosphate

Nucleophilic serine
amino acid in AChE

Phosphate ester of serine
amino acid in AChE

"Phosphate Aging"

Loss of alkyl on phosphate ester
increases resistance to hydrolysis

Very slow
hydrolysis

HO—Ser——AChE

Regenerated AChE

AChE not regenerated

Fig. (29). Inhibition of AChE by phosphoric acid derivatives. Hydrolysis of serine phosphate ester on AChE is very slow and becomes impossible when the ester "ages" *in vitro*.

Before a phosphate ester "ages" and irreversibly inhibits enzyme activity, a patient may be given pharmacologic agents designed to reverse the mechanism of action of phosphorous-based covalent AChE inhibitors. Pralidoxime (2-pyridine aldoxine methyl chloride, or 2-PAM) contains quaternary ammonium nitrogen that associates with the AChE active site and positions its highly nucleophilic oxime oxygen atom for maximum effect near the AChE active site serine hydroxyl functional group (Fig. **31**). Rescue therapy with 2-PAM accelerates the decomposition of the phosphate ester and allows for regeneration of the AChE enzyme. If the phosphate esters have aged, however, rescue agents are incapable of effectively promoting hydrolysis of the serine phosphate ester and the AChE enzyme is thereafter permanently deactivated [40].

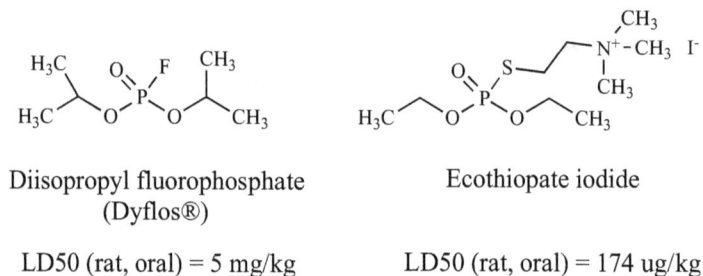

Diisopropyl fluorophosphate
(Dyflos®)

Ecothiopate iodide

LD50 (rat, oral) = 5 mg/kg

LD50 (rat, oral) = 174 ug/kg

Fig. (30). Dyflos and ecothiopate LD_{50} information.

Phosphate ester of serine
amino acid in AChE

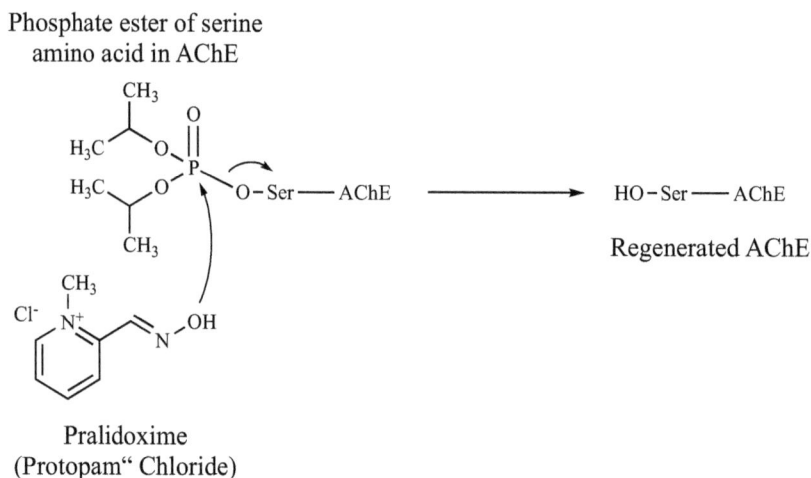

Regenerated AChE

Pralidoxime
(Protopam" Chloride)

Fig. (31). Pralidoxime contains a nucleophilic oxime hydroxyl group capable of accelerating the decomposition of AChE phosphate ester, regenerating the enzyme.

When an AChE inhibitor is overdosed, ACh is not degraded at the synapse and the synapse becomes hyperstimulated, leading to serious adverse effects. Atropine may be administered to prevent overstimulation of muscarinic receptors in AChE inhibitor poisoning. Also, co-administration of diazepam as a sedative and antiseizure agent may be indicated.

Due to their extreme duration of the activity, phosphoric acid derivatives are not clinically useful therapeutics. They have significant toxicities and therefore have seen the most use as pesticides or as chemical warfare agents designed to incapacitate living things. There are many examples of pesticides and "G- and V-series" organophosphorus "area denial" chemical weapons that have been designed for these uses (Fig. **32**) [41].

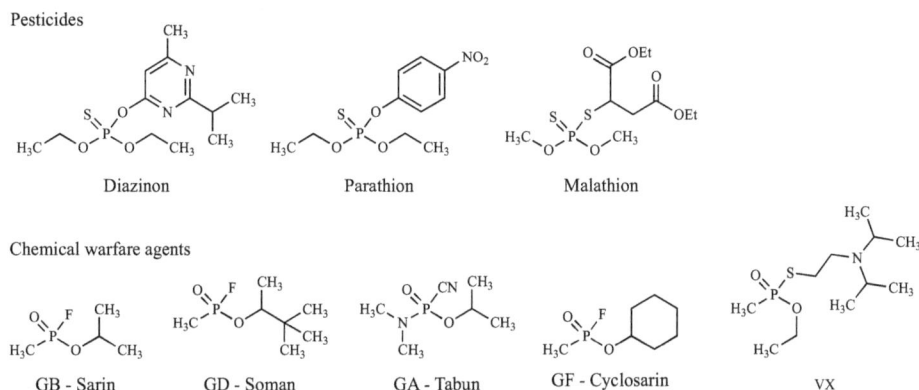

Fig. (32). Examples of pesticides and chemical warfare agents that are phosphoric acid-derived acetylcholinesterase inhibitors.

NEUROMUSCULAR BLOCKING AGENTS

- *Depolarizing muscle nicotinic receptor neuromuscular blocking agents*
- *Non-depolarizing muscle nicotinic receptor neuromuscular blocking agents*
- *Ganglionic-nicotinic receptor blocking agents*

The neuromuscular junction (Fig. **33**) contains mostly nAChR and therefore agonists and antagonists of nicotinic receptors are used to affect muscle function. Clinically, they are most often employed for peripheral muscle paralysis during surgical procedures.

Depolarizing Muscle Nicotinic Receptor Neuromuscular Blocking Agents

Only a single depolarizing agent, succinylcholine, is regularly used in clinical settings. Succinylcholine is an agonist of nAChR, stimulating the opening of the receptor and causing depolarization of the cell membrane. Succinylcholine persists at the nAChR and continuously activates it, preventing normal stimulation from presynaptically released ACh and halting further action potentials in the muscle cell (Fig. **34**). Succinylcholine, therefore, causes a "depolarizing" blockade of the neuromuscular junction. It is a very short-acting drug that is metabolized by plasma cholinesterase to pharmacologically inactive succinylmonocholine [42].

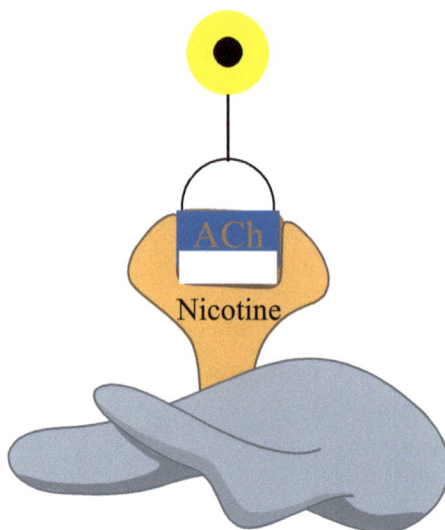

Neuromuscular junction

Fig. (33). Nicotinic acetylcholine receptors at the neuromuscular junction.

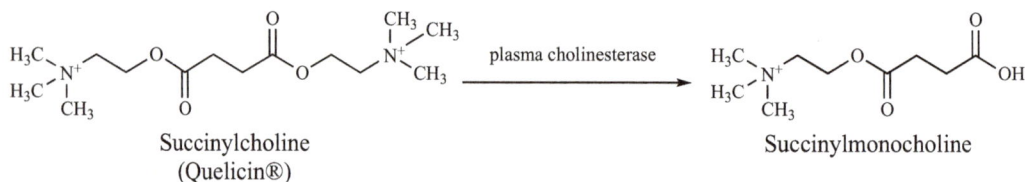

Succinylcholine
(Quelicin®)

Succinylmonocholine

Fig. (34). Rapid hydrolysis of succinylcholine by plasma cholinesterase.

Non-depolarizing Muscle Nicotinic Receptor Neuromuscular Blocking Agents

Nicotinic receptor antagonists may prevent endogenous ACh binding and therefore inhibit muscle cell depolarization by preventing nAChR activation. These antagonists are referred to as competitive "nondepolarizing" neuromuscular blocking agents (Fig. **35**). They are generally categorized by the duration of action as short-acting (5-20 min), intermediate (30-80 min), and long (80-180 min), agents. They are further defined by an onset of action that is either short (~1 minute) or long (4-6 minutes) [43].

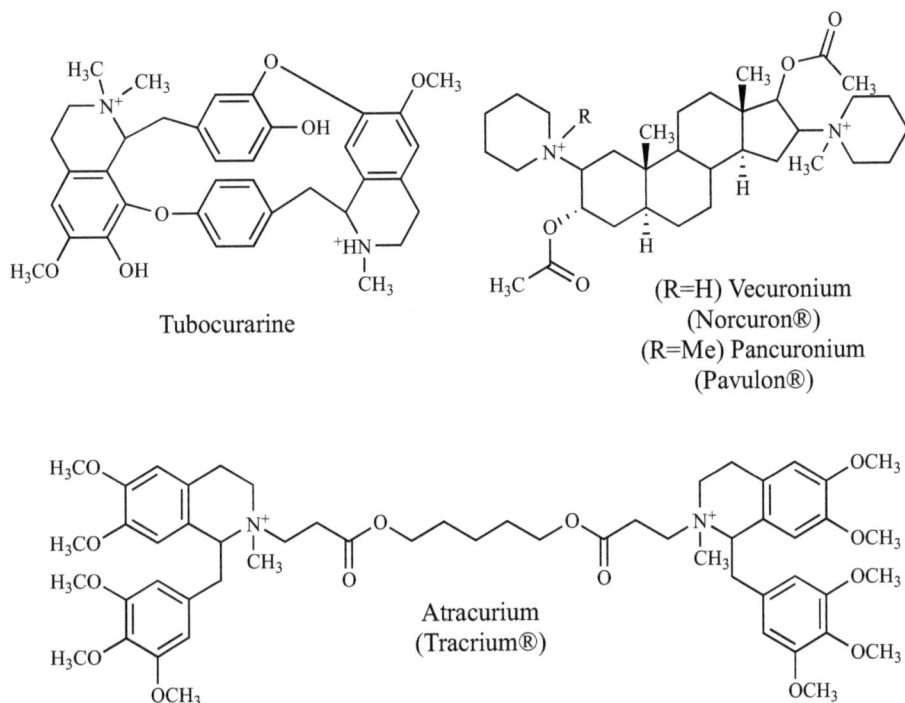

Fig. (35). Long- and intermediate-duration neuromuscular blocking agents.

Originally derived from the *curare* arrow poisons used by South American Indians, tubocurarine is a long-acting agent which causes a persistent neuromuscular blockade that is difficult to completely reverse. Both tubocurarine and the ammonia steroid pancuronium instigate a prolonged blockade with a long onset of action. Intermediate-acting agents such as atracurium and short-duration derivatives such as mivacurium offer more control during blockade reversal (Fig. 36). Enzymatic hydrolysis by plasma cholinesterase is the primary mechanism for inactivation of short-acting mivacurium and yields a quaternary alcohol and a quaternary monoester metabolite. The clearance of this drug is very high and extremely dependent on the concentration of plasma cholinesterases [44].

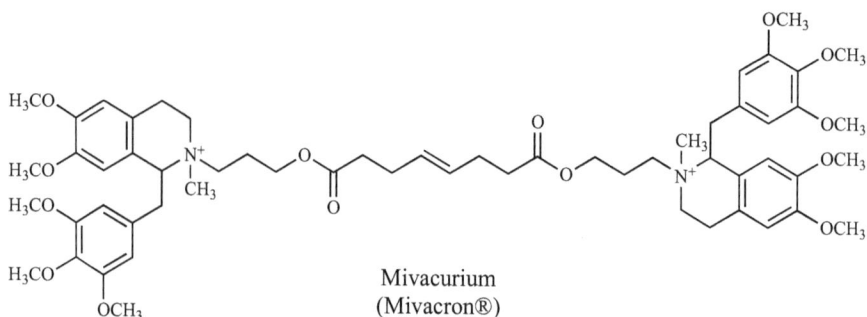

Fig. (36). Mivacurium short-duration neuromuscular blocking agent.

Because nAChR is expressed in autonomic ganglia as well as the neuromuscular junction, adverse effects from ganglionic blockade may be seen.

Ganglionic-Nicotinic Receptor Blocking Agents

Certain nAChR antagonists with specificity for ganglionic nicotinic receptors are used as ganglionic blockers. Mecamylamine is indicated for use to reduce blood pressure in instances of aortic dissection while also reducing the sympathetic reflexes that would result from increases in pressure at the site of vascular injury. Mecamylamine concentrates in the liver and kidneys and is excreted slowly in the urine unchanged. The rate of renal elimination is influenced markedly by urinary pH, and acidification promotes renal excretion of the secondary amine (Fig. **37**) [45].

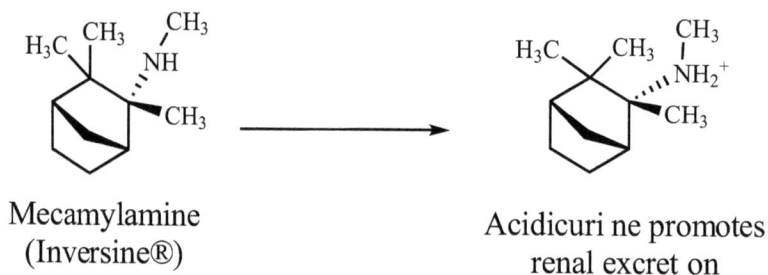

Mecamylamine
(Inversine®)

Acidicuri ne promotes
renal excret on

Fig. (37). Mecamylamine renal excretion is enhanced by acidic urine.

TREATMENT OF ALZHEIMER'S DISEASE (AD)

Alzheimer's Disease (AD) is the most common type of dementia. It is a progressive and debilitating disease that has a significant clinical impact on both the patient, family members, and caregivers. Dementia associated with AD has been termed organ failure of the brain; it is a failure of cognition, function, and behavior [46]. AD is classified as late-onset, usually occurring in patients ≥ 65 years of age, or as early-onset if diagnosed in patients < 65 years of age. Early signs and symptoms of the disease include short-term memory loss, such as names or events. Additionally, early symptoms displayed by patients include the appearance of being withdrawn or depression and anxiety. With further decline, patients will often be confused or disoriented; they show signs of impaired judgment with behavioral changes like agitation and irritability in addition to potential delusions and hallucinations. In the later stages of the disease, patients exhibit impairment of activities of daily living (ADL) such as hygiene activities, dressing, eating, *etc.* and patients will likely have difficulty speaking and walking. As the disease progresses and complications ensue, family members often become overwhelmed with providing care, requiring nursing home placement [46].

Epidemiology

According to the 2019 Alzheimer's Disease Facts and Figures, 5.6 million Americans ≥ 65 years of age have AD; additionally, there are 200,000 Americans with younger-onset AD to a total of 5.8 million Americans of all ages diagnosed with AD [47]. In 2010, the reported incidence of AD worldwide was more than 35 million people [48]. Alzheimer's disease affects women more than men. Of the 5.2 million Americans older than 65 years of age, 3.4 million (about 65%) are women and 1.8 million (about 35%) are men. When evaluating ethnicity, older African-Americans are about 2 times more likely than older whites to have AD while older Hispanics are about 1.5 times as likely as older whites to have AD [47].

Pathophysiology

Although we do not know of one definitive cause of Alzheimer's Disease, there are several potential etiologies reported that include the amyloid hypothesis, cholinergic deficit, appearance of neurofibrillary tangles (NFT) and neuronal cell death, most notably in the areas of the brain that are important for memory (the cortex and especially the hippocampus) and cognitive functions. Important pathophysiological consequences of the disease include a decline in cholinergic activity as well as other neurotransmission abnormalities such as sustained excitatory glutamate activity, both of which are target areas for current drug therapy. Other additional pathophysiological components that potentially increase the risk of AD include inflammatory or immunologic alterations, hypercholesterolemia, and cerebrovascular disease, with genetics playing a key role in AD progression [48 - 50].

β-Amyloid Hypothesis

AD is characterized by the deposition of amyloid β peptide (Aβ) plaques. Amyloid precursor protein (APP) is found on chromosome 21; it is a cellular membrane protein that is highly concentrated in neuronal synapses, functioning in cell adhesion and signal transduction [51]. APP undergoes proteolysis by either α-secretase or β-secretase and then by γ-secretase. APP that is sequentially cleaved by α-secretase and then by γ -secretase yields p3 fragment, a small, soluble peptide. If APP is sequentially cleaved by β-secretase and then by γ-secretase, it yields β-amyloid protein fragment, a small insoluble peptide that is neurotoxic with effects seen at neuronal synapses. Aβ peptides are degraded by two proteases: insulin-degrading enzymes and neprilysin. Accumulation results when the formation is greater than clearance of Aβ protein peptides, allowing aggregation with resultant formation of Aβ protein plaques; the "amyloid hypothesis" of Alzheimer's Disease [48 - 50].

Accumulation of Aβ peptides also has a deleterious effect on tau, a phosphorylated protein found in cell membranes. Tau attaches to and helps stabilize microtubules, which are important in nutrient transport, and propagation of signaling along the axon. Hyperphosphorylated tau, thought to occur after Aβ peptide accumulation and plaque formation, is an insoluble protein that lacks affinity for microtubules. The resultant impairment in the ability of hyperphosphorylated tau to attach and stabilize the microtubule allows the tubule to "unravel," thereby impairing axonal transport with eventual neuronal cell death. Furthermore, hyperphosphorylated tau proteins can aggregate to one another, causing them to twist with the formation of neurofibrillary tangles (NFT). NFT formation is believed to be a major contributing factor to AD and cognitive impairment with a correlation seen between dementia and quantity of NFTs; higher concentrations of NFTs are associated with a higher degree of cognitive decline and severity of AD [48 - 50].

Cholinergic Hypothesis

Aβ protein plaques destroy multiple neuronal pathways, the most prominent of which involves the cholinergic pathway, with a decline in cholinergic activity correlating with cognitive impairment and AD severity. The "cholinergic hypothesis" is believed to be a consequence and not an etiology of AD. As AD progresses, there are fewer cholinergic neurons and fewer nicotinic receptors in the hippocampus and cortex. Neurotrophin receptors on cholinergic neurons are also significantly reduced in the late stages of AD. The decline in neurotrophins may help explain some of the cognitive and behavioral decline seen in AD as they play a role in learning and memory as well as behavior; they are also involved in proliferation and differentiation of neurons [48]. Presynaptic nicotinic receptor stimulation regulates the release of neurotransmitters important in memory and mood, including ACh, glutamate, serotonin, and norepinephrine. Aβ peptides have the potential to bind to nicotinic receptors and cause a decrease in ACh release, also decreasing cholinergic activity [49, 50, 52].

Other Hypothesis

Glutamate, serotonin, and norepinephrine are neurotransmitters that have been identified with altered activity in AD patients. Glutamate is an excitatory neurotransmitter involved in >60% of brain synapses, including many neuronal transmissions important to learning and memory. The N-methyl-D-aspartate (NMDA) receptor, one of the three postsynaptic glutamate receptors, has been linked to AD pathophysiology. When left in synapses for extended periods, glutamate becomes neurotoxic, destroying nerves by allowing an influx of calcium with altered neuronal signal transduction; it appears there is a continual low-level stimulation of this receptor in the brains of AD patients. Abnormal glutamate activity may also be linked to the development of NFT by an increase in APP production, hyperphosphorylated tau protein and plaques [49]. Serotonin receptors may be altered in AD, leading to the depression and anxiety that is often observed in AD patients. A decrease in norepinephrine, as well as its receptors, is likely associated with the aggression and agitation seen with the disease.

Other risk factors (Table 5) that contribute to AD progression have been identified as well. Apolipoprotein E (APOE) is a gene carrying the code for the synthesis of proteins that function to transport cholesterol in the blood. Possession of apolipoprotein E-ε4 (APOE- ε4), one of three of the alleles for APOE, is the greatest genetic risk factor (especially if the patient inherits an APOE- ε4 allele from each parent) for the development of late-onset AD. APOE- ε4 may lead to increased production of Aβ [47]. Additionally, Aβ peptide production is believed to increase in the presence of hypercholesterolemia; lower Aβ levels have been observed with inhibition of cholesterol synthesis in patients receiving statin therapy. Cerebrovascular disease causes decreased perfusion to the brain leading to degenerative changes and cognitive impairment, thereby resulting in vascular dementia. Besides previously mentioned actions, Aβ peptides in the brain are involved in biochemical reactions that yield oxidized free radicals; this oxidative stress is believed to be important early in the progression of the disease as it has been linked to plaque and NFT formation. Aβ peptides, NFT, and neuronal cell damage stimulate an inflammatory response which precipitates further damage, one of which is cell apoptosis via cytokine release [48 - 50].

Table 5. AD Risk Factors.

Risk Factors for Developing Alzheimer's Disease	
Non-modifiable	**Modifiable**
Age*	Hypertension
Apolipoprotein E-ε4 (APOE-ε4)[§]	Hypercholesterolemia
Family history[¥]	Diabetes Mellitus
Head trauma or brain injury	Obesity
	Smoking

*Advancing age (usually in adults ≥ 65 years old) is the overall greatest risk factor for developing AD; [§]Apolipoprotein E-ε4 (APOE-ε4) is the main genetic risk factor for developing late-onset AD, with risk increasing further if an individual has inherited an APOE-ε4 allele from each parent; [¥]Especially if first-degree relatives – parents and/or siblings with AD.

Pharmacotherapy

While there are no drugs currently available to cure the disease or stop its progression, there are two classes of medications available that help improve symptoms and cognitive function, as well as slow disease progression and patient decline associated with AD. The two classes are AChE inhibitors and N-Methy--D- Aspartate (NMDA) receptor antagonists.

Acetyl Cholinesterase (AChE) Inhibitors

Loss of cholinergic activity in the central nervous system; decline in ACh levels and degeneration of cholinergic neurons, has been linked to impaired memory and cognition associated with Alzheimer's dementia [55 - 57]. Based on this "cholinergic hypothesis", AChE inhibitors alone or in combination with Memantine are currently FDA approved for the treatment of cognitive symptoms of AD [58, 59]. The AChE inhibitors act by inhibiting the rapid hydrolysis of ACh and thereby increasing synaptic concentrations of this neurotransmitter. It should be noted that even though the clinical benefits of AChE inhibitors are dose-dependent, increased doses also increase the risk of side effects. The side effects associated with the use of AChE inhibitors are mostly due to cholinergic stimulation and include gastrointestinal (GI) symptoms such as diarrhea and flatulence. Because of their side effects on the GI tract, AChE inhibitors should be used with caution in patients with active peptic ulcer disease or active GI bleed, and concurrent administration with NSAIDs, which can also aggravate GI bleed, should be avoided. Their cholinergic effects may aggravate asthma or chronic obstructive pulmonary disease and may affect bladder outflow with urinary incontinence/obstruction. These agents should also be used with caution in individuals with cardiovascular disease or cardiac arrhythmias; AChE inhibitors may cause bradycardia, atrioventricular heart block, or Torsades de Pointes. CNS effects seen by AChE inhibitors warrant that they be used with caution in patients with epilepsy, a seizure may occur with increased cholinergic activity, unexplained syncope, and cholinesterase (ChE) inhibition may exacerbate extrapyramidal symptoms (EPS) [46].

Donepezil (Aricept®)

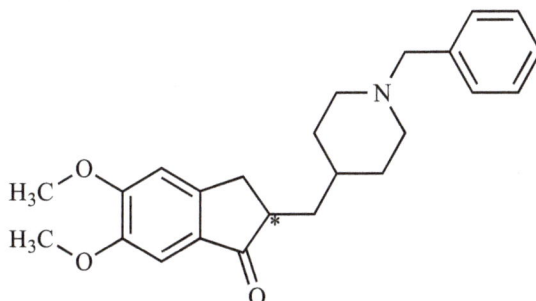

Donepezil (Aricept®)

Donepezil is FDA-approved for the treatment of mild to moderate or moderate to severe dementia associated with AD [46]. A combination product Namzaric⁺, with Memantine, is indicated for the treatment of moderate to severe dementia of the Alzheimer's type. Donepezil, a piperidine derivative, is marketed as its racemic mixture. Both the R- and S-enantiomers inhibit AChE with the R-enantiomer being more potent than the S-enantiomer *in vitro*. Donepezil is a noncovalent, non-competitive, reversible inhibitor of AChE. Donepezil is classified as a short-acting agent since it binds to AChE via hydrogen bonds and inhibits the enzyme for a short duration of time. However, relative to tacrine, donepezil is considered to be more potent with a high degree of selectivity for AChE (~1250-fold) than for butyrylcholinesterase (BuChE). Additionally, donepezil exhibits greater selectivity for central AChE than for non-neuronal AChE [60 - 62].

Pharmacokinetics

Donepezil exhibits good oral absorption (100% relative oral bioavailability) and may be given with or without food. Peak plasma concentrations are reached in about 3-4 hours. Donepezil is highly protein bound (about 96%) with ~75% bound to albumin and ~21% bound to α_1-acid glycoprotein.[60] Donepezil undergoes hepatic metabolism via CYP3A4 and CYP2D6 with CYP3A4 being the primary metabolizing enzyme (Fig. **38**) [63, 64]. The 6-O-desmethyl metabolite is pharmacologically active and inhibits AChE to the same extent as the parent compound *in vitro* [65].

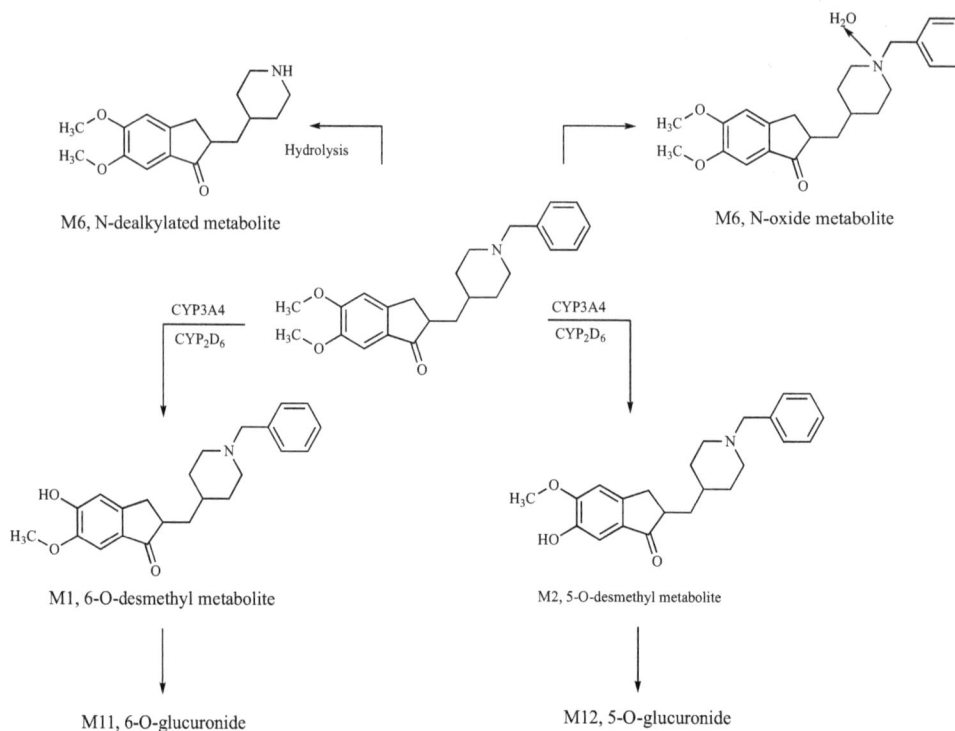

Fig. (38). Metabolism of Donepezil.

The half-life of donepezil is about 70 hours [50]. It is initiated at a dose of 5 mg orally once daily and may be titrated after 4-6 weeks to a maximum dose of 10 mg orally once daily. Dosage forms available are tablets and orally disintegrating tablets (ODT); furthermore, generic dosage forms are available in the United States.

Side effects/Drug Interactions

Additional side effects to the ones previously mentioned include nausea, hypertension, dizziness, headache, insomnia or somnolence, fatigue, and depression. Potential drug-drug interactions include donepezil and succinylcholine where prolongation of neuromuscular blockade may be seen. When combined with bethanechol, cholinergic adverse effects, such as bradyarrhythmias, bronchospasm, hyperhidrosis (excessive sweating), diarrhea, and vomiting may be observed. Decreased efficacy of donepezil may be seen when combined with oxybutynin or tolterodine (due to their anticholinergic effects). Ketoconazole and quinidine increase donepezil's bioavailability (due to CYP enzyme inhibition) whereas; donepezil causes increased exposure to ramelteon when these two drugs are administered concurrently [46, 50, 53].

Rivastigmine (Exelon∘) 2000, Oral; 2008, Patch

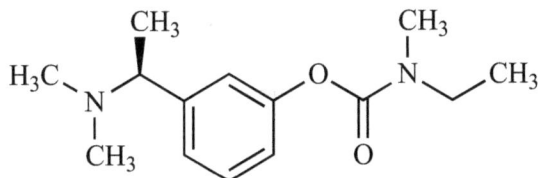

Rivastigmine (Exelone)

Rivastigmine, a carbamate derivative, forms a covalent bond with the OH group of Ser200 of AChE resulting in a carbamylated esteratic site (Fig. **39**). The regeneration of active AChE is extremely slow and results in prolonged inhibition of AChE's activity, for ~10 hours. Therefore, rivastigmine is classified as a pseudo-irreversible or intermediate-acting agent relative to the other AChEIs [66 - 68]. It should also be noted that rivastigmine not only inhibits acetylcholinesterase activity but also inhibits BuChE to an equal extent, this is the cholinesterase inhibitor with the highest degree of BuChE inhibition. However, it does exhibit selectivity for CNS enzyme inhibition over peripheral enzyme inhibition [66]. Rivastigmine is FDA-approved for the treatment of mild to moderate dementia.

Pharmacokinetics

Rivastigmine is a lipophilic agent with excellent blood-brain barrier penetration. Oral rivastigmine is well absorbed and is recommended to be taken with food to potentiate absorption and GI tolerability [66]. Peak plasma concentration is reached in about one hour. Rivastigmine is about 40% protein bound. Esterases, such as cholinesterase, hydrolyze rivastigmine to the phenolic derivative which then undergoes N-demethylation and/or sulfate conjugation with the metabolites undergoing renal excretion predominantly, 97%. The half-life of oral rivastigmine is about 1.5 hours and about 3 hours for the transdermal route [50]. Initial doses of the oral dosage form are 1.5 mg orally twice daily. If doses are tolerated, oral rivastigmine may be titrated every two weeks to 3 mg, then 4.5 mg then up to a maximum dosage of 6 mg orally twice daily.

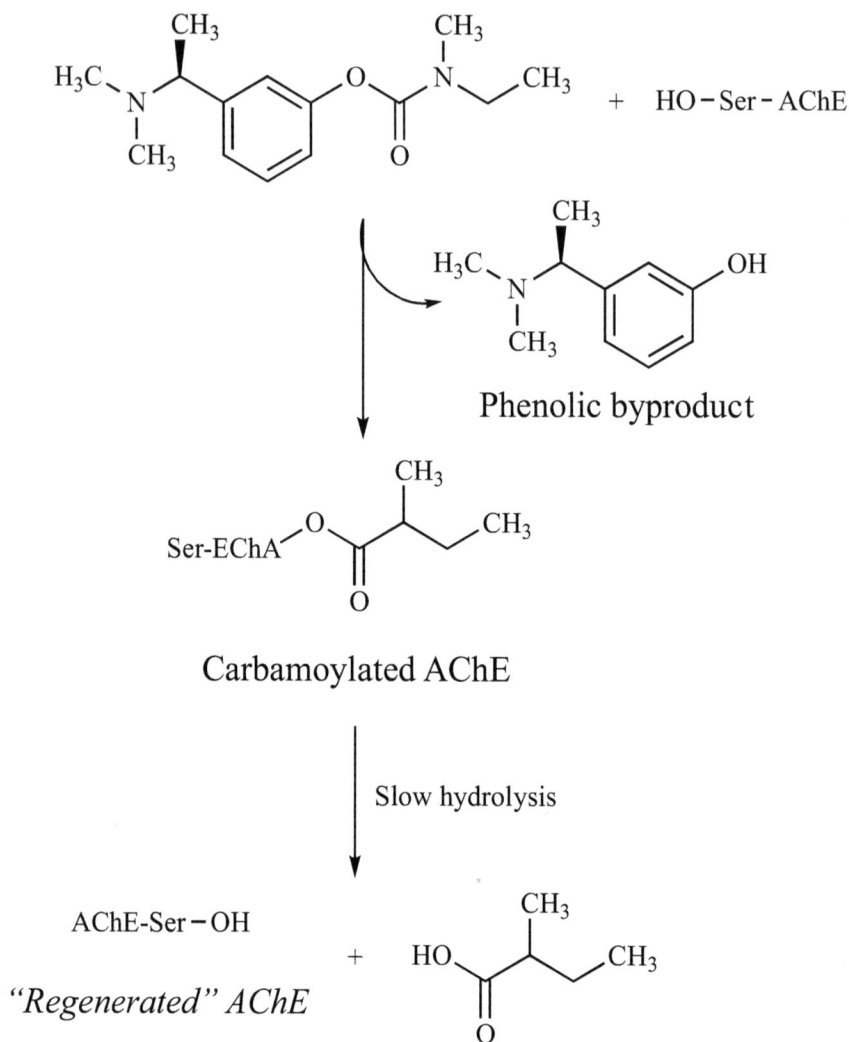

Fig. (39). Mechanism of action of rivastigmine.

Rivastigmine is also available as a transdermal patch with extended-release of the medication. The patch allows titration to maximal doses while diminishing or eliminating intolerable side effects. The initial starting dose of the transdermal formulation is 4.6 mg/24 hr patch applied once daily and after tolerating for at least four weeks, it may be increased to a maximum dose of 9.5 mg/24 hr patch applied once daily. For patients who have trouble tolerating an oral ChEI due to GI side effects, the transdermal patch of rivastigmine is a good option.

Side effects/Drug Interactions

Since rivastigmine does not undergo hepatic metabolism via the CYP mediated pathways, the potential for clinically significant drug interactions when co-administered with other CYP enzyme substrates is low. Immediate switching from an oral AChEI to rivastigmine does not require a washout period and is generally safe and well-tolerated in AD patients; minimal adverse events have been reported but may include skin lesions, erythema or itching, and some may still experience the GI side effects [54]. For patients switching from oral to patch on a daily dose < 6 mg of PO rivastigmine, the patient should be started on the 4.6 mg/24 hr patch. If the daily dose is 6-12 mg, the patient should be switched to 9.5 mg/24 hr patch. The patch should be applied the day after the last oral dose is taken. The patch should be applied to hairless skin free of cuts, preferably on the upper back, arm, or chest, and the application sites should be rotated. There are currently no generics available of either dosage form. Additional side effects to the once previously mentioned include weight loss and dizziness. Rivastigmine in combination with metoclopramide may result in increased extrapyramidal side effects (EPS). Concurrent use with tolterodine and oxybutynin may result in decreased efficacy of rivastigmine [46, 50, 53].

Galantamine (Razadyne®) 2001

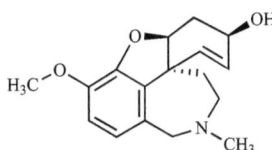

Galantamine (Rezadyne)

Galantamine is a tertiary amine alkaloid that inhibits AChE in a competitive reversible manner. However, reports indicate that its ability to allosterically potentiate neuronal nicotinic receptors (nAChRs), by binding to the α-subunit, is primarily responsible for its therapeutic effects [69]. Galantamine also exhibits greater selectivity (~53-fold) for AChE *in vitro* than for BuChE which may explain the better tolerability, decreased peripheral adverse effects, observed with galantamine use [70, 71]. Galantamine is FDA-approved for the treatment of mild to moderate Alzheimer's Disease.

Pharmacokinetics

Galantamine has good absorption after oral administration and should be taken with food. Peak plasma concentration is reached in about one hour with immediate release formulations and about 5 hours with extended-release formulations. Galantamine exhibits much less protein binding than observed with other cholinesterase inhibitors, about 20%. It is hepatically metabolized by CYP3A4 to norgalantamine and by CYP2D6 to O-desmethyl galantamine followed by glucuronidation. Other metabolic outcomes include N-demethylation, N-oxidation, and epimerization (Fig. **40**) [72]. Almost all pharmacological activity is attributed to unchanged galantamine in plasma with none of the unconjugated plasma metabolites found to exhibit appreciable AChE activity (considered to be inactive) [71 - 73].

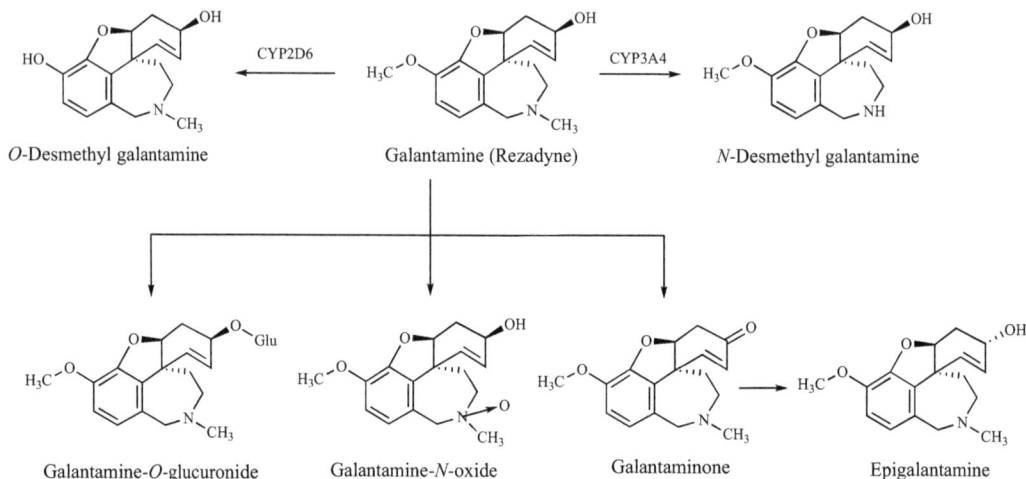

O-Desmethyl galantamine   Galantamine (Rezadyne)   *N*-Desmethyl galantamine

Galantamine-*O*-glucuronide   Galantamine-*N*-oxide   Galantaminone   Epigalantamine

Fig. (40). Galantamine metabolism.

The half-life of galantamine is about seven hours.[50] Initiation of galantamine is usually with the extended-release (ER) product at a dose of 8 mg orally once daily and is titrated at four-week intervals to 16 mg and then to a maximum dose of 24 mg orally once daily. It is also available as an immediate-release tablet and as an oral solution, the initiating doses of these formulations are 4 mg orally twice daily and it may be titrated at four-week intervals up to 8 mg twice daily and then to 12 mg twice daily. For patients with moderate renal impairment or moderate hepatic impairment, the maximum daily dose should not exceed 16 mg and for severe renal impairment or severe hepatic impairment, galantamine should not be used. There are generic formulations available for each of these dosage forms.

Side effects/Drug-interactions

Additional side effects to the once previously mentioned include weight loss, dizziness, and headache. Thrombocytopenia is a rare adverse effect that may be observed with galantamine. Potential drug-drug interactions include decreased efficacy of galantamine if given with oxybutynin or tolterodine (anticholinergic agents). Concurrent administration with quinidine, ketoconazole, fluoxetine, paroxetine, amitriptyline, or fluvoxamine may result in increased galantamine concentrations [46, 50, 53].

NMDA Receptor Antagonist: Memantine (Namenda◦) 2003

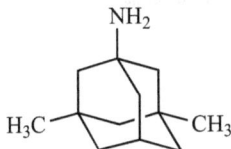

Memantine (Namenda®)

The N-methyl-D-aspartate (NMDA) receptors are a subtype of glutamate receptors and mediate a number of physiological neuronal functions. These ligand-gated ion channel (ionotropic) receptors are composed of four subunits with the NR2 and NR1 subunits required for the receptor's activity. NMDA receptor activation has immense functional significance; normal physiological activation results in beneficial effects like neuronal survival whereas sustained excessive activation (glutamate-mediated "Excitotoxicity") results in neuronal death, a characteristic feature observed in acute and chronic neurological disorders. These differential effects observed with NMDA receptor activation can be attributed to NMDA receptor location with postsynaptic receptor activation associated with favorable outcomes whereas extrasynaptic receptor activation leads to neuronal cell death. Therefore, it is imperative that NMDA receptor blockers differentiate between extrasynaptic and postsynaptic receptors; block pathological activation of NMDA receptors without affecting their normal physiological function [74 - 77].

Memantine is the only FDA-approved NMDA antagonist currently available for the treatment of moderate to severe Alzheimer's disease. Namzaric◦, a donepezil combination product, is indicated for the treatment of moderate to severe dementia of the Alzheimer's type in patients stabilized on 10 mg of donepezil hydrochloride once daily. Memantine exhibits an excellent safety profile whereas the use of other NMDA receptor blockers like ketamine is associated with deleterious effects like memory loss and symptoms of schizophrenia. This unusual safety profile of memantine can be explained by its ability to preferentially block extrasynaptic NMDA receptors with a rapid off-rate. Additional reasons include the ability of memantine to act as an open-channel blocker (is only able to enter the channel and block current flow after the channel opening) and block the NMDA receptor in an un-competitive manner [74, 75].

Pharmacokinetics

Memantine exhibits good oral absorption and can be given with or without food.

It reaches peak plasma concentrations in about 3-8 hours for the immediate release formulation and in 9-12 hours for the extended release formulation. It is ~45% protein bound and is predominantly excreted renally in its unchanged form. The half-life of memantine is 60-80 hours [50]. The metabolism of memantine is independent of the CYP enzyme system and undergoes partial hepatic metabolism. Memantine is available as oral tablets, capsules and as a liquid formulation. Patients initiated on the immediate release formulations, tablets, and solution, may begin at a dose of 5 mg orally once daily or divided as 2.5 mg orally twice daily. The dose may be titrated at one-week intervals to a total daily dose of 10 mg, then a total daily dose of 15 mg up to a maximum of 20 mg orally once daily or divided as 10 mg orally twice daily. The extended release formulation, capsules, the initial dose is 7 mg orally once daily and titration of 7 mg at 1-week intervals may be given up to a maximum dose of 28 mg once daily as tolerated. For patients with severe renal impairment, the maximum doses of the immediate release formulation are 10 mg daily or 5 mg twice daily and for the extended release formula, the maximum dose recommended is 14 mg once daily. There are no generic formulations available.

Side effects/Drug interactions

Patients may experience side effects, especially while the dose is titrated, which include confusion, dizziness, headache, and somnolence.[46] Other potential side effects include hypertension or hypotension, syncope, diarrhea, constipation, and vomiting. Serious side effects include Stevens-Johnson syndrome, deep vein thrombosis, liver impairment or hepatitis, acute renal failure, cerebral infarction, cerebrovascular accident or transient ischemic attack, intracranial hemorrhage, and seizures. Potential drug-drug interactions include carbonic anhydrase inhibitors and sodium bicarbonate, which may decrease memantine clearance. Interactions that may alter the serum concentrations of both memantine and the interacting drug include nicotine polacrilex, quinidine, ranitidine, cimetidine, and hydrochlorothiazide [52].

Table 6. PK/PD Summary of AChEIs

	Donepezil (Aricept·)	Rivastigmine (Exelon·)		Galantamine (Razadyne·)		Memantine (Namenda·)	
Dosage Forms	Tablet and orally disintegrating tablet	Capsule & solution	ER transdermal Patch	Tablet & solution	ER capsule	Tablet & solution	ER capsule
Initial Dose	5 mg QD	1.5 mg BID	4.6 mg/24 hr patch applied QD	4 mg BID	8 mg QD	5 mg QD or 2.5 mg BID	7 mg QD

(Table 6) cont.....

	Donepezil (Aricept•)	Rivastigmine (Exelon•)		Galantamine (Razadyne•)		Memantine (Namenda•)	
Max Dose	10 mg QD	6 mg BID	9.5 mg/24 hr patch applied QD	12 mg BID	24 mg QD	20 mg QD or 10 mg BID	28 mg QD
FDA Indication	Mild to moderate AD Moderate to severe AD	Mild to moderate AD		Mild to moderate AD		Moderate to severe AD	
Mechanism of action (MOA)	AChEI	AChEI BuChEI		AChEI Nicotinic agonist		NMDA receptor antagonist	
Half-life ($T_{1/2}$)	70 hours	1.5 hours	3 hours	7 hours		60-80 hours	
Protein Binding	96%	40%		18%		45%	
Clearance/ Metabolism	Hepatic CYP 3A4/2D6	Urinary		Hepatic CYP 3A4/2D6		Urinary	

Place in Therapy

Initial management of Alzheimer's disease should include a review of current medications and discontinuation of any that are unnecessary, especially those that may affect mental status. A cholinesterase inhibitor should be initiated in mild dementia associated AD. For moderate dementia AD, a cholinesterase inhibitor or memantine may be initiated; once titrated to maximum tolerated dose, the other agent is usually added to complement treatment. There are two medications currently with FDA-approval for severe dementia associated AD, donepezil and memantine. As patients reach the severe stage of AD, therapy may be continued but with no further benefit in the prevention of the decline in cognition or memory. Patients who reach the terminal stage of AD have essentially no quality of life left; at this point, AD therapy should be withdrawn and palliative care with comfort measures should be initiated.

CASE STUDY

RR is a 72-year-old obese female who is a retired high school teacher. At a routine physical examination, she is accompanied by her daughter who reports that her mother seems more sad, withdrawn and has forgotten several planned engagements, *e.g.* grand-daughter's birthday party, bake sale event at church, haircut appointment, *etc.* She also arrived at her son's house recently (2.5 hrs from her home) after going the wrong direction when trying to go to a friend's house. [mild-moderate AD]

Past Medical History (PMH): depression, hypertension, seasonal rhinitis, alcoholic cirrhosis, overactive bladder, type II diabetes mellitus, and back pain

SH: smokes 1/2 a pack per day for 40yrs, negative for alcohol consumption now, but drank heavily in the past.

Current Meds: carvedilol, diphenhydramine, lisinopril, pioglitazone, paroxetine, sitagliptin, oxybutynin, daily multivitamin, and ibuprofen

1. List AD risk factors that RR has.
2. Describe the two main pathophysiologic etiologies of Alzheimer's Disease.
3. Which of the following agents would you initiate and why?

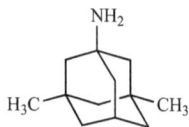

Memantine (Namenda®)   Galantamine (Razadyne®)   Rivastigmine (Exelon®)

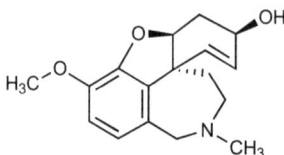

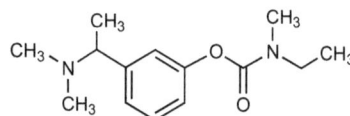

4. Which of the following agents exhibits a relatively longer duration of enzyme inhibition and explain your rationale?
5. What therapeutic modifications would you recommend?

Either in agreement with or contrary to your recommendation, RR was initiated on rivastigmine 1.5 mg BID with an increase in dose every 2 weeks to 3 mg BID, then to 4.5 mg BID up to 6 mg BID. At the 4.5 mg BID dose, she and her daughter report back to your clinic due to intolerable side effects RR is experiencing. Based on RR's complaints, the physician decides to change RR to topical therapy instead of an alternate oral medication in the same class.

1. Identify the medication-related adverse effects RR is most likely complaining about?
2. What are the other potential side effects of rivastigmine?
3. Please provide a recommendation and state how you would counsel RR.

RR has been maintained for two years on the topical therapy, but now her daughter reports at her appointment that RR is more easily agitated. She has called the police on several occasions stating that she has been robbed: a television, radio, and various other items. Furthermore, she tells her son that she thinks his sister is stealing from her- jewelry, baking pans, a sewing machine, *etc*. She is also having difficulty with activities of daily living and the decision is made that RR will move in with her daughter. [moderate-severe AD]

What therapeutic modifications would you make at this time and why?

RR does moderately well for the next three years, but she has now lost the ability to care for herself, she cannot walk and her daughter has injured her back while providing care; it is decided to place RR in a nursing home. She stops eating and she has lost a significant amount of weight (she weighs 38.6 kg, about 85% IBW), RR now has to be fed parenterally. [End stage AD]

Drug Discovery Case Study

The Quaternary Advantage – Ipratropium and the Kinetic Selectivity of Tiotropium

Currently, the two most widely used cholinergic drugs in the United States are albuterol/ipratropium (Combivent®), and tiotropium (Spiriva®), used in the management of allergic rhinorrhea and COPD respectively. Both ipratropium and tiotropium are quaternary ammonium derivatives of atropine that will not penetrate the CNS and have effects at the muscarinic receptor subtypes M1, M2, and M3.

Tertiary amines atropine and scopolamine are distributed widely in tissues and suffer from unfavorable side-effect profiles since the M3 receptor subtype is broadly expressed in the human body. Clinically useful quaternary ammonium derivatives of atropine and scopolamine began to come into use in disease state therapies where poorly absorbed, CNS inactive compounds are acceptable [78]. The first three of note were scopolamine butyl bromide, ipratropium bromide, and oxitropium bromide (Fig. **41**).

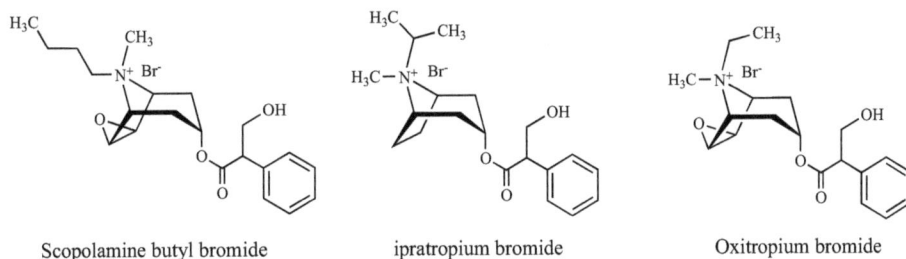

Scopolamine butyl bromide   ipratropium bromide   Oxitropium bromide

Fig. (41). Quaternary ammonium therapeutic derivatives of atropine and scopolamine.

Scopolamine butyl bromide was registered in Germany in 1951 and is used for the treatment of abdominal pain caused by gastrointestinal spasms and menstrual cramps. After oral administration, it has very low (<1%) bioavailability, but it is available for binding to muscarinic receptors in the intestinal lumen. Ipratropium bromide and oxitropium bromide are both used as inhaled bronchodilators in the management of COPD and reduce airway mucus secretion [79]. Again, since these drugs have very low systemic absorption; they exhibit no other pharmacologic effects at therapeutic doses.

Table 7. Receptor affinity and dissociation half-life of ester modifications of NMS.

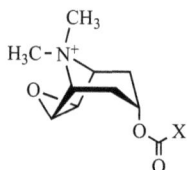

Compound	X	M3 pK_i	M3 $t_{1/2}$ (h)
N-methyl scopolamine (NMS)		10.2	0.77
A		8.98	
B		8.93	0.04
C		9.9	0.12
D		10.0	
E		10.6	0.92

The usefulness of these medications is limited by their lack of selectivity for a muscarinic receptor subtype, yet all three exhibit a significantly longer duration of effect and higher bronchospasmolytic potency than atropine [80, 81]. The reason for this extended effect may be the increased residence time of the quaternary drug structure in bronchial or intestinal tissues.

The M2 subtype of the muscarinic receptor is present in presynaptic locations that may control the release of ACh into the synapse in a negative feedback effect. A blockade of M2 would, therefore, be expected to increase the release of ACh and counteract the bronchodilatory effect or duration of an antimuscarinic drug. It would be beneficial, then, to design a compound with a prolonged duration of action at the M3receptor, while maintaining selectivity for the M3 over the M2 subtype. In order to extend the dissociation kinetics of the drug from the receptor, the M3 receptor dissociation half-life must be evaluated concurrently with M3 receptor binding data.

In an evaluation of receptor affinity and dissociation kinetic parameters of scopolamine analogues, N-methylscopolamine (NMS) exhibited a receptor affinity and dissociation half-life that was similar to ipratropium [82]. Analogues of NMS were evaluated for M3 muscarinic receptor affinity and the half-life of dissociation from the M3 receptor subtype. Initially, a series of ester modifications were evaluated (Table 7) [83]. The removal of the methylene unit of phenylpropionic acid in NMS and the exchange of the phenyl group for a thienyl (A and B) immediately lowered the pKi by an order of magnitude, but subtle improvements are seen in the binding affinity once a bulkier two-ring substituent was added. (C and D). A dithienyl substitution pattern (E) gave consistent binding affinities >10 and half-lives longer than NMS.

Once the dithienyl ester was identified as an active component, other areas of the molecule were evaluated for binding affinity and half-life at the M3 receptor subtype (Table 8). Evaluation of groups at R_3 between the thienyl rings showed that any deviation from a hydroxyl group (F-I) yielded a pK_i that hovered around 10, and half-lives that were <1h. A larger substituent on the axial nitrogen position R_2 always caused a decrease in binding affinity (J-L), and the epoxide ring was also a necessary feature, as its removal significantly reduced the M3 half-life (M) of tiotropium.

Both ipratropium and tiotropium have a robust binding affinity to the muscarinic receptor subtypes M1-M3 (Table 9). Tiotropium binds to the M3 receptor much longer than to the M1 and M2 receptors. The sustained occupancy of tiotropium at the M3 receptor clearly explains the long-lasting bronchodilation of tiotropium that allows for once-daily dosing. In contrast, binding at the M2 receptor is 10 times shorter, reducing the likelihood of M2-mediated side effects. These properties of tiotropium result in a "kinetic selectivity" toward the M3 receptor subtype, the pharmacological target responsible for bronchoconstriction and mucus hypersecretion in chronic airway diseases [84, 85].

Table 8. Dithienyl analogue receptor affinity and dissociation half-life.

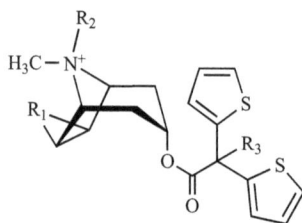

Compound	R_1	R_2	R_3	M3 pK_i	M3 $t_{1/2}$ (h)
F	O	Me	OMe	8.91	0.17
G	O	Me	CH_2OH	10.0	0.76
H	O	Me	Me	10.6	0.92
I	O	Me	H	10.3	0.32
J	O	Et	OH	10.7	4.45
K	O	iPr	OH	9.7	
L	O	nPr	OH	8.9	
M	-	Me	OH	10.5	3.3
Tiotropium	O	Me	OH	11.2	27.0

STUDENT SELF STUDY GUIDE

1. Describe the biosynthesis, storage, and degradation of ACh *in vivo*.
2. Discuss the potential inhibitory and excitatory effects of acetylcholine in the synaptic area.
3. Distinguish the effects of ACh on nicotinic and muscarinic acetylcholine receptors.

4. Differentiate the structural characteristics of nAChR and mAChR.
5. Highlight the structural similarities of acetylcholine and acetylcholine receptor agonists.
6. Summarize the properties and efficacy of mAChR antagonists in the treatment of COPD and asthma.
7. Summarize the properties and efficacy of mAChR antagonists in the treatment of urinary incontinence.
8. Relate the advantages of M_3-subtype selective mAChR antagonists in the treatment of urinary incontinence.
9. Categorize AChE inhibitors by the mechanism of action as reversible noncovalent, reversible noncovalent, and irreversible covalent
10. Discuss medication strategies that may allow for the reversal of AChE blockade *in vivo*.
11. What are the potential etiologies reported for AD?
12. Describe the characteristic features of β-amyloid hypothesis and Cholinergic hypothesis
13. List the risk factors for developing AD
14. Discuss the mechanism of action of acetyl cholinesterase inhibitors (AChEIs), and highlight their characteristic modes of inhibition
15. Summarize the pharmacokinetic profile, side effects, and drug interactions of donepezil
16. Summarize the pharmacokinetic profile, side effects, and drug interactions of rivastigmine
17. Summarize the pharmacokinetic profile, side effects, and drug interactions of galantamine
18. Describe the mechanism of action of memantine, its pharmacokinetic profile, side effects, and drug interactions

Table 9. Receptor affinity and dissociation half-life of ipratropium and tiotropium at M1-M3 receptor subtypes.

	M1 pK_i	M2 pK_i	M3 pK_i	M1 $t_{1/2}$ (h)	M2 $t_{1/2}$ (h)	M3 $t_{1/2}$ (h)	$t_{1/2}$ Ratio M3/M2
ipratropium	9.4	9.53	9.58	0.1	0.03	0.22	7.3
tiotropium	10.8	10.69	11.02	10.5	2.6	27	10.4

PRACTICE QUESTIONS

1. Endogenous biosynthesis of ACh is catalyzed by the (choline acetyltransferase) enzyme and the *in vitro* degradation of ACh is catalyzed by the (acetyl cholinesterase) enzyme.

2. Cholinergic receptors may be differentiated by their responses to the alkaloid small molecules muscarine and _____.

a. caffeine

b. nicotine

c. adenine

d. xylazine

3. Any muscarinic effect in the body may be blocked by the administration of _____.

a. atropine

b. muscarine

c. caffeine

d. nicotine

4. Muscarinic acetylcholine receptors are classified as:

a. G-protein coupled receptors

b. ligand-gated ion channels

c. Irreversible inhibitors

d. partial agonists

5. Nicotinic acetylcholine receptors are classified as:

a. G-protein coupled receptors

b. ligand-gated ion channels

c. Irreversible inhibitors

d. partial agonists

6. Unmodified acetylcholine is used as a selective muscarine receptor antagonist. (true/false)

7. Active muscarinic receptor agonists contain a positively charged nitrogen atom, preferably a

a. secondary amine

b. carboxamide

c. quaternary ammonium salt

d. sodium salt

8. Compared to uncharged drug forms, cholinergic medications containing quaternary salts will likely have _____ CNS penetration.

a. less

b. more

c. the same amount of

9. Oxybutynin administered in a/an _____ formulation promotes steady plasma concentrations of the active desethyloxybutynin metabolite.

a. transdermal

b. oral

c. intravenous

d. extended-release

e. a and d

f. a and b

10. The metabolic pathway of fesoterodine differs from tolterodine because it does not rely on _____ for *in vivo* production of the active 5-HMT metabolite.

a. CYP 2D6 enzymes

b. CYP 3A4 enzymes

c. nonspecific esterases

d. acetylcholinesterase

11. If an irreversible covalent AChE inhibitor is allowed to "age", then the activity of the AChE enzyme will be:

a. enhanced

b. unchanged

c. transiently deactivated

d. permanently deactivated

12. When treating AD with donepazil or rivastigmine, decreased efficacy is likely if the patient is taking a/an _____.

a. anticholinergic

b. beta-blocker

c. statin

d. benzodiazepine

NOTES

Historical Perspective: Further Reading:

[1] Sneader W. Drugs from naturally occurring prototypes: Biochemicals – Neurohormones. In: Sneader W ed. *Drug Discovery. A History*. West Sussex, England: John Wiley & Sons Ltd; 2005.

[2] Sneader W. Drugs from naturally occurring prototypes: Phytochemicals – Alkaloids. In: Sneader W ed. *Drug Discovery. A History*. West Sussex, England: John Wiley & Sons Ltd; 2005.

[3] Sneader W. Synthetic drugs: Drugs discovered through serendipitous observations involving humans. In: Sneader W ed. Drug Discovery. A History. West Sussex, England: John Wiley & Sons Ltd; 2005.

CONSENT FOR PUBLICATION

Not applicable.

CONFLICT OF INTEREST

The authors confirm that the contents of this chapter have no conflict of interest.

ACKNOWLEDGEMENTS

Declare none.

REFERENCES

[1]   Standing Committee on the Scientific Evaluation of Dietary Reference Intakes and its Panel on Folate OBV, and Choline and Subcommittee on Upper Reference Levels of Nutrients. Food and Nutrition Board Institute of Medicine Dietary Reference Intakes for Thiamin, Riboflavin, Niacin, Vitamin B6, Folate,   Vitamin   B12,   Pantothenic   Acid,   Biotin,   and   Choline 2012.https://download.nap.edu/openbook.php?record_id=6015&page=390

[2]   Cohen EL, Wurtman RJ. Brain acetylcholine: increase after systemic choline administration. Life Sci 1975; 16(7): 1095-102.
        [http://dx.doi.org/10.1016/0024-3205(75)90194-0] [PMID: 1134185]

[3]   Haubrich DR, Wedeking PW, Wang PF. Increase in tissue concentration of acetylcholine in guinea pigs in vivo induced by administration of choline. Life Sci 1974; 14(5): 921-7.
        [http://dx.doi.org/10.1016/0024-3205(74)90081-2] [PMID: 4828407]

[4]   Wecker L. Neurochemical effects of choline supplementation. Can J Physiol Pharmacol 1986; 64(3): 329-33.
        [http://dx.doi.org/10.1139/y86-054] [PMID: 3708441]

[5]   Nothnagel Gv. Ueber Cholin und verwandte Verbindungen, mit besonderer beriucksichtigung des Muscarins. Arch Pharm (Berl) 1894; 232: 261.
        [http://dx.doi.org/10.1002/ardp.18942320405]

[6]   Ewins AJ. Acetylcholine, a New Active Principle of Ergot. Biochem J 1914; 8(1): 44-9.
        [PMID: 16742288]

[7]   Raju TN. The Nobel chronicles. 1936: Henry Hallett Dale (1875-1968) and Otto Loewi (1873-1961). Lancet 1999; 353(9150): 416.
        [http://dx.doi.org/10.1016/S0140-6736(05)75001-7] [PMID: 9950485]

[8]   Koelle GB. Acetylcholine--current status in physiology, pharmacology and medicine. N Engl J Med 1972; 286(20): 1086-90.
        [http://dx.doi.org/10.1056/NEJM197205182862006] [PMID: 4336251]

[9]   The Nobel Prize in Physiology or Medicine. 2012.http://www.nobelprize.org/ nobel_prizes/ medicine/laureates/1936/

[10]   Hall JE. Guyton and hall textbook of medical physiology. 12th ed., Pennsylvania: Saunders Elsevier 2011.

[11]   Papke RL. Merging old and new perspectives on nicotinic acetylcholine receptors. Biochem Pharmacol 2014; 89(1): 1-11.
        [http://dx.doi.org/10.1016/j.bcp.2014.01.029] [PMID: 24486571]

[12]   Numa S, Noda M, Takahashi H, *et al.* Molecular structure of the nicotinic acetylcholine receptor. Cold Spring Harb Symp Quant Biol 1983; 48(Pt 1): 57-69.

[http://dx.doi.org/10.1101/SQB.1983.048.01.008] [PMID: 6586363]

[13]   Changeux JP, Bertrand D, Corringer PJ, *et al.* Brain nicotinic receptors: structure and regulation, role in learning and reinforcement. Brain Res Brain Res Rev 1998; 26(2-3): 198-216.
[http://dx.doi.org/10.1016/S0165-0173(97)00040-4] [PMID: 9651527]

[14]   Millar NS, Harkness PC. Assembly and trafficking of nicotinic acetylcholine receptors (Review). Mol Membr Biol 2008; 25(4): 279-92.
[http://dx.doi.org/10.1080/09687680802035675] [PMID: 18446614]

[15]   Holladay MW, Dart MJ, Lynch JK. Neuronal nicotinic acetylcholine receptors as targets for drug discovery. J Med Chem 1997; 40(26): 4169-94.
[http://dx.doi.org/10.1021/jm970377o] [PMID: 9435889]

[16]   Philip NS, Carpenter LL, Tyrka AR, Price LH. Nicotinic acetylcholine receptors and depression: a review of the preclinical and clinical literature. Psychopharmacology (Berl) 2010; 212(1): 1-12.
[http://dx.doi.org/10.1007/s00213-010-1932-6] [PMID: 20614106]

[17]   Miochol E. (Acetylcholine Chloride) Kit [Package insert] 2012.http://dailymed.nlm.nih.gov/ dailymed/ drugInfo.cfm?id=18455

[18]   Ing HR, Kordik P, Williams DP. Studies on the structure-action relationships of the choline group. Br J Pharmacol Chemother 1952; 7(1): 103-16.
[http://dx.doi.org/10.1111/j.1476-5381.1952.tb00696.x] [PMID: 14904909]

[19]   Ing HR. The Structure-Action Relationships to the Choline Group. Science 1949; 109(2828): 264-6.
[http://dx.doi.org/10.1126/science.109.2828.264-b] [PMID: 17774885]

[20]   NIH. Miostat-carbechol solution

[21]   Bethanechol   Chloride   NIH.   DailyMed   2014.http://dailymed.nlm.nih.gov/   dailymed/ drugInfo.cfm?setid=45285692-de51-413e-8a51-7fb792eccc81

[22]   NIH.   Evoxac™.   DailyMed   2014.http://dailymed.nlm.nih.gov/   dailymed/ drugInfo.cfm?setid=0679dd4c-fece-4c6d-b273-2c62237e8973

[23]   Noaiseh G, Baker JF, Vivino FB. Comparison of the discontinuation rates and side-effect profiles of pilocarpine and cevimeline for xerostomia in primary Sjögren's syndrome. Clin Exp Rheumatol 2014; 32(4): 575-7.
[PMID: 25065774]

[24]   NIH.   Atropen™.   DailyMed   2014.   http://dailymed.nlm.nih.gov/   dailymed/ drugInfo.cfm?setid=e2d4307d-da8f-49f5-aac0-02355dd9ffb7

[25]   Hansel TT, Barnes PJ. Tiotropium bromide: a novel once-daily anticholinergic bronchodilator for the treatment of COPD. Drugs Today (Barc) 2002; 38(9): 585-600.
[http://dx.doi.org/10.1358/dot.2002.38.9.696535] [PMID: 12582447]

[26]   Busch-Petersen J, Lainé DI. Inhaled long-acting muscarinic antagonists in chronic obstructive pulmonary disease. Future Med Chem 2011; 3(13): 1623-34.
[http://dx.doi.org/10.4155/fmc.11.127] [PMID: 21942252]

[27]   NIH.   Spiriva™.   DailyMed   2014.http://dailymed.nlm.nih.gov/   dailymed/ drugInfo.cfm?setid=820839ef-e53d-47e8-a3b9-d911ff92e6a9

[28]   NIH.   Atrovent™.   Dailymed   2014.http://dailymed.nlm.nih.gov/ dailymed/drugInfo.cfm?setid=f07439a7-1d1c-468f-8fd7-149e3d959a32

[29]   Zobrist RH, Schmid B, Feick A, Quan D, Sanders SW. Pharmacokinetics of the R- and S-enantiomers of oxybutynin and N-desethyloxybutynin following oral and transdermal administration of the racemate in healthy volunteers. Pharm Res 2001; 18(7): 1029-34.
[http://dx.doi.org/10.1023/A:1010956832113] [PMID: 11496941]

[30]   NIH.   Detrol   LA™.   DailyMed   2014.http://dailymed.nlm.nih.gov/   dailymed/

drugInfo.cfm?setid=c98eb213-9c80-4698-9710-a9855059b8bb

[31] Malhotra B, Gandelman K, Sachse R, Wood N, Michel MC. The design and development of fesoterodine as a prodrug of 5-hydroxymethyl tolterodine (5-HMT), the active metabolite of tolterodine. Curr Med Chem 2009; 16(33): 4481-9.
[http://dx.doi.org/10.2174/092986709789712835] [PMID: 19835561]

[32] NIH.   Enablex™.   DailyMed   2014.http://dailymed.nlm.nih.gov/   dailymed/ drugInfo.cfm?setid=a712f252-16d9-47df-b2bf-6794228f3a88

[33] NIH.   Vesicare™.   DailyMed   2014.http://dailymed.nlm.nih.gov/   dailymed/ drugInfo.cfm?setid=9acee910-cdb2-4052-b8b3-c26aff1c8716

[34] Olanow CW, Stern MB, Sethi K. The scientific and clinical basis for the treatment of Parkinson disease (2009). Neurology 2009; 72(21) (Suppl. 4): S1-S136.
[http://dx.doi.org/10.1212/WNL.0b013e3181a1d44c] [PMID: 19470958]

[35] Propantheline   Bromide   NIH.   DailyMed   2014.http://dailymed.nlm.nih.gov/   dailymed/ drugInfo.cfm?setid=84a920c8-b637-4741-b9b2-fc607e245ce0

[36] Glycopyrrolate   NIH.   DailyMed 2014.
http://dailymed.nlm.nih.gov/dailymed/drugInfo.cfm?setid=62267afe-1a73-4623-984e-646db590ec5b

[37] Fürst S, Friedmann T, Bartolini A, *et al*. Direct evidence that eseroline possesses morphine-like effects. Eur J Pharmacol 1982; 83(3-4): 233-41.
[http://dx.doi.org/10.1016/0014-2999(82)90256-4] [PMID: 6293841]

[38] Ecothiopate NIH. Toxnet ChemIDPlus http://chem.sis.nlm.nih.gov/ chemidplus/rn/513-10-0

[39] NIH. Diisopropyl difluorophosphate iodide. Toxnet ChemIDPlus http://chem.sis.nlm.nih.gov/ chemidplus/ rn/ 55-91-4

[40] Education CAEHaM. Cholinesterase Inhibitors: Including Insecticides and Chemical Warfare Nerve Agents. Part 4 - Section 11 Management Strategy 3: Medications 2-PAM (2-Pyridine Aldoxime Methylchloride)   (Pralidoxime)   accessed   2014.http://www.atsdr.cdc.gov/   csem/ csem.asp?csem=11&po=23

[41] Response CEP. Chemical Weapons Categories 2015.http://emergency.cdc.gov/agent/ agentlistchem-category.asp

[42] NIH.   Succinylcholine   chloride.   DailyMed™   2015.http://dailymed.nlm.nih.gov/ dailymed/drugInfo.cfm?setid=c06156ae-b889-4250-bc85-1435b2635829

[43] Golan DE, Tashjian AH, Armstrong EJ, Armstrong AW. Principles of pharmacology: The pathophysiologic basis of drug therapy. 3rd ed., Wolters Klower/LWW 2012.

[44] NIH.   Mivacurium   chloride.   DailyMed™   2015.http://dailymed.nlm.nih.gov/ dailymed/drugInfo.cfm?setid=98ca2c17-43e2-49af-abbc-f870877e5786

[45] NIH.   Mecamylamine   hydrochloride.   DailyMed™   2015.http://dailymed.nlm.nih.gov/ dailymed/drugInfo.cfm?setid=b87994ee-26a5-4d00-99e7-796bc17961f12015.

[46] Atri A. Effective pharmacological management of Alzheimer's disease. Am J Manag Care 2011; 17 (Suppl. 13): S346-55.
[PMID: 22214392]

[47] 2019 Alzheimer's Disease Facts and Figures. https://www.alz.org/ media/ documents/alzheimers-facts-and-figures-2019-r.pdf

[48] Querfurth HW, LaFerla FM. Alzheimer's disease. N Engl J Med 2010; 362(4): 329-44.
[http://dx.doi.org/10.1056/NEJMra0909142] [PMID: 20107219]

[49] Morrison AS, Lyketsos C. The pathophysiology of alzheimer's disease and directions in treatment. Adv Studies in Nursing 2005; 3(8): 256-70.

[50] Massoud F, Gauthier S. Update on the pharmacological treatment of Alzheimer's disease. Curr Neuropharmacol 2010; 8(1): 69-80.
[http://dx.doi.org/10.2174/157015910790909520] [PMID: 20808547]

[51] Mattson MP. Cellular actions of β-amyloid precursor protein and its soluble and fibrillogenic derivatives. Physiol Rev 1997; 77(4): 1081-132.
[http://dx.doi.org/10.1152/physrev.1997.77.4.1081] [PMID: 9354812]

[52] Parihar MS, Hemnani T. Alzheimer's disease pathogenesis and therapeutic interventions. J Clin Neurosci 2004; 11(5): 456-67.
[http://dx.doi.org/10.1016/j.jocn.2003.12.007] [PMID: 15177383]

[53] Micromedex. Obtained on-line February 2 2012.https://www.thomsonhc.com/ home/ dispatch/CS/21CC6C/PFActionId/pf.HomePage/ssl/true

[54] Han HJ, Lee JJ, Park SA, *et al.* Efficacy and safety of switching from oral cholinesterase inhibitors to the rivastigmine transdermal patch in patients with probable Alzheimer's disease. J Clin Neurol 2011; 7(3): 137-42.
[http://dx.doi.org/10.3988/jcn.2011.7.3.137] [PMID: 22087207]

[55] Anand A, Patience AA, Sharma N, Khurana N. The present and future of pharmacotherapy of Alzheimer's disease: A comprehensive review. Eur J Pharmacol 2017; 815: 364-75.
[http://dx.doi.org/10.1016/j.ejphar.2017.09.043] [PMID: 28978455]

[56] Bartus RT, Emerich DF. Cholinergic markers in Alzheimer disease. JAMA 1999; 282(23): 2208-9.
[http://dx.doi.org/10.1001/jama.282.23.2208] [PMID: 10605966]

[57] Auld DS, Kornecook TJ, Bastianetto S, Quirion R. Alzheimer's disease and the basal forebrain cholinergic system: relations to beta-amyloid peptides, cognition, and treatment strategies. Prog Neurobiol 2002; 68(3): 209-45.
[http://dx.doi.org/10.1016/S0301-0082(02)00079-5] [PMID: 12450488]

[58] Terry AV Jr, Buccafusco JJ. The cholinergic hypothesis of age and Alzheimer's disease-related cognitive deficits: recent challenges and their implications for novel drug development. J Pharmacol Exp Ther 2003; 306(3): 821-7.
[http://dx.doi.org/10.1124/jpet.102.041616] [PMID: 12805474]

[59] Birks J. Cholinesterase inhibitors for Alzheimer's disease. Cochrane Database Syst Rev 2006; (1): CD005593
[PMID: 16437532]

[60] Wilkinson DG. The pharmacology of donepezil: a new treatment of Alzheimer's disease. Expert Opin Pharmacother 1999; 1(1): 121-35.
[http://dx.doi.org/10.1517/14656566.1.1.121] [PMID: 11249555]

[61] Rogers SL, Yamanishi Y, Yamatsu K. E2020: the pharmacology of a piperidine cholinesterase inhibitor.Cholinergic basis for Alzheimer therapy. Boston: Birkhauser 1991; pp. 315-20.
[http://dx.doi.org/10.1007/978-1-4899-6738-1_33]

[62] Sherman KA. Pharmacodynamics of oral E2020 and tacrine in humans: novel approaches.Cholinergic basis for Alzheimer therapy. Boston: Birkhauser 1991; pp. 321-8.
[http://dx.doi.org/10.1007/978-1-4899-6738-1_34]

[63] Matsui K, Mishima M, Nagai Y, Yuzuriha T, Yoshimura T. Absorption, distribution, metabolism, and excretion of donepezil (Aricept) after a single oral administration to Rat. Drug Metab Dispos 1999; 27(12): 1406-14.
[PMID: 10570021]

[64] Tiseo PJ, Perdomo CA, Friedhoff LT. Metabolism and elimination of 14C-donepezil in healthy volunteers: a single-dose study. Br J Clin Pharmacol 1998; 46 (Suppl. 1): 19-24.
[http://dx.doi.org/10.1046/j.1365-2125.1998.0460s1019.x] [PMID: 9839761]

[65]   65 Aricept (donepezil hydrochloride) [Eisai Inc], Drug Label Information accessed from DailyMed Current Drug Information http://dailymed.nlm.nih.gov/ dailymed/lookup.cfm?setid=98e451e1-e4d--4439-a675-c5457ba20975Accessed June 3, 2013.

[66]   Jann MW. Rivastigmine, a new-generation cholinesterase inhibitor for the treatment of Alzheimer's disease. Pharmacotherapy 2000; 20(1): 1-12.
[http://dx.doi.org/10.1592/phco.20.1.1.34664] [PMID: 10641971]

[67]   Anand R, Gharabawi G. Clinical development of Exelon (ENA 713): the ADENA programme. J Drug Dev Clin Pract 1996; 8: 9-16.

[68]   Enz A, Floersheim P. Cholinesterase inhibitors: an overview of their mechanism of action.Alzheimer's disease Therapeutic strategies. Boston: Birkhauser 1994; pp. 211-5.

[69]   Samochocki M, Höffle A, Fehrenbacher A, *et al.* Galantamine is an allosterically potentiating ligand of neuronal nicotinic but not of muscarinic acetylcholine receptors. J Pharmacol Exp Ther 2003; 305(3): 1024-36.
[http://dx.doi.org/10.1124/jpet.102.045773] [PMID: 12649296]

[70]   Thomsen T, Kewitz H. Selective inhibition of human acetylcholinesterase by galanthamine in vitro and in vivo. Life Sci 1990; 46(21): 1553-8.
[http://dx.doi.org/10.1016/0024-3205(90)90429-U] [PMID: 2355800]

[71]   Lilienfeld S. Galantamine--a novel cholinergic drug with a unique dual mode of action for the treatment of patients with Alzheimer's disease. CNS Drug Rev 2002; 8(2): 159-76.
[http://dx.doi.org/10.1111/j.1527-3458.2002.tb00221.x] [PMID: 12177686]

[72]   Mannens GSJ, Snel CA, Hendrickx J, *et al.* The metabolism and excretion of galantamine in rats, dogs, and humans. Drug Metab Dispos 2002; 30(5): 553-63.
[http://dx.doi.org/10.1124/dmd.30.5.553] [PMID: 11950787]

[73]   Bachus R, Bickel U, Thomsen T, Roots I, Kewitz H. The O-demethylation of the antidementia drug galanthamine is catalysed by cytochrome P450 2D6. Pharmacogenetics 1999; 9(6): 661-8.
[http://dx.doi.org/10.1097/00008571-199912000-00001] [PMID: 10634129]

[74]   Johnson JW, Kotermanski SE. Mechanism of action of memantine. Curr Opin Pharmacol 2006; 6(1): 61-7.
[http://dx.doi.org/10.1016/j.coph.2005.09.007] [PMID: 16368266]

[75]   Xia P, Chen HS, Zhang D, Lipton SA. Memantine preferentially blocks extrasynaptic over synaptic NMDA receptor currents in hippocampal autapses. J Neurosci 2010; 30(33): 11246-50.
[http://dx.doi.org/10.1523/JNEUROSCI.2488-10.2010] [PMID: 20720132]

[76]   Simoni E, Daniele S, Bottegoni G, *et al.* Combining galantamine and memantine in multitargeted, new chemical entities potentially useful in Alzheimer's disease. J Med Chem 2012; 55(22): 9708-21.
[http://dx.doi.org/10.1021/jm3009458] [PMID: 23033965]

[77]   Danysz W, Parsons CG. Alzheimer's disease, β-amyloid, glutamate, NMDA receptors and memantine--searching for the connections. Br J Pharmacol 2012; 167(2): 324-52.
[http://dx.doi.org/10.1111/j.1476-5381.2012.02057.x] [PMID: 22646481]

[78]   Analogue-based Drug Discovery II. Hoboken, NJ, USA: Wiley-VCH 2010.

[79]   Barnes PJ. The role of anticholinergics in chronic obstructive pulmonary disease. Am J Med 2004; 117 (Suppl. 12A): 24S-32S.
[PMID: 15693640]

[80]   Bauer VR. [Pharmacology of the bronchospasmolytic oxitropium bromide]. Arzneimittelforschung 1985; 35(1A): 435-40.
[PMID: 4039183]

[81]   Bauer R, Püschmann S, Wick H. The effect of (8r)-3alpha-hydroxy-8-isopropyl-1alphaH,5a-phaH-tropaniumbromide-(+/-)-tropate ((ipratropiumbromide) on tracheobronchial spasm, bronchial

and salivary secretions, ECG and heart rate (author's transl). Arzneimittelforschung 1976; 26(5a): 981-5.
[PMID: 134728]

[82]   Motulsky HJ, Mahan LC. The kinetics of competitive radioligand binding predicted by the law of mass action. Mol Pharmacol 1984; 25(1): 1-9.
[PMID: 6708928]

[83]   Disse B, Reichl R, Speck G, Traunecker W, Ludwig Rominger KL, Hammer R. Ba 679 BR, a novel long-acting anticholinergic bronchodilator. Life Sci 1993; 52(5-6): 537-44.
[http://dx.doi.org/10.1016/0024-3205(93)90312-Q] [PMID: 8441333]

[84]   Casarosa P, Bouyssou T, Germeyer S, Schnapp A, Gantner F, Pieper M. Preclinical evaluation of long-acting muscarinic antagonists: comparison of tiotropium and investigational drugs. J Pharmacol Exp Ther 2009; 330(2): 660-8.
[http://dx.doi.org/10.1124/jpet.109.152470] [PMID: 19478135]

[85]   Tautermann CS, Kiechle T, Seeliger D, *et al.* Molecular basis for the long duration of action and kinetic selectivity of tiotropium for the muscarinic M3 receptor. J Med Chem 2013; 56(21): 8746-56.
[http://dx.doi.org/10.1021/jm401219y] [PMID: 24088171]

CHAPTER 2

Drugs Affecting Adrenergic System

M. O. Faruk Khan[1,*] and **Les Ramos**[2]

[1] *School of Pharmacy, University of Charleston, Charleston, WV, USA*

[2] *College of Pharmacy, Southwestern Oklahoma State University, Weatherford, OK, USA*

Abstract: This chapter is a comprehensive account of medicinal chemistry of drugs affecting the adrenergic system. It provides the mechanisms of action of drugs and detail of structure-activity relationships of the adrenergic drugs to give the knowledge base for pharmacists. After the study of this chapter students will be able to:

• Comprehend the historical background of adrenergic neurochemistry and drugs acting on this system

• Explain adrenergic neurotransmitters and their functions

• Classify adrenergic receptors and their structures and binding

• Discuss direct and indirect acting sympathomimetic (adrenergic agonists) and sympatholytic (adrenergic antagonists) drugs

• Explain SAR for direct and indirect acting adrenergic receptor agonists and antagonists

• Delineate the clinical significance of these classes of drugs

• Identify the discovery process of these agents

Keywords: Adrenergic agonists and antagonists, Adrenergic drugs, Clinical use of adrenergic drugs, Drug receptor interaction, Epinephrine and norepinephrine, Structure activity relationship, Sympathomimetic agents.

HISTORICAL BACKGROUND

As early as 3000 BC the Chinese used ephedrine, a sympathomimetic agent obtained from plant *Ephedra vulgaris*, to make the asthma medicine ma huang [1]. In 1894, Oliver and Schäfer of University College in London for the first time

---

* **Corresponding author M. O. Faruk Khan**: School of Pharmacy, University of Charleston, Charleston, WV, USA; Tel: 304-357-4860; E-mail: mdomarkhan@ucwv.edu

reported the presence of a substance in water, alcohol and glycerin extracts of the adrenal gland with compelling action on the blood vessels, skeletal muscles and heart [2]. The substance was mistakenly identified by Moore [3], a colleague of Schäfer, as a pyridine or piperidine compound; however, Fränkel [4] of Vienna correctly concluded it to be a catechol and amine-containing substance (catecholamine). Abel of Johns Hopkins University obtained it as a stable benzoate in almost pure form and termed as "epinephrine" [5]. Takamine, a New Jersey based industrial chemist, patented the process of crystallizing the pure epinephrine base and marketed it through Parke Davis & Company as Adrenalin® [6].

Wilson [7] coined the term "adrenaline" and later Slotz and Dakin independently synthesized adrenaline and noradrenaline ('nor' stands for *nitrogen öhne radikal* that is the absence of methyl on nitrogen) [8] and tested for the pharmacological activity. Noradrenaline (norepinephrine; NE in the US) was shown by von Euler in 1946 [9] to be the principal chemical transmitter for the sympathetic nervous system. The hormone is now officially known in the US as epinephrine (and NE for the neurotransmitter) but in the UK and British Commonwealth as adrenaline (and noradrenaline for the neurotransmitter).

In 1948, Ahlquist tested the activity of the catecholamines adrenaline, noradrenaline and isoproterenol on different tissues and suggested the presence of two distinct types of adrenergic receptors (ARs), α and β [10]. In most tissues, except for the intestine, the α receptor was associated with an excitatory function (in the intestine it is associated with inhibitory function). On the other hand, β receptor was associated with the inhibitory function in most tissues except in myocardium where it was excitatory. Land *et al* [11] later subdivided β receptor into β_1 and β_2. Most recently β_3 receptor, found firstly in adipose tissues, has also been reported [12]. Langer [13] and Starke *et al* [14] in 1974 independently subdivided α receptors into α_1 and α_2. The α_1 receptors are those found in the vascular smooth muscles and the α_2 receptors are those found in the sympathetic neuron, central nervous system and melanocytes [15].

Epinephrine was first used in 1903 to treat asthma by the oral route, and more advantageously, by the subcutaneous route due to its vasoconstrictive and bronchodilator effects. It was also used for its vasoconstrictive effects to control bleeding in surgery and postpartum hemorrhage. Epinephrine was shown to be effective as an aerosol for the treatment of asthma in 1910, and 30 years later isoproterenol was used as a bronchodilator due to its selective β agonist effects. Isoetharine was synthesized in 1936 but came into clinical practice as a bronchodilator in 1951 as a more selective β agonist.[16] Terbutaline came into the clinical practice in the 1970s with a major advantage that it is a selective β_2

agonist thus causing no unwanted cardiac effects but is short-acting. The real advance in asthma treatment came in the 1990s with the introduction of salmeterol, a long-acting selective β_2 agonist (LABA) [16].

The widespread use of β blockers in cardiovascular diseases, including angina, arrhythmia and hypertension, emerged with the revolutionary discovery of propranolol in 1964 by the 1988 Nobel laureate Sir James Black [17]. Propranolol and related lipophilic and nonselective β blockers exhibit bronchospasm or CNS side effects. In the 1970s, selective β_1 blockers with relatively less lipophilicity were introduced (*e.g.*, atenolol), which are cardioselective and devoid of unwanted effects on the airways and CNS and are now most frequently prescribed drugs for hypertension and other cardiac problems [18]. Drugs that selectively block the α_1 ARs or selectively activate the α_2 ARs are now commonly used as antihypertensive agents [19].

Some of the historically significant drug structures are shown in Fig. **1**. Today, drugs affecting the adrenergic system comprise one of the largest classes of clinical agents and many of these frequently occur in the top 200 drug list, a few occurring in the last few years are shown in Fig. **2**.

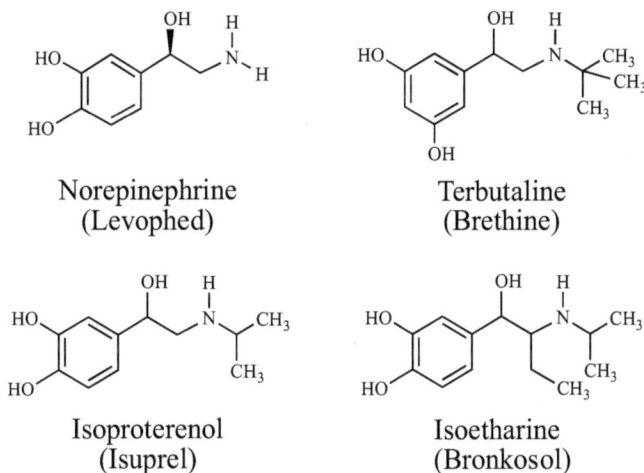

Norepinephrine
(Levophed)

Terbutaline
(Brethine)

Isoproterenol
(Isuprel)

Isoetharine
(Bronkosol)

Fig. (1). Few historic drugs affecting the adrenergic system.

A. Adrenergic Agonists

Epinephrine (Epipen)

L-(+)-Pseudoephedrine
(Sudafed)

Albuterol (Accuneb)
Levalbuterol (Xopenex)

D-(-)-Ephedrine

Salmeterol (Advair;
with fluticasone)

Brimonidine
(Alphagan)

Clonidine
(Catapres)

Tizanidine
(Zanaflex)

B. Beta-Adrenergic Blockers

Bisoprolol (Zebeta)

Propranolol (Inderal)

Sotalol (Betapace)

Atenolol (Tenormin)

Metoprolol (Toprol)

Nadolol (Corgard)

Carvedilol (Coreg)

Timolol (Betimol)

Labetalol (Normodyne)

C. Alfa-Adrenergic Blockers

Terazosin (Hytrin); R =   Doxazosin (Cardura); R =

Alfuzosin (Uroxatral)

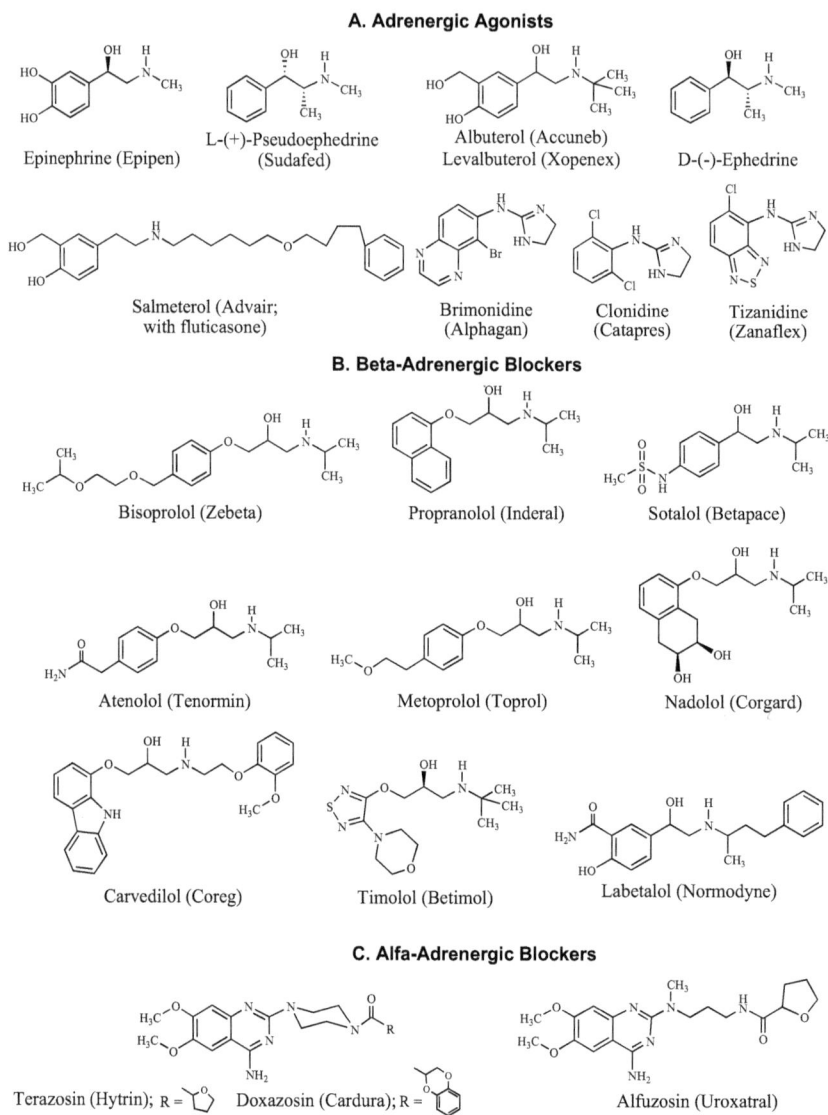

Fig. (2). Adrenergic agents frequently occur in the top 200 drug list.

THE INTRODUCTORY CONCEPTS

Drugs affecting the adrenergic system are chemical agents that exert their principal pharmacological effects either by enhancing or reducing the activity of various components of the sympathetic division of the autonomic nervous system. These agents may act through adrenergic neurotransmitters or directly on various types of ARs.

Adrenergic Neurotransmitters

NE is the neurotransmitter of postganglionic sympathetic neurons, which is released from the sympathetic nerve endings to the synaptic cleft. Epinephrine is synthesized and stored in the adrenal medulla, from where it is released into circulation and acts as an adrenergic hormone. The solutions of epinephrine and NE become colored due to oxidative degradation to corresponding *ortho*-quinone form (Fig. 3), which is usually stabilized by reducing agents, ascorbic acid or sodium bisulfites.

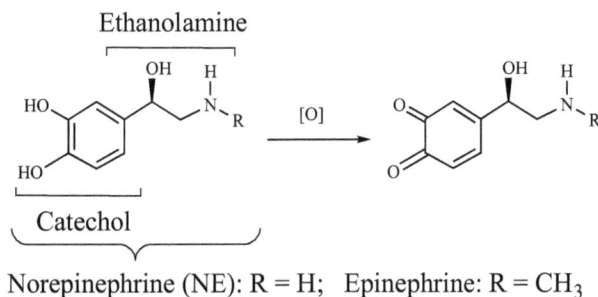

Fig. (3). Structures of epinephrine and norepinephrine showing different functional groups.

The biosynthesis of epinephrine from tyrosine (and also from phenylalanine) is shown in Chapter 8 (Volume 1). It is also biosynthesized along with NE in certain neurons in CNS. The rate-limiting step is the conversion of tyrosine to dihydroxyphenylalanine (DOPA) in the presynaptic terminal by the action of tyrosine hydroxylase, which is then decarboxylated to dopamine. Finally, in the synaptic vesicle, dopamine is converted into NE by the stereoselective enzyme β-hydroxylase and is held in the bound form (Fig. 4). The (R) enantiomer is biosynthesized and possesses biological activity. In response to an impulse at the presynaptic terminals, NE is released from several vesicles into the synaptic cleft where it activates the ARs. Within milliseconds, a large portion of the NE is reabsorbed into presynaptic terminals from where it may be re-uptaken into the vesicles for further release by the rapidly firing fibers. Catechol-*O*-methyl transferase (COMT) may methylate a small portion of NE at the synaptic cleft to the inactive form. If the storage of NE in the vesicles is adequate, the excess NE at the presynaptic terminals can be oxidative deaminated (inactivated) by mitochondrial monoamine oxidase (MAO) [20].

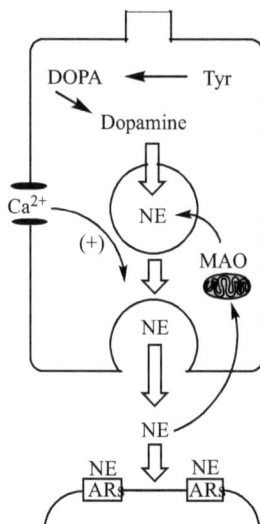

Fig. (4). Adrenergic neurochemistry: synthesis, releasing, reuptake and actions.

Adrenergic Receptors (ARs)

The ARs are the group of membrane-bound G protein coupled hormones or neurotransmitter receptors of 7TM family, β_2 AR being the first to be cloned. As mentioned in the previous sections, there are two types of ARs – α and β ARs. The α AR is divided into α_1 and α_2 which are further subdivided into α_{1A}, α_{1B}, α_{1C} and α_{2A}, α_{2B}, α_{2C}; and β is subdivided into β_1, β_2 and β_3. Using β_2 AR as the model, it has been hypothesized that amino terminal to the middle of the third intracellular loop form the major *domain A* and from the middle of the third intracellular loop to the carboxyl terminal form the major *domain B*. The two domains are flexible and may stay in two conformations – active and inactive – inactive being the more stable. Agonists stabilize a specific arrangement of the two domains that is recognized by the G protein (active form) and the antagonists stabilize a different conformation that is not recognized by the G protein (inactive conformation). It should be clear that ligand recognition and activation or inactivation are dynamic processes (Fig. **5**) [21].

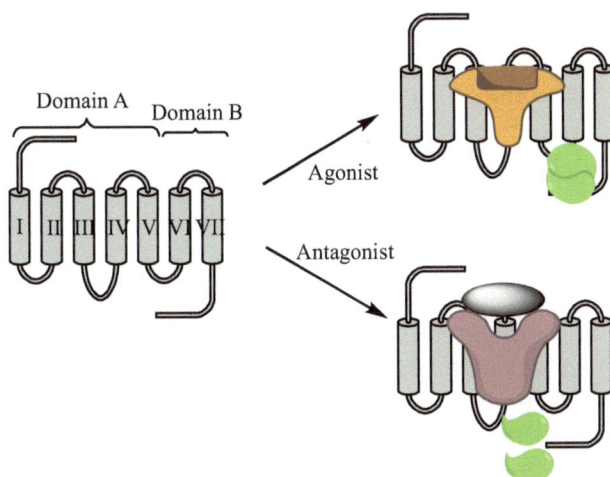

Fig. (5). Model showing the agonist and antagonist binding to the β_2 adrenoceptor.

The detail binding study of the catecholamines with the β_2-receptor supported the Easson-Stedman hypothesis of binding of (-)-NE with its receptor through *three-point interactions* with ARs. The protonated ammonium function of the catecholamines (*e.g.* NE) causes an ionic interaction with the Asp113 in the TM3 of the receptor. The residues Ser204 and Ser207 present in the TM5 of the receptor cause hydrogen bonding interaction with the *meta-* and *para*-hydroxyl groups of the catecholamines, respectively (Fig. **6A**) [22]. Ser165 (TM4), Asn292 (TM6) and Ser319 (TM7) are suggested to be the potential sites for hydrogen bonding interaction of the β-hydroxyl group of the catecholamines with β ARs (Fig. **6A**). However, it is also possible that such interaction with α ARs involves Ser90 (TM2) as shown using α_{2A} as the model (Fig. **6B**). The (+)-catecholamines or β-desoxy catecholamines cannot participate in such three-point interactions [22].

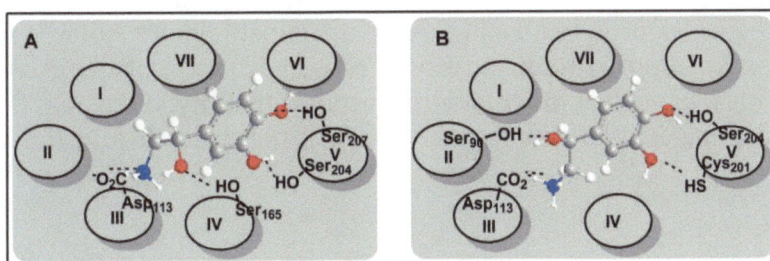

Fig. (6). Norepinephrine binding to the β_2 (A) and α_{2A} adrenoceptors.

Overall, the three points of both α and β ARs include:

- An anionic site, which binds the positive ammonium group
- One hydrogen bonding area for the β-hydroxyl group
- A flat non-polar area with two hydrogen bonding sites for catechol hydroxyl groups.

Epinephrine stimulates both α and β receptors equally and NE stimulates mainly α receptors (and only slightly to β receptors). Thus, epinephrine has a much stronger effect on the heart expressing mainly β receptors. (Table **1**) shows a few important effects on effector organs in response to α and β receptor stimulations. Some effector organs express only α receptor and others express β receptors; and the net effect depends on the ratio of these two in a particular effector organ. The inotropic (strength) and chronotopic (rate) effects of the heart are associated with β_1 stimulation, while the vasodilation and bronchial relaxation are associated with the β_2 stimulation [20].

Table 1. The Effects of Adrenergic Stimulations.

α Stimulation (α_1 and α_2)	β Stimulations (β_1 and β_2)
Vasoconstriction (α_1)	Vasodilatation (β_2)
Mydriasis (α_1)	Increased heart rate & strength (β_1)
Intestinal relaxation (α_1)	Bronchial relaxation (β_2)
Glycogenolysis (α_1)	Glycogenolysis (β_2)

The nonselective agonist, NE, has very limited therapeutic application due to following reasons: a) nonselectiveness, b) orally ineffective as rapidly metabolized and if given IV is effective only for 1-2 minutes. The most commonly clinically used agents acting through the adrenergic mechanism include: a) selective α_1 agonists (vasoconstrictors) used as nasal decongestants, b) α_2 agonists used as antihypertensive agents, c) α_1 antagonists used as antihypertensive agents as well as prostatic hyperplasia treating agents, d) β agonists used as bronchodilator, β_2 selective agonist is more suitable for asthma (bronchial relaxation) without cardiac effects, e) β_3 selective agonist for overactive bladder, and f) the β blockers used to treat hypertension, β_1 selective ones are advantageous in this respect that will not exacerbate asthmatic attack [20].

DRUGS AFFECTING ADRENERGIC SYSTEM: STRUCTURES, ACTIVITY, METABOLISM AND RELATED THERAPEUTIC CONSIDERATIONS

The Antiadrenergics Affecting Synthesis, Storage, or Release of NE (Fig. 7)

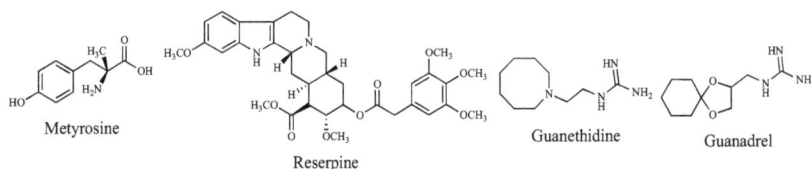

Fig. (7). Representative structures of antiadrenergics affecting synthesis, storage, or release of NE.

Metyrosine

Mechanism of Action: Metyrosine (Demser) is α-methyl-L-tyrosine. Because of the structural similarity of metyrosine with tyrosine, the precursor of NE and epinephrine biosynthesis, the drug competitively inhibits *tyrosine hydroxylase* (Fig. **8**), the first and rate limiting step of catecholamine biosynthesis. Thus, it significantly lowers the catecholamine production (35 to 80%). The (-) isomer of metyrosine is biologically active, but the racemic mixture is clinically used for controlling hypertensive episodes associated with the rare disease pheochromocytoma [23].

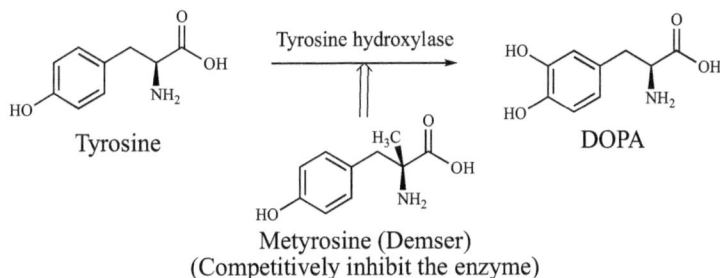

Fig. (8). First step in catecholamine synthesis; inhibited by metyrosine.

Pharmacokinetics: Metyrosine is well absorbed after oral administration and largely excreted in the urine as unchanged drug. Some catechol metabolites are the minor metabolites in the urine (<1%) [24].

Reserpine

Mechanism of Action

It is a prototypical drug affecting the vesicle storage of catecholamine. It binds extremely tightly with the Mg-ATPase that transports catecholamines from cytoplasm into storage vesicles. Thus, the circulating catecholamines are metabolized by MAO, with resulting depletion of NE and epinephrine in sympathetic and serotonergic neurons and adrenal medulla. Deserpidine and rescinnamine are similar drugs, which are all obtained from plant, *Rauwolfia serpentina* [20].

Pharmacokinetics

Reserpine has slow onset but sustained effects even after the withdrawal of the therapy. It is about 50% orally bioavailable compared with IV dose. It is highly plasma protein bound (96%). Its metabolism is not well known [24].

Guanethidine and Guanadrel

These drugs enter the adrenergic neuron by way of uptake-1, accumulate within the neuronal storage vesicle, stabilize the vesicle making them less responsive to nerve impulse and thus the ability to burst and release the catecholamines [20]. The resulting inhibition of NE release and storage in the neuron causes the blockade of activity. All these drugs contain a guanidine moiety [$CNHC(=NH)NH_2$], which is attached to either an alicyclic or an aromatic lipophilic group. Due to side effects these drugs are rarely used in clinical practice.

Direct-Acting Sympathomimetic Agents

Drugs that stimulate selectively or nonselectively α and/or β ARs or their subtypes fall under this category. These agents carry closely related pharmacophoric groups as NE. There are two different pharmacophoric classes of compounds: a) the β-phenylethylamine derivatives, and b) the imidazoline derivatives. The detail structure activity relationships (SAR) and ADMET parameters of the individual drugs in these two classes are discussed below.

The General Mechanism and SAR of β-Phenylethylamine Derivatives (Direct and Indirect Acting Agonists)

The β-phenylethylamines are the structural analogs of epinephrine and NE. The minimum pharmacophoric requirements for agonist activity at the adrenergic receptor sites include a basic protonatable amine, a β-hydroxyl function, and a hydrogen bonding group on the aromatic ring (Fig. **9**), all of which together cause a *three-point interaction* with the receptors (Fig. **6**). The slight differences in the substitution patterns on the amine function (R_1), aromatic ring (R_3) and the ethyl side chain (R_2) that will change the molecules' physicochemical characteristics including lipid-water partition coefficients (LWPC) as well as stereochemistry, will have impact on its receptor selectivity (α, β or their subtypes), potency, mode of action (direct or indirect) and metabolic stability and thus the duration of action. The overall SAR can be summarized as follows [20, 25]:

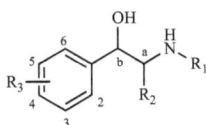

Fig. (9). The β-Phenyl- ethylamine pharmacophore.

Sar 1

The maximal activity is seen in β-phenylethylamine derivatives with OH in *meta* and *para* positions (3,4-disubstitution), and a β-OH of correct stereochemical configuration as in NE, epinephrine and isoproterenol (i.e., *R* configuration) that cause *three-point interaction* at the receptor site (Fig. **6**).

Sar 2

The amino group is essential for direct agonist activity, which should be optimally separated from the aromatic ring by two carbon atoms. Both 1°, and 2° amines are found among the potent drugs but 3° or quaternary amines tend to be poor direct agonists and are not used clinically.

Sar 3

Bulkier substituent on the N atom decreases the α-receptor activity and increases the β-receptor activity possibly due to the presence of a large lipophilic pocket in the vicinity of the amine-binding Asp113 of only βARs, which is absent in the αARs. Thus, isoproterenol, which has a bulky *N*-substituent (isopropyl), is a potent β-agonist, but poor α agonist. *N-tert*-butyl group provide more β_2 selectivity, *e.g.*, colterol is 9-10 times more potent at β_2 receptor than β_1 receptor.

Sar 4

Large substituents on N atom also protect it from metabolism by MAO. However, it does not have much clinical significance in terms of duration of action if the drugs also have a catechol function, which is deactivated by COMT. If the compound is stable against COMT (*e.g.* the non-catechol drugs), then the MAO stability will significantly increase the duration of action of the drug.

Sar 5

Methyl or ethyl substitution on α-carbon reduces both α and β agonist activity, at the same time reduces MAO-metabolism. They also have greater selectivity for β_2 over β_1 and α_2 over α_1 (the greater α_2 effect is advantageous in getting centrally acting antihypertensive methyldopa). Stereochemically, the *erythro* (*e.g.*, β*R*,α*S*-α-methylnorepinephrine) isomer possesses significant activity at α receptor. The ethyl substitution abolishes α activity keeping some β activity and thus providing a selective β agonist, *e.g.*, isoetharine.

Sar 6

The catechol moiety can be replaced with resorcinol (*e.g.*, metaproterenol) or the 3-OH of the catechol structure can be replaced with a hydroxymethyl (*e.g.*, albuterol), which shows β_2 selectivity and stability against COMT, and thus improved oral bioavailability and longer duration of action. Adding a large lipophilic group on the amine function (*e.g.* salmeterol) will provide drug with even longer duration of action both due to its partitioning into the lipid barrier of bronchial membrane as well as improved β_2 receptor binding, *e.g.*, salmeterol has duration of 12h vs 4h for albuterol.

Sar 7

Removal of the 4-OH from catechol (*e.g.*, phenylephrine) increases α selectivity while removal of the 3-OH increases β selectivity. Removal of the both OH groups provides both direct and indirect acting agents depending on the stereochemistry of the alkyl chain (SAR 5 and 8). Thus, the eythro analog of β*R*,α*S*-α-methylnorepinephrine lacking a OH group on the aromatic ring, ephedrine, has both direct and indirect activity and its enantiomer has primarily indirect effect. Its *threo* diastereomers, pseudoephedrine (both enantiomers), have virtually no direct effect and fewer CNS side effects.

Sar 8

The removal of β-hydroxyl group decreases and the addition of α-methyl group increases indirect agonist effects through stimulation of NE release from the vesicles. However, the stereochemistry has tremendous role in these effects. While the *erythro* isomer of α-methylnorepinephrine possesses direct effect (SAR 5), its *threo* isomer (R,R-α-methylnorepinephrine) possesses primarily indirect effects.

Sar 9

N-Substituent decreases indirect, NE-releasing activity with substituents larger than methyl rendering the compound virtually inactive, and tertiary amines are inactive.

Therapeutic Evaluation of the β-Phenylethylamine Direct Acting Adrenergic Agonists

The structures of a few important direct acting adrenergic agonists of the β-phenylethylamine derivative class are shown in Fig. (**10**) (as well as in (Figs. **1** and **2**). The physicochemical characteristics, the metabolism and related therapeutic evaluations of the individual agents are discussed below.

Epinephrine mimics most actions of the sympathetic nervous system by activating both α and β ARs (SAR 1 of phenylethylamine). It is administered by rapid IV injection if needed to rapidly raise blood pressure. It relaxes the bronchial smooth muscles, an action beneficial in asthmatic attack. It is not orally effective, and the IV dose is rapidly metabolized to inactive form. Metanephrine or normetanephrine are the chief metabolites in the urine. These can also be sulfate- and glucuronide-conjugated and excreted in the urine. 3-methoxy-4-hydroxy-mandelic acid (vanillyl-mandelic acid: VMA)is also detectable in the urine (Fig. **11**) [24].

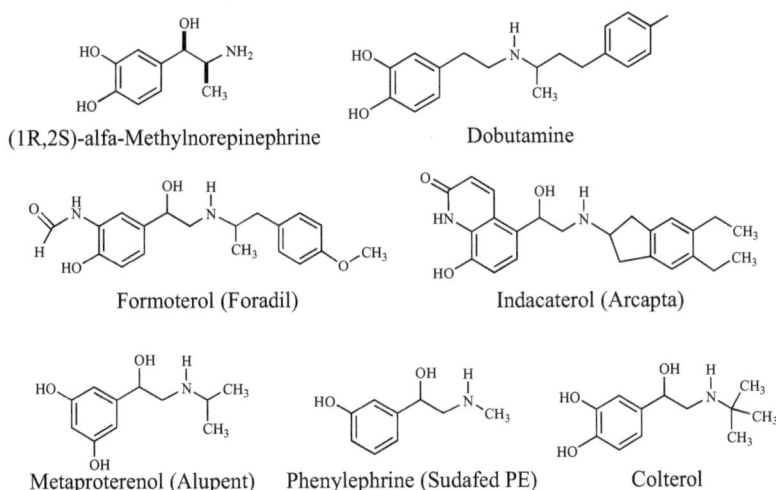

(1R,2S)-alfa-Methylnorepinephrine   Dobutamine

Formoterol (Foradil)   Indacaterol (Arcapta)

Metaproterenol (Alupent)   Phenylephrine (Sudafed PE)   Colterol

Fig. (10). Structures of a few direct acting adrenergic agonist of β-phenylethylamine class.

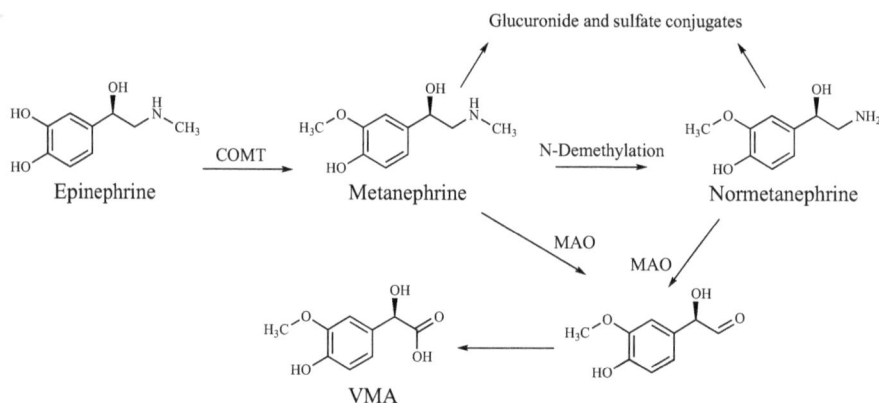

Fig. (11). Metabolic transformations of epinephrine.

Methyldopa is an antihypertensive agent that works by a dual mechanism: 1) aromatic amino acid decarboxylase inhibition, and 2) its conversion into an active metabolite ***α-methylnorepinephrine*** that centrally stimulates $α_2$ ARs (SAR 5 of phenylethylamine). The net result of both is the reduction in tissue concentrations of the sympathetic neurotransmitters thus causing reduced blood pressure. Only the L-α-methyldopa is active as the antihypertensive agent. It reduces both standing and supine blood pressure. It is now mainly used in pregnancy-induced hypertension (PIH) where other safer alternatives are contraindicated.

About 70% of the drug is absorbed and is extensively metabolized forming sulfate conjugate and other oxidative products (Fig. **12**) [24]. ***Phenylephrine*** on the other hand is a locally active $α_1$ adrenergic agonist (SAR 7 of phenylethylamine) and is thus used as a nasal decongestant due to its vasoconstrictive action. It is quickly metabolized both by MAO as well as sulfate and glucuronide conjugations, thus has little or no bioavailability in the brain [24].

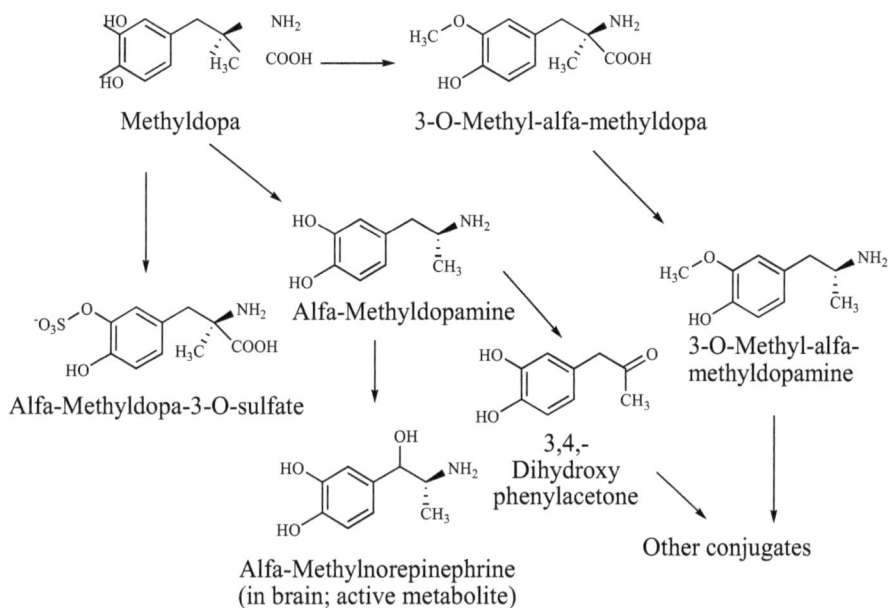

Fig. (12). Metabolic biotransformations of methyldopa.

Dobutamine, developed as a structural analogue of the nonselective β agonist ***isoproterenol*** without a β-OH group, is a selective β_1 agonist [26]. It is used to treat acute heart failure related to surgery, or congestive heart failure due to its positive inotropic action. The (+) isomer of dobutamine is a potent β_1 agonist and α_1 antagonist, while the (−) isomer is an α_1 agonist. Thus, the racemic dobutamine is clinically used, which has overall β_1 agonist activity. It is readily metabolized by COMT but not MAO and thus has a short half-life and is orally ineffective [20, 24].

Albuterol (also known as salbutamol in non-US territory) is a relatively selective β_2 adrenergic bronchodilator (SAR 3 of phenylethylamine) and thus more effective than isoproterenol at comparable doses in treating bronchial asthma with fewer cardiovascular effects. Also, because its *m*-OH group is replaced with a hydroxymethyl group, it is not a substrate for COMT (SAR 6 of phenylethylamine) and is longer acting than isoproterenol. Unlike isoproterenol, it is orally effective. It is extensively metabolized by sulfate conjugation and is excreted primarily through urine [20, 24].

The other selective β_2 adrenergic agonist ***metaproterenol*** is an orcinol derivative (SAR 6 of phenylethylamine). Less than 10% of metaproterenol is absorbed intact. Like albuterol, it is neither metabolized by COMT nor converted to glucuronide conjugates but is primarily converted to sulfate conjugates in the GUT and excreted in the urine.

Terbutaline is similar to metaproterenol except that it has a *tert*-butyl side chain on the amine instead of isopropyl side chain. It exhibits similar pharmacologic and pharmacokinetic behaviors like metaproterenol but higher potency as well as β_2 selectivity, which are comparable to albuterol [27].

β_2 Adrenergic Agonist and Cardiac Function

Although β_2 AR is main type in the bronchial muscle, convincing evidences support that 10% to 50% of β_2 ARs may be present in the human heart with unknown function. The sulfate conjugates of all these β_2 agonists produce a clinically significant cardiovascular effect in some patients when the drug should be discontinued. These may also have some effects on the QTc interval and other cardiac functions and should be used with caution in patients with cardiovascular disorders, especially coronary insufficiency, cardiac arrhythmias, and hypertension [24].

Long Acting β2-Adrenoceptor Agonists (LABAs)

Salmeterol

Salmeterol (Serevent Discus) is a derivative of albuterol with a 11-atom long bulky and lipophilic arylalkyl ether chain that makes it a β_2-adrenoceptor agonist (LABA) (SAR 6 of phenylethylamine) [28, 29]. It is available as dry powder inhaler for the treatment of asthma and chronic obstructive pulmonary disease (COPD). It is used both as a single agent as well as in combination with fluticasone. However, in June 2010, the FDA released a health advisory that contraindicated the use of LABA alone and should be used in combination with corticosteroids for the treatment of asthma [30]. This warning is not applicable for COPD treatments. The other LABA, *formoterol*, which is less lipophilic, has similar efficacy as salmeterol, but with faster onset and higher potency. *Arformoterol* (Brovana) is an *(R,R)-(−)*-enantiomer of formoterol, the active isomer, thus has better potency than formoterol. The solution of its tartrate salt is approved for treatment of COPD, which is administered twice daily (morning and evening) by nebulization.

Salmeterol is administered as xinafoate (pharmacologically inert, but with long half-life) salt, which is dissociated in solution and are absorbed, distributed, metabolized, and eliminated independently. Salmeterol acts in the lung with insignificant systemic level/effects. Salmeterol base is highly plasma protein bound (96%). It is completely metabolized *via*. hydroxylation by CYP3A4 enzyme and is eliminated primarily in the feces [24].

Indacaterol

(Arcapta) is another inhaled LABA approved for the long term, once-daily maintenance bronchodilator treatment of airflow obstruction in patients with COPD, including chronic bronchitis and/or emphysema. However, it is not indicated to treat acute deteriorations of COPD nor is approved for the treatment of asthma. Its prescribing information contains a Black Box Warning for increased risk of asthma-related death, as with any LABA.

Indacaterol should be used with caution in patients taking xanthine derivatives, steroids, diuretics or non-potassium sparing diuretics due to increased risk of hypokalemia. It should be used with caution or avoided in patients receiving MAOIs, TCAs, or any drug known to cause QT interval prolongation. As with any β_2-adrenergic agonist bronchodilator, concomitant use of beta-blocker, particularly a non-selective agent, may diminish its effectiveness.

Indacaterol is available in capsules containing powder for inhalation and should only be administered using the supplied Neohaler. It is not to be used for quick or rescue relief of symptoms and is only intended for once-daily maintenance treatment of COPD. After inhalation, it attains 43-45% absolute bioavailability as it is possibly a low-affinity substrate of P-glycoprotein. The majority of the drug in serum is unchanged and phenolic O-glucuronides (by UGT1A1) and hydroxylated products (by CYP3A4) are the major metabolites. Other minor metabolites include *N*-glucuronide, and C- and *N*-dealkylated products. The renal elimination plays a minor role, while serum clearance and/or clearance of the unchanged drug or its metabolites through feces play a major role [24].

Olodaterol (Striverdi Respimat)

(Fig. **13**) is an ultra-long-acting β adrenoreceptor agonist (ultra-LABA) used as an inhalation for treating patients with COPD. It is a full β_2 agonist with a higher in vitro selectivity for β_2 receptors than formoterol and salmeterol accounting for less incidence of cardiac side effects. Since it is bound to the receptor tightly with a very long dissociation half-life (17.8 hours), it allows a once-a-day application. It is administered as soft mist inhaler (Respimat) in patients with COPD, bronchitis and/or emphysema, but not indicated for asthma. Olodaterol is metabolized by glucuronidation and CYP2C8- & CYP2C9- mediated O-demethylation [31 - 33]. *Vilanterol* is another ultra-LABA approved in combination with fluticasone furoate (*Breo Ellipta*) for the treatment of (COPD). Vilanterol is also available with muscarinic antagonist umeclidinium bromide (*Anoro Ellipta*).

β₃ Adrenergic Receptor Agonist

Mirabegron (Myrbetriq) is the first ever β₃ adrenergic receptor agonist approved for the treatment of overactive bladder with symptoms of urge urinary incontinence, urgency, and urinary frequency. The mechanism of action of mirabegron represents a novel approach to the treatment of this condition. It directly stimulates the bladder β₃ adrenergic receptors leading to detrusor muscle relaxation and increased bladder capacity. (Fig. **14**) shows the SAR of the different functional groups of mirabegron.

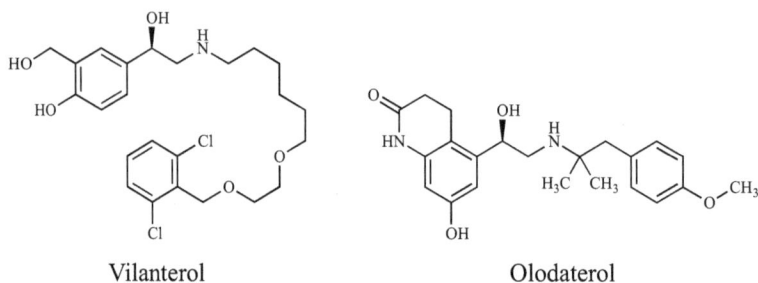

Vilanterol   Olodaterol

Fig. (13). Structures of ultra-long-acting LABAs.

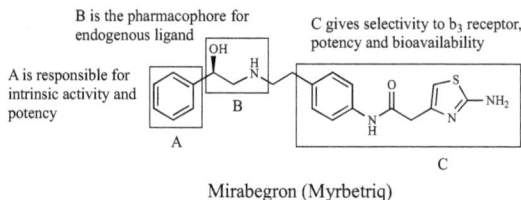

Mirabegron (Myrbetriq)

Fig. (14). Structure of mirabegron showing the different functional groups and their significance.

In clinical trials, the most commonly reported adverse effects of mirabegron were tumors, hypertension, nasopharyngitis, urinary tract infection, headache, and hypersensitivity reactions.

Mirabegron metabolism includes dealkylation, oxidation, glucuronidation, and amide hydrolysis resulting in two principal pharmacologically inactive metabolites. The major hepatic isozyme for its metabolism is CYP2D6. Since mirabegron also inhibits CYP2D6, co-administration of a CYP2D6 substrate (*e.g.*, metoprolol) may require dosage adjustments of the interacting drug. Mirabegron may also lead to excessive plasma levels of digoxin. It is recommended to use the lowest digoxin dose in patients also receiving mirabegron. The maximum daily dose in patients with severe renal impairment and moderate liver dysfunction should be reduced. Mirabegron should not be administered to patients with end-stage renal disease or severe liver impairment [34].

The General SAR of Imidazolines (α Adrenergic Agonist and Antagonists)

The pharmacophoric group of the imidazoline α-adrenergic receptor agonists and antagonists are shown in (Fig. **15**). X is usually a single amino or methylene group. The general SAR can be summarized as follows [20, 25].

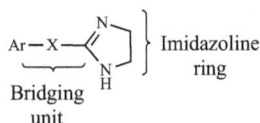

Fig. (15). Pharmacophoric group of imidazoline derivatives.

Sar 1

A lipophilic group like Cl or small alkyl group like methyl in *ortho* position of the aromatic ring of the methylene bridged derivatives (X = -CH$_2$-) is required for α agonist (α$_1$ and α$_2$) activity. The *meta* or *para* substitutions with bulky lipophilic groups provide selectivity for α$_1$ over α$_2$.

Sar 2

The methylene bridged imidazolines with no lipophilic substitution on the aromatic ring lack agonist activity providing α antagonists.

Sar 3

The aminoimidazolines (X = -NH-) with Cl- or Br- substitution at the *ortho* position of the aromatic ring provide α$_2$ selective agents. The imidazoline ring can be replaced with a ring-opened guanidine ring to provide agents with similar mechanism of action.

Therapeutic Evaluation of the Imidazoline α Adrenergic Agonists

Naphazoline*, *tetrahydrozoline*, *xylometazoline* and *oxymetazoline (Fig. **16**) are α$_1$ adrenergic agonists (SAR 1 for imidazolines) and are used for their vasoconstrictive effects as nasal and ophthalmic decongestants. These agents mimic the molecular shape of epinephrine and bind to α adrenergic receptors in the nasal mucosa. They have limited access to CNS (pKa = 9-10) thus are not used for systemic effects.

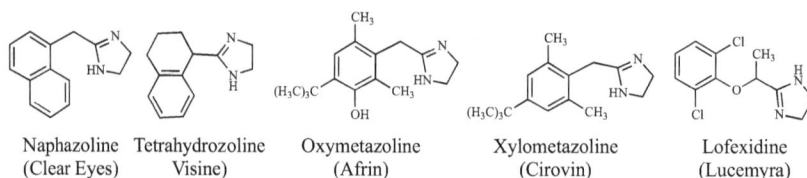

Fig. (16). Some imidazoline α_1 and α_2 adrenergic agonists.

Clonidine (Catapres; Fig. **2**) is α_2-selective and used as an antihypertensive due to its CNS effect. Because dichlorophenyl is attached to the guanidine N atom, its pKa decreases to 8.0 (pKa of guanidine 13.6), and thus is not extensively ionized at physiologic pH and can enter CNS. About 50% of the absorbed immediate-release oral dose of clonidine is metabolized in the liver producing 2,6-dichlorophenylguanidine as the principal metabolite along with few minor metabolites [24].

Brimonidine (Alphagan P; Fig. **2**) is also a selective α_2 agonist like clonidine. However, it is used mainly in ophthalmic preparations for the treatment of primary open angle glaucoma as an alternative first-line therapy or as an adjunct to other first-line drugs. It is extensively metabolized primarily by the liver enzymes *via*. *N*-oxidation to 2,3-dioxobrimonidine, as well as oxidative cleavage of the imidazoline ring to 5-bromo-6-guanidinoquinoxaline [24, 35].

Tizanidine (Fig. **2**) is another member of this class that is used for its central α_2 adrenergic effect as a muscle relaxant to treat the spasms, cramping, and tightness of muscles caused by multiple sclerosis, spastic diplegia or back pain. About 95% of the dose of tizanidine is metabolized to inactive metabolites primarily by CYP1A2.

Lofexidine *(Lucemyra®;* Fig. **(16)** is the newest α_{2A}-adrenergic receptor agonist with anti-short hypertensive effect (half-life 11h), but less effective than clonidine. It was approved in the United Kingdom in 1992, and in the USA in May 2018, as the first non-opioid medication for the symptomatic management and treatment of opioid withdrawal. The activation of α_{2A}-adrenergic receptor inhibits the synthesis of cAMP, as is the case with chronic opioid use. Abrupt discontinuation of opioid use produces a rise in the level of cAMP and NE through compensatory mechanisms of continuous negative feedback, producing numerous withdrawal symptoms. Lofexidine replaces the opioid-driven inhibition of cAMP and NE production by activating the α_{2A}-adrenergic receptor thus inhibiting the compensatory negative feedback to moderate the symptoms of opioid withdrawal. It does not interact with the opioid receptor in moderating the withdrawal symptoms [36].

Lofexidine has good oral bioavailability (>72%) undergoing about 30% first pass metabolism. The peak plasma concentration occurs after 2-5 hours of administration. About 94% of the administered dose of lofexidine is eliminated through the renal system, about 10% is unchanged drug and 5% is the hydrolysis product, N-(2-aminoethyl)-2-(2,6-dichlorophenoxy)propanamide. The *O*-dealkylated product, 2,6-dichlorophenol, is the major metabolite (about 80% of administered dose) in the urine (Fig. **17**). Both of these metabolites, in addition to a third metabolite, 2-(2,6-dichlorophenoxy) propionic acid (deamidated product), are inactive. The enzymes involved in these metabolic changes include CYP2D6 (major) and CYP1A2 & CYP2C19 (minor) [37].

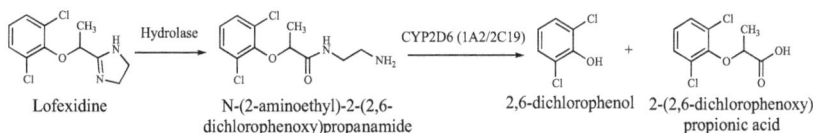

Fig. (**17**). Metabolic transformation of lofexidine.

Indirect-Acting Sympathomimetics (Figs. 2 and 18)

Amphetamine and *p-tyramine* are prototypical indirect acting adrenergic agonists (SAR 7 & 8 of phenylethylamine). Amphetamine is the least polar and has the highest delivery to the brain with enormous stimulating effects through indirect adrenergic, dopaminergic and serotonergic actions. It stimulates the secretion of all these neurotransmitters in the brain. Thus, it is highly popular for recreational use as a performance enhancer and has much addictive potential. However, *p*-tyramine that occurs in cheese has little delivery to the brain has primarily local adrenergic effects and is metabolized by MAO-A.

The clinically useful drug *4-hydroxyamphetamine* has little or no ephedrine-like, CNS-stimulating action, and is used for dilating pupil. *Pseudoephedrine* is also an indirect-acting drug with β-OH, with the carbon at (*S*) configuration, which is in wrong stereochemistry for the direct acting drugs. In *D-(-)-ephedrine*, β-OH has correct configuration (*R*) for direct activity and possesses mixed effects. Its *erythro* enantiomer, L-(+)-ephedrine, is not clinically used. The *threo* racemate, L-(+)-pseudoephedrine hydrochloride or sulfate, is clinically used as a nasal/sinus decongestant and stimulant as a single ingredient or in combination with antihistamines and/or NSAIDs in many OTC preparations.

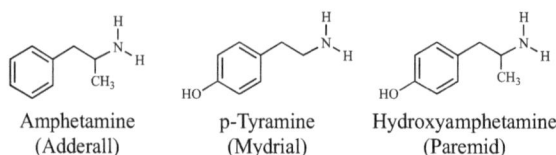

Amphetamine   p-Tyramine   Hydroxyamphetamine
(Adderall)   (Mydrial)   (Paremid)

Fig. (18). Structures of a few indirect acting adrenergic agonists.

Adrenergic Receptor Antagonists

The α Adrenergic Antagonists

The Imidazoline Derivatives

Tolazoline and *phentolamine* (Fig. **19**) are nonselective competitive α-receptor antagonists, which are structurally similar to the imidazoline α-agonists. Tolazoline lacks a lipophilic substitution on the aromatic ring that makes it an antagonist (**SAR 2** of imidazolines). However, among two aromatic rings of phentolamine, one contains a lipophilic group, but it is still an antagonist through an unknown mechanism [20, 25]. For their vasodilator effects these agents are used to treat spasms of peripheral blood vessels and as antidotes to reverse the severe peripheral vasoconstriction [38]. Phentolamine is also used to reverse the effects of local anesthetics in dental practices [39].

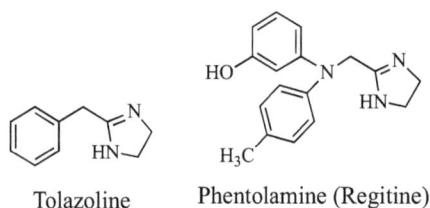

Tolazoline   Phentolamine (Regitine)

Fig. (19). Structures of α adrenergic antagonists.

The Irreversible α-Blocker

β-Haloalkylamines are *irreversible* α-receptor blockers through the mechanism shown in Fig. (**20**), *e.g.*, *phenoxybenzamine*. The cysteine molecule at the active site of αAR in TM3 is likely to involve in making the nucleophilic attack to form the stable linkage [40]. This causes vasodilatation of the blood vessel, which is useful as an antihypertensive.

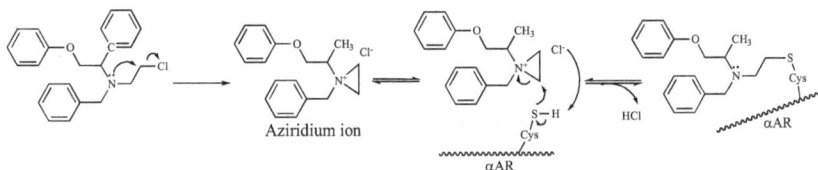

Fig. (20). Mechanism of irreversible αAR blockade by phenoxybenzamine.

Although it is the first α-blocker to be used for the treatment of benign prostatic hyperplasia [40], due to unwanted side effects its current use in the treatment of hypertension is restricted mainly to that caused by pheochromocytoma. It has a slower onset and a longer duration of action compared with other α-blockers.

$α_1$ and $α_2$ Selective Antagonists

The quinazolines, prazosin (Minipress®), terazosin (Hytrin®) and doxazosin (Cardura®), are the group of highly selective $α_1$-receptor antagonists (Fig. 2). All these agents contain three components: quinazoline ring, piperazine ring, and acyl moiety. The amino group on the quinazoline ring is very important for $α_1$-selectivity. The piperazine ring can be replaced with piperidine or an acyclic alkylamine moiety, *e.g.* alfuzosin, (Uroxatral®; (Fig. 2), without loss of affinity. The acyl group has pharmacokinetic significance. Prazosin has oral bioavailability of 50-70%, terazosin has 90%, and Doxazosin has 65%. The half-life and duration of action are for prazosin 2-3 and 4-6, terazosin 9-12 and 18, and doxazosin 22 and 36 hours, respectively. Terazosin and doxazocin are used to lower BP especially if associated with BPH. Prazosin can also be used but need frequent dosing.

Yohimbine and ***corynanthine*** (Fig. **21**) are two indole alkaloids differing only in the relative stereochemistry of carbon containing the carbomethoxy substituent as shown in structures. Yohimbine is an $α_2$-antagonist while corynanthine is an $α_1$-antagonist. Yohimbine increases heart rate and blood pressure as a result of its blockade of the $α_2$ receptors in the CNS. It has been used experimentally to treat male erectile impotence.

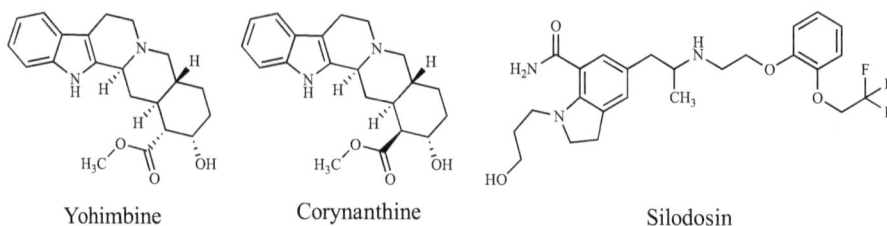

Yohimbine   Corynanthine   Silodosin

Fig. (21). Representative structures of a few $\alpha_{1 \text{ and}}\alpha_2$-selective antagonists.

Silodosin (Rapaflo; Fig. **21**) is a highly selective inhibitor of the α_{1A} AR and thus in contrast to other α_1-blockers causes no orthostatic hypotension but seems to cause more problems with ejaculation.

β-Adrenergic Receptor Antagonists (β-Blockers)

Agents that antagonize the β ARs are more commonly known as β-blockers. Many equally effective beta-blockers are now available, which differ only in lipophilicity, bioavailability PK parameters and thus the duration of actions that affect the choice of agents. The β-blockers with a relatively short duration of action need two- or three-times daily dosing. However, their sustained-release dosage forms may be used once daily for hypertension and twice daily for angina treatment. Atenolol, bisoprolol, carvedilol, celiprolol, and nadolol are long acting and need only once daily.

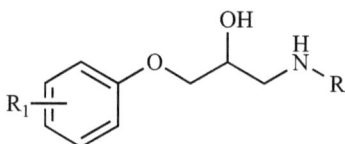

Fig. (22). Pharmacophoric group of β blockers.

Propranolol was the first clinically used β-blocker in which the catechol moiety of the phenylethylamine derivatives is replaced with a naphthyloxy function thus comprising a new class of *aryloxypropanolamines*. The pharmacophoric group of the aryloxypropanolamine is shown in Fig. (**22**). The nature of the aromatic ring and its substituents (R1) as well as the nature of side chain amine and its substituents (R) determine the β-blocker activity and the pharmacokinetics of the new derivatives in this class. The general SAR of this class of compounds can be summarized as follows:

Sar 1

The aryloxy and the hydroxyl ethylamine groups (Fig. **22**) are the minimum requirements for the antagonistic property. Replacement of the ethereal oxygen with S, CH_2 or $N-CH_3$ decreases the β-blocking activity.

Sar 2

The aryloxy propanolamines are more potent than the aryl ethanolamines. The three-carbon side chain having hydroxyl group with *S*-configuration exhibits optimum affinity to β receptor. Alpha methyl substitution at the side chain decreases activity. They interact with the receptor site in the similar way as the agonists.

Sar 3

SAR 3*N,N*-disubstituted tertiary amines have little β-blocking activity and isopropyl, tertiary butyl, phenylethyl, hydroxyl phenyl ethyl or methoxy phenyl ethyl substituted secondary amines are more potent β-blockers.

Sar 4

The aromatic ring can be a substituted phenyl, naphthyl or equivalent group to have optimal activity; phenanthrene or anthracene decreases the activity. The aromatic portion appears to perturb the receptor to inhibit it.

Sar 5

para-Substituent of sufficient size on aromatic ring along with the absence of *meta*-substituent give rise to $β_1$-blockers, practolol is the prototypical. Selective $β_1$-blockers are commonly referred as cardio-selective β-blockers.

Nonselective β-Blockers

The structures of a few nonselective β blockers are shown in Fig. (**23**). The discovery of ***propranolol*** in 1960s as the first nonselective β-blocker (SAR 4 of β-blockers) led James Black (see latter in drug discovery case story) to win the 1988 Nobel Prize and the use of this drug by North Korean Olympic medalist pistol shooter Kim Jong Su led to disqualify him from the Olympic 2008. Although the racemic propranolol is used clinically its *S*(-)-isomer is more potent and also less rapidly metabolized than the *R*(+)-isomer (SAR 1 & 2 of β-blockers). Decreased cardiac output, inhibition of renin release, and inhibition of tonic sympathetic nerve outflow in the brain are thought to be the contributing factors for its antihypertensive effect. By blocking the catecholamine induced heart rate it reduces the oxygen requirements of the heart, which is beneficial in angina pectoris. However, abrupt discontinuation of propranolol therapy may exacerbate angina and myocardial infarction (MI) and is suggested to reduce its dose gradually over at least a few weeks. Its β-blocking effect also exerts antiarrhythmic action and at higher dosages exerts a quinidine-like or anesthetic-like membrane action affecting cardiac action potential.

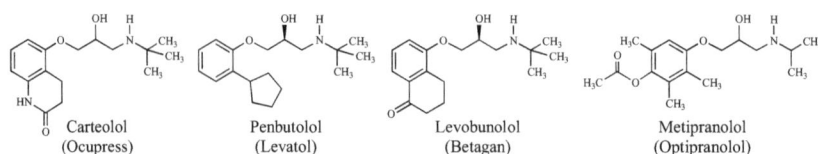

Fig. (23). Structures of few nonselective β adrenergic blockers.

Propranolol is highly lipophilic and thus well absorbed orally but undergoes first-pass metabolism with ~25% bioavailability. Due to lipophilicity it also exerts high CNS bioavailability as well as CNS side effects especially sleep disturbances and nightmares. Aromatic hydroxylation (*para*), *N*-dealkylation and deamination, and direct glucuronidation/sulfate conjugation are the major metabolic routes (Fig. **24**). The major oxidative enzymes are CYP2D6 and CYP1A2 [25].

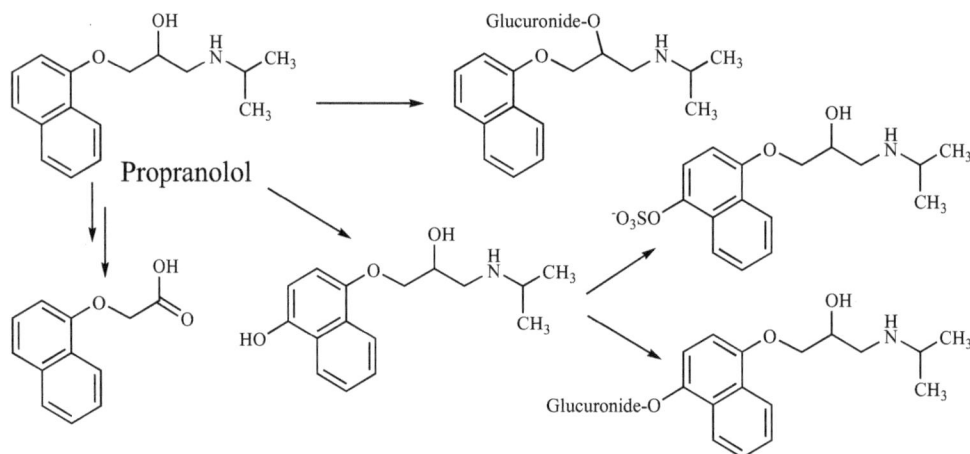

Fig. (24). The major metabolic routes of propranolol.

Nadolol is another nonselective β-blocker (SAR 1, 2 & 4) with similar activity but with more polarity than propranolol and thus imparts less brain delivery and negligible CNS side effects including sleep disturbances and nightmares [41]. It reduces heart rate and cardiac output and thus both systolic and diastolic blood pressures at rest and on exercise. The competitive antagonism at peripheral adrenergic sites (especially cardiac) leads to decreased cardiac output. It also suppresses renin secretion from the kidneys.

The average absolute bioavailability of nadolol after oral administration is about 30% and ~30% of it is plasma protein bound. Due to low lipophilicity it enters the liver cells less and thus less metabolized ensuring longer duration of action than most β-blockers [42]. It is excreted in the urine mostly unchanged. Due to metabolic stability and long half-life (20 to 24 hours), it is administered once daily [25].

Sotalol is a phenyl ethanolamine derivative with side chain similar to isoproterenol. However, it lacks the important aromatic hydroxyl functions required for agonist activity and contains a bulky 4-(methyl) sulfonamide group which gives the antagonist activity. It imparts a dual action, a non-selective β-block (SAR 1, 2 & 4) as well as potassium channel block. It is thus a class III anti-arrhythmic agent, used to treat ventricular tachycardias [42] and atrial fibrillation [43]. The abrupt discontinuation of sotalol dosages may lead to induced arrhythmia. It is absorbed completely after oral administration and due to polarity is poorly delivered to the brain. It is not bound to plasma proteins and excreted mostly unchanged in the urine [25].

(±)-Carvedilol is used clinically; however, the S(-) enantiomer possesses β-blocking activity (SAR 2) and both R(+) and S(-) enantiomers possess α-blocking activity. Its β-blocking activity is seen within 1h of dosages leading to similar pharmacological action like other β-blockers, notably reduced cardiac output and reflex orthostatic tachycardia. The α_1-blocking activity is characterized by the attenuated pressor effects of phenylephrine, vasodilation, and reduced peripheral vascular resistance. All these effects contribute to the reduction of blood pressure.

Carvedilol has a tricyclic ring system with additional aromatic ring making it highly lipophilic that allows it to be rapidly and completely absorbed orally. However, because it undergoes extensive, stereospecific, first-pass metabolism, it has only 25% - 35% bioavailability. It is highly plasma protein (albumin) bound (>98%). The aromatic ring hydroxylation and subsequent glucuronidation and sulfate conjugation are the primary metabolic routes, which are excreted primarily into the feces. The *O*-demethylation and 4'-hydroxylation at the phenol ring lead to 3 active metabolites, which are more potent β-blockers than carvedilol. CYP2D6 and CYP2C9 and, to a lesser extent, CYP2D6 and to some extent CYP3A4, are the enzymes responsible for the 4'- and 5'-hydroxylation of both isomers, and CYP2C9 is the primary enzyme for *O*-demethylation of *S*(---carvedilol. Genetic polymorphism is evident with CYP2D6. The poor metabolizers may experience 2- to 3-fold higher plasma concentrations of *R*(+)-

carvedilol exhibiting only 20 - 25% more plasma concentration of S(+)-carvedilol than the fast metabolizers [25].

Timolol has a *tert*-butyl side chain and entirely different aromatic system from most β-blockers and exerts similar pharmacological activity like other nonselective β-blockers [44]. It is used to treat hypertension and to prevent heart attacks. It is relatively lipophilic and thus can cross BBB. This is advantageous to control migraine headaches. It is also useful in ophthalmic practice to treat glaucoma in nonasthmatic patients. It is well absorbed after oral administration and only slightly plasma protein bound. It undergoes about 50% first-pass metabolism and along with the metabolites, it is excreted by the kidneys [25].

Labetalol, like carvedilol, is a mixed α/β adrenergic antagonist with an estimated α- to β-blockade ratio of 1:3 and 1:7 following oral and IV administration, respectively. It is used to treat hypertension. However, if used by IV infusion in refractory hypertension it may lead to severe orthostatic hypotension (due to $α_1$-blockade) and bradycardia [25, 45].

Labetalol is completely absorbed following oral administration; however, due to extensive first-pass metabolism it has only 25% absolute bioavailability, which may increase if administered with food. The phenolic hydroxyl group undergoes extensive glucuronidation and the metabolites are excreted in the urine as well as into the feces. Although it crosses the placental barrier, due to polarity it only negligibly crosses the blood-brain barrier [25].

Carteolol is a long-acting, nonselective, β-blocker with intrinsic sympathomimetic activity and is useful in glaucoma, because it reduces intra ocular pressure possibly through reduced aqueous production. It is well absorbed following oral administration with an absolute bioavailability of ~85%. It is partially metabolized to 8-hydroxycarteolol (an active metabolite) and its glucuronide conjugates, and ~50 to 70% of the dose is eliminated unchanged by the kidneys. *Levobunolol*, which is structurally similar to carteolol (amide of carteolol is replaced with keto function), is >60 times more potent than its dextro isomer in nonselective β-blocking activity and is devoid of significant local anesthetic or intrinsic sympathomimetic activity. It is thus useful in hypertension and glaucoma like other β-blockers, however, is not suitable for patients with asthmatic symptoms. *Metipranolol* is similar to levobunolol in terms of pharmacological activity and is used mainly for the treatment of glaucoma [25].

Penbutolol also has some intrinsic agonist activity and is more potent than propranolol in nonselective β-blocking activity when taken orally. It is well-absorbed after oral administration and extensively metabolized in the liver by hydroxylation and glucuronidation. It has a duration of antihypertensive effects of about 24 hours and thus administered once a day. The side effect profile is similar to other nonselective β-blockers [46].

Selective β₁-Blockers (Cardioselective β-Blockers)

All the β₁-blockers (Fig. **25**) have the same mechanism of action in the management of primary open angle glaucoma (POAG). Both nonselective and β₁-selective blockers can be used to control POAG. However, if the patients also suffer from bronchial obstruction the nonselective β-blockers are contraindicated and the selective β₁-blockers are the first line treatments in these cases at therapeutic doses. Similar generalization stands for the treatment of hypertension and other cardiac problems including angina.

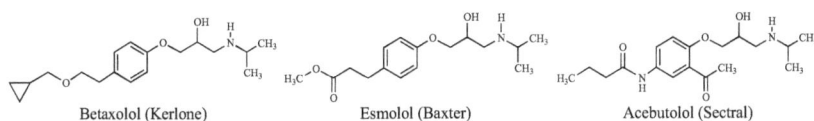

Betaxolol (Kerlone)   Esmolol (Baxter)   Acebutolol (Sectral)

Fig. (25). Structures of few selective β₁ blockers.

Bisoprolol is relatively more β₁-selective (SAR 5 of β-blockers) compared to other commonly used selective β₁-blockers [47, 48]. It is more selective at lower doses. At higher doses it also inhibits β₂-receptors of bronchial and vascular muscles. It is a potent antihypertensive as well as cardioprotective agent. The inhibition of renin secretion by about 65% also contributes in its antihypertensive activity [51]. Because it has long lipophilic chain as well as hydrophilic functional groups, it is well absorbed orally, undergoes partial first pass metabolism and exhibits about 80% absolute bioavailability. It is only partially bound to serum proteins (~30%). Bisoprolol, that accounts for about 50%, and its inactive metabolites (non CYP2D6 mediated metabolism) are eliminated equally by renal and non-renal routes [25].

Atenolol is a selective β₁-blocker (SAR 5 of β-blockers) introduced in 1976, and since it does not cross the blood-brain barrier (BBB) due to polarity it avoids various CNS side effects [52]. Following oral administration, it is rapidly but incompletely (~50%) absorbed and the remainder is excreted unchanged in the feces. The absorbed drug is excreted primarily unchanged in the urine. It is slightly bound to plasma protein (~6-16%) [25].

The selective β₁-blocking antihypertensive drug *(±)-metoprolol* (SAR 5) is employed orally either as prolonged-release or conventional-release formulation. It is moderately lipophilic with a short half-life, therefore needs at least twice daily administration or as a prolonged-release dosage form. At higher doses it also inhibits β_2 ARs of the bronchial and vascular muscles. It is rapidly and completely absorbed after oral administration. However, due to first-pass metabolism it has only ~50% absolute bioavailability. Only a small fraction of the drug (about 12%) is bound to human serum albumin. Metoprolol undergoes extensive, stereospecific metabolism primarily by CYP2D6 and is excreted primarily in urine, <5% of which is unchanged drug. About 8% of whites and about 2% of most other populations are devoid of CYP2D6 and are known as poor metabolizers and need lower doses of metoprolol [25].

Esmolol, a cardioselective β-blocker (SAR 5) at therapeutic doses, has rapid onset [50] and a very short duration of action. It is also considered to be a class II antiarrhythmic agent [51]. It is commonly used in surgical patients to prevent tachycardia by slow intravenous injection. The ester-methyl side chain at *para* position of aromatic ring makes it a *soft drug* that is rapidly hydrolyzed (half-life ~9 minutes) by plasma esterases to an inactive carboxylic acid (Fig. 26), which is primarily excreted in the urine. Esmolol is about 55% bound to plasma protein but its carboxylic acid metabolite is only 10% bound [25].

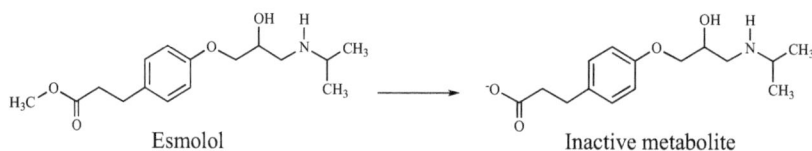

Fig. (26). Metabolic inactivation of esmolol.

Betaxolol, at therapeutic doses, has greater affinity for β_1 ARs than metoprolol with cardioprotective and glaucoma protective effects. Both oral and ophthalmic preparations are available for the management of hypertension and glaucoma, respectively. It is considered as a first line treatment for POAG. It is lipophilic and completely absorbed after oral administration and undergoes small first-pass effect rendering an absolute bioavailability of ~89%. It is ~50% bound to plasma proteins, metabolized by liver enzymes and excreted in the urine, 15% of which is unchanged parent drug [25].

Acebutolol contains an *ortho*-acetyl substitution in addition to the typical *para* substitution of the selective β_1-blockers and exerts less cardioselectivity than most selective β_1-blockers [52]. Unlike many other β-blockers it does not decrease HDL. Although it is well absorbed after oral administration, it undergoes substantial first pass metabolism leading to low (35-50%) absolute bioavailability. The hepatic metabolism produces active metabolites including desbutyl amine acetolol which is readily acetylated to the equipotent diacetolol (Fig. 27). It is about 26% plasma protein bound. Acebutolol and diacetolol are relatively hydrophilic allowing minimal crossing of the BBB. It is eliminated in both urine (30-40%) and feces (50-60%) [25].

Black Box Warning with Systemic Use β-Blockers

Patients abruptly withdrawn from both cardioselective and noncardioselective β-blocker therapy may experience exacerbation of angina and, in some cases, myocardial infarction. When discontinuing chronically administered β-blockers in patients with ischemic heart disease, gradually reduce the dosage over a period of one to two weeks and carefully monitor the patient.

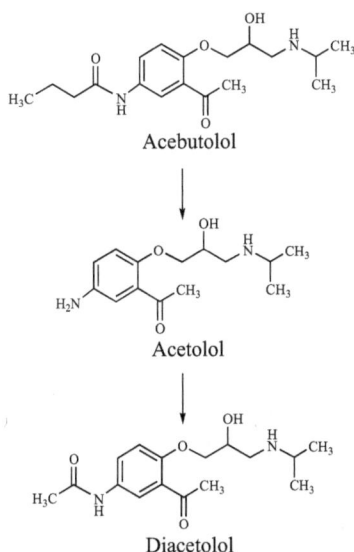

Fig. (27). Metabolism of acebutolol.

CASE STUDIES

Case 1. SL, a 50-year-old African American man is under antihypertensive, CHF and asthma medication. Having a family history of POAG, being an African American a group where POAG is prevalent, and his ophthalmic symptoms led his optometrist to diagnose him with POAG. The optometrist is trying to decide on a suitable initial therapy for SL and asks your opinion. You are the pharmacist on duty for both SL and his optometrist. You have the following structures to choose from.

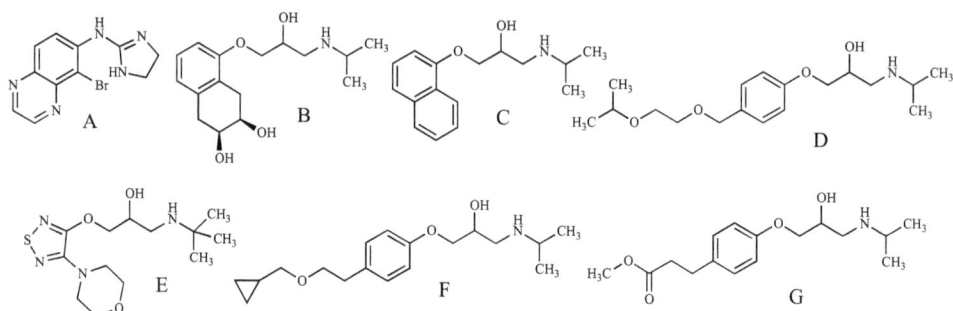

1. Which structure(s) is/are suitable for starting an initial therapy for SL? Justify your answer by considering SAR, mechanism and duration of action of the drug structures.
2. Which structure(s) should not be used for SL? Why?
3. After two weeks of initial therapy if you want to add an adjunct to better control his glaucoma, which structure would be the best and why?
4. If the patient had no asthma or any bronchial dysfunction and you wanted a drug with minimal CNS effect, which one would you prefer. Explain by applying the pharmacokinetic parameters of the drug.

Case 2. RT, a 12-year-old boy, has been coughing occasionally for the last two days with some breathing difficulties. Before that he was suffering from viral flu and upper respiratory tract infection for 3 days. After physical examination his physician is considering that he has moderate respiratory distress with audible wheezes, occasional coughing, and a hyperinflated chest. After a thorough examination of all his related parameters the physician is positive that RT is suffering from an acute asthma attack. RT is given O_2 and the physician is considering starting with a suitable nebulizer. You have the following drug structures for use in nebulizer.

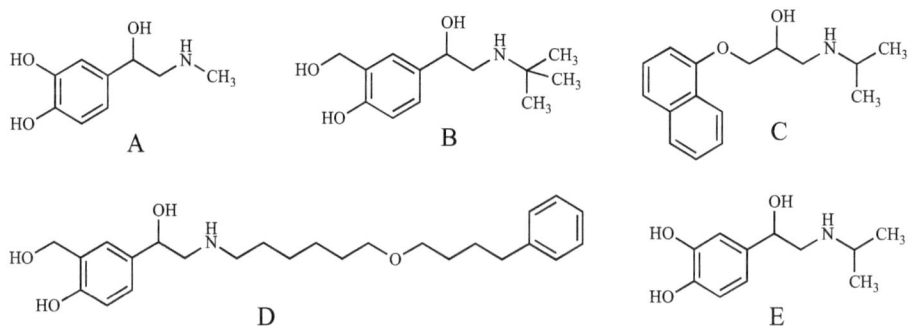

1. Which structure(s) is/are suitable for starting an initial therapy for RT? Justify your answer by considering SAR, mechanism and duration of action of the drug structures.
2. Why you did not choose the other structures?
3. Which structure is contraindicated for RT? Why?
4. If RT was suffering from a severe asthma attack during the springtime but mild during the rest of the year, and that he often has sleep disturbances during nighttime due to this attack during spring, which structure would be most suitable for him and why?
5. Would you use the drug you chose in question 4 alone or in combination with a corticosteroid? Explain.

Case 3. SK a 60-year-old male car mechanic with a history of 2-pack/day cigarette smoking is coughing intermittently on a daily basis with increasing shortness of breath. He used to have a chronic cough, which is lessened now after quitting smoking for about a year. He has been using a short acting β_2-agonist by inhalation on a PRN basis, yet his dyspnea is worsened. He has mild wheezing and the spirometry demonstrated that he is suffering from a moderate (GOLD Stage II) COPD. A long-term treatment is sought and following drug options are available.

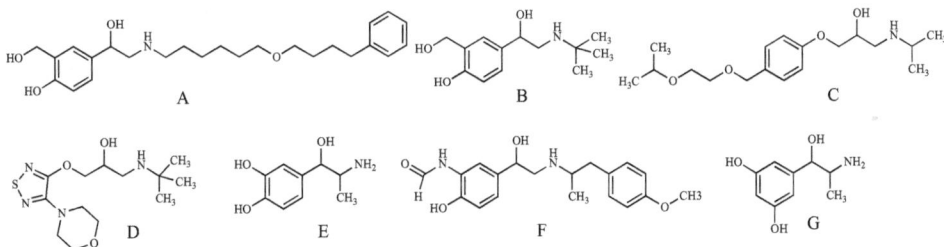

1. Select the most appropriate structure(s) for SK. Justify your choices on the basis of the pharmacology and SAR of the available structures.
2. Would you use the drug chosen in question 1 alone or in combination with a corticosteroid? Explain.
3. Would you use the drug chosen if the COPD were severe or very severe (GOLD stage III or IV)?
4. Which one of the structures is contraindicated in this patient and why?

Case 4. LR is a 49-year-old male with history of hypertension and is hospitalized due to acute MI. He is having a left ventricular dysfunction. He is also an asthmatic patient which is worsening during springtime. He uses a bronchodilator on PRN basis to control his acute asthma attacks. To control his hypertension as well as the cardiac dysfunction, in addition to an ACE inhibitor, a suitable β-

blocker is sought. You have the following structures to choose from.

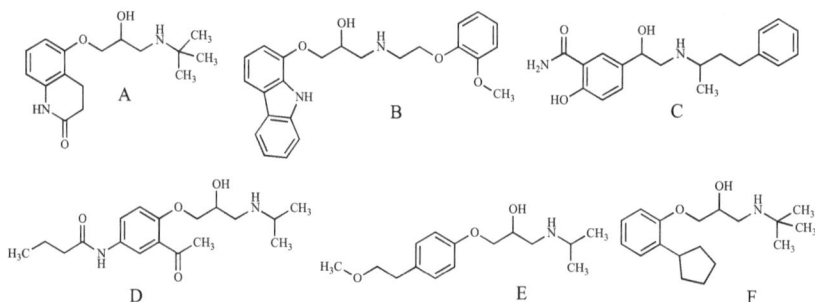

1. Explain the pros and cons for each of the structures. Include SAR.
2. Which structure is the best for LR? Why?
3. Why are other drugs not suitable?
4. Which drugs are mixed α/β-blockers? Are they suitable for this patient?

Case 5. DC is a 55-year-old male with hypertension currently under control (BP 138/84) with a diuretic and a calcium channel blocker for a year. For the last few weeks he has been experiencing difficulty in starting urination and also low urinary flow, symptoms consistent with BPH. His physician is considering adding a new antihypertensive agent to control his BP as well as BPH.

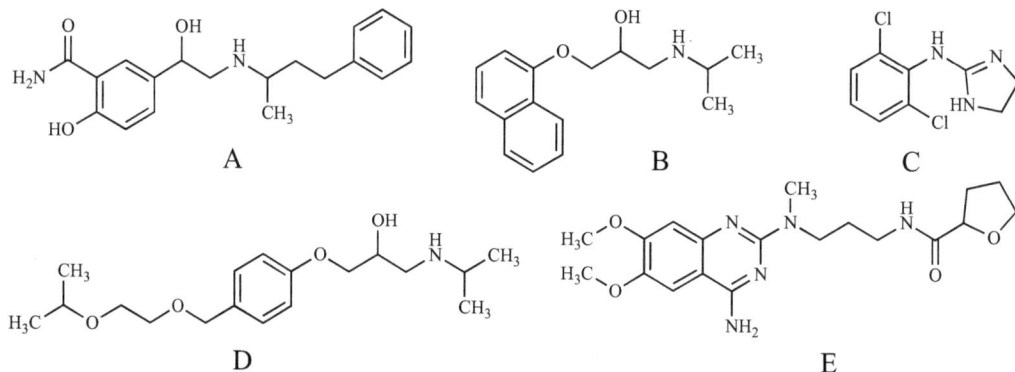

1. Which drug is the most suitable for DC? Why?
2. What therapeutic aims must you keep in mind when selecting an agent for DC?
3. Why did you not choose the other agents?

Case 6. MM, a 45-year-old man with a 1.5-pack-day smoking history is experiencing chronic angina. He has a 5-year history of diabetes mellitus. His ability to walk is limited by peripheral vascular disease and quick tiredness. A suitable β-blocker should be initiated for the treatment of his angina.

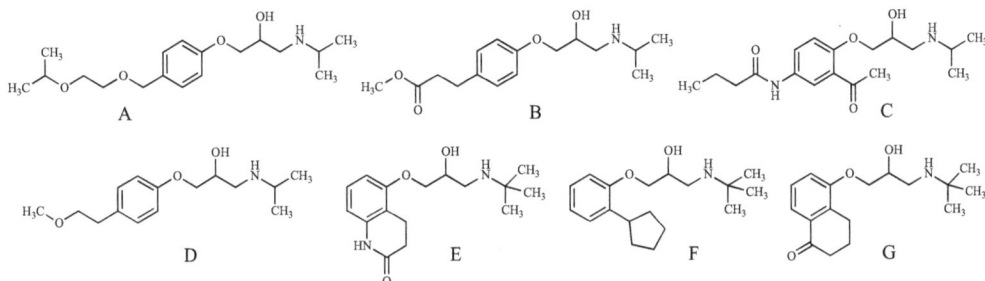

1. Which of the structures provided would be viable candidates for antianginal therapy? Take into consideration the therapeutic window, SAR and mechanism of action?
2. Has the history of smoking, and/or diabetes and peripheral vascular disease any influence in this choice of agent?
3. Which agent will have minimal peroral activity? Why?

DRUG DISCOVERY CASE STUDIES

Discovery of Adrenergic Agonists [48]

The discovery of the adrenergic agonists (Fig. **28**) is an excellent example of the introduction of the structurally related analogs of hormones as therapeutic agents. Barger and Dale in 1910 [53] investigated the bioisosteres epinephrine and tyramine and variety of structural analogs and described them as sympathomimetic amines. Adrenalone, a synthetic intermediate of epinephrine, was marketed as topical haemostatic agent and deoxyepinephrine was marketed as vasoconstrictor and pressor agent. Removal of 4-OH from epinephrine furnished phenylephrine and removal of the 3-OH furnished oxedrine in 1927. Phenylephrine was marketed as nasal decongestant and oxedrine as vasoconstrictor in 1930 [53].

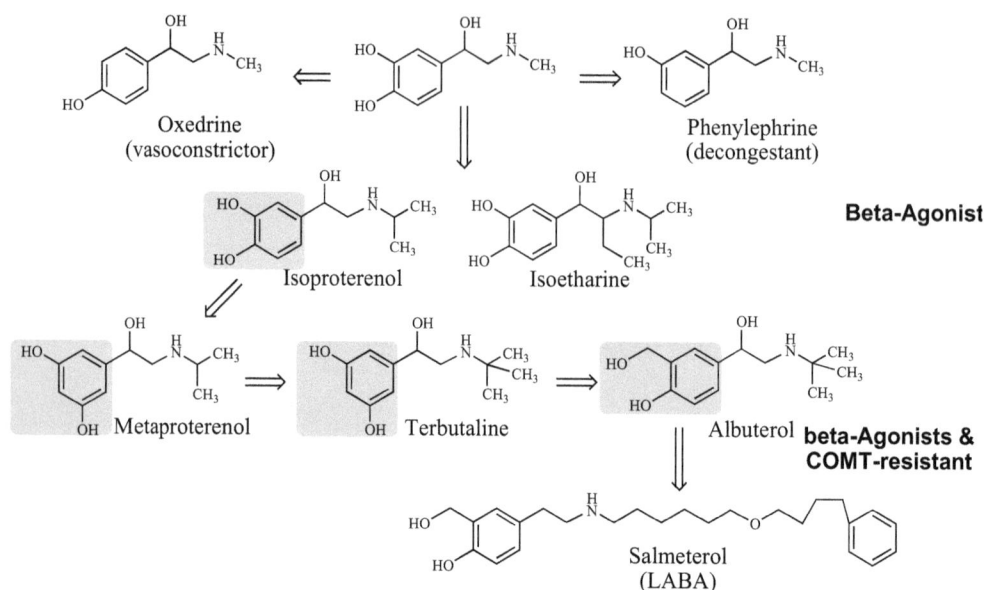

Fig. (28). Development of adrenergic agonists based on the techniques of hormone analogs.

The continuous innovation over epinephrine to incorporate more lipophilicity led to the discovery of isoetharine (in 1934) at the Höchst laboratories and many years later isoproterenol (marketed in 1941 as Aludrin) at the University of Vienna as potent bronchodilators without hypertensive effects. Both of these were later found to be selective β agonists. However, these drugs, being catecholamines, showed metabolic instability thus low oral bioavailability as well as short duration of action. The innovation continued for decades starting from the 1940s [53].

In 1961, laboratories of the Boehringer introduced metaproterenol, where the catechol moiety of isoproterenol is replaced with orcinol moiety. Not only it retained the activity of isoproterenol, but it was also later found to be somewhat β_2-selective as well as resistant against destruction by catechol *O*-methyltransferase (COMT) and, to some extent, by sulfokinase. Within 5 years Astra introduced terbutaline (in 1966) by replacing the *N*-isopropyl group of metoproterenol with *N*-*tert*-butyl, which showed both enhanced potency and higher β_2-selectivity. Ware, a division of Glaxo, developed albuterol in 1967 by replacing the *meta* hydroxyl group of catechol moiety with a hydroxymethyl group and using the similar side chain as terbutaline. It retained high potency, high β_2-selectivity as well as the expected longer duration of action and soon became the drug of choice to control asthma. Glaxo researchers later attached a long lipophilic chain on the amine nitrogen to discover salmeterol, which is 5-10 times more potent than albuterol, very long acting and has introduced a new class termed LABA (Fig. **28**) [53].

Discovery of Adrenergic Antagonists – The Discovery of Propranolol [49]

Slater of Eli Lilly, Indianapolis first reported the AR antagonistic activity of dichloroisoproterenol on tracheal strips in 1957 [54]. In search of a long acting bronchodilator (β-agonist), they replaced the two hydroxyl groups with chlorine groups, but it serendipitously turned out to be antagonist. Later, Moran of Emory University by experimenting on cardiac muscles showed it to be a partial agonist [55].

James Black became interested in these findings. He was working at ICI Pharmaceutical (now AstraZeneca) at Alderley Park in Cheshire for antianginal therapy. He had the hypothesis that it would be advantageous to reduce the oxygen demand for the heart instead of increasing oxygen supply by nitrates or other vasodilators in treating angina. It could be performed by blocking the β AR of the heart muscle that will reduce the heart rate and thus the oxygen demand. In the early 1960s, he tested pronethalol, an analog of dichloroisoproterenol where bulky dichloro functions were replaced with a benzene ring and confirmed it to be a β-blocker [56]. It was shown to be beneficial in preventing tachycardia and angina and also reducing blood pressure in hypertension and was marketed in 1963. However, long term toxicology study revealed its cancer producing potential to the thymus gland and was soon taken off the market. Then he modified the structure by increasing the distance between the alcoholic hydroxyl group on the side chain and the aromatic ring to furnish propranolol (Fig. **29**). Propranolol was licensed in 1964 as a general use β-blocker. It is the first nonselective β-blocker to be created as an entirely new class of therapeutic agent for the treatment of angina, arrhythmia and hypertension, an innovation indebted to Sir James Black's 1988 Nobel Prize. Now series of nonselective as well as cardio selective β-blockers are in the market [57].

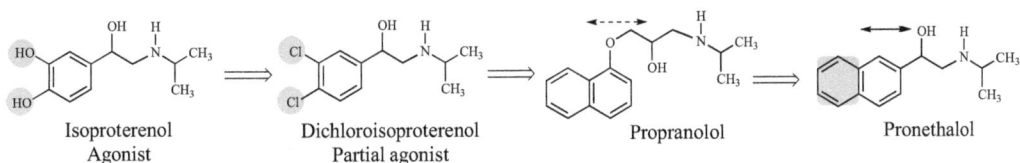

Fig. (29). Discovery process of β blocker propranolol.

STUDENT SELF-STUDY GUIDE

1. Which stereoisomer of norepinephrine is biologically active? Why based on the SAR content of this chapter? Currently, there are several hypotheses about

this phenomenon?

2. Key enzymes in the biosynthesis of NE that are drug targets.
3. Structures of DOPA, NE and epinephrine.
4. Types of interaction of NE at the receptor site (both α and β) and the key amino acids involved in it.
5. Mechanism of action of metyrosine. Which isomer is active? Is it sympathomimetic or sympatholytic?
6. Which drug (with structure) works on ATP-driven monoamine transporter and what is its effect?
7. What are the drugs that contain guanidine moiety? How do they work and what is the effect?
8. How do you differentiate from structures between the direct, indirect or mixed mechanisms?
9. The structure activity relations (SAR) of phenylethylamine based adrenergic agonists and antagonists including stereochemistry.
10. What key structural features make a phenylethylamine derivative agonist or antagonist; direct, indirect or mixed; α or β selective; α_1 or α_2 and β_1 or β_2 selective?
11. What are imidazoline-based drugs (both agonists and antagonists)? Why clonidine is active in the brain better than other imidazoline analogs?
12. What are irreversible α-receptor blockers? How do they work?
13. What are highly selective α_1-receptor antagonists? What are key structural features for their receptor selectivity and PK parameters?
14. Which stereoisomer of yohimbine is α_1 antagonist and which one is a_2 antagonist?
15. What is the development process of β-adrenergic agonists? How do you differentiate between nonselective, β-selective and β_2-selective agonists? How short acting and long acting bronchodilators are differentiated structurally?
16. What are the pros and cons of SABA and LABA in the treatment of asthma?
17. What is the development process of β-blockers? How can you differentiate between nonselective and β_1 selective agents?
18. What are the pros and cons of cardioselective and nonselective β-blockers in the treatment of hypertension, tachycardia and POAG?

STUDENT SELF-ASSESSMENT QUESTIONS

Part I:

Directions: Each of the numbered items or incomplete statements in this section is followed by answers or by completions of the statements. Select the **one** lettered answer or completion that is **best** in each case.

The duration of action of X,Y,Z is in the order (longest to shortest)

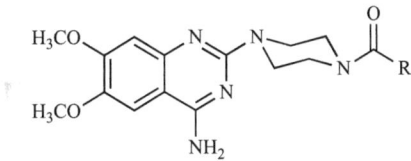

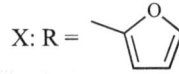

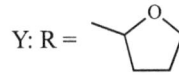

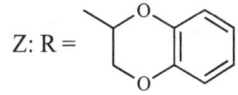

A. $X \rightarrow Y \rightarrow Z$

B. $X \rightarrow Z \rightarrow Y$

C. $Z \rightarrow X \rightarrow Y$

D. $Y \rightarrow X \rightarrow Z$

E. $Z \rightarrow Y \rightarrow X$

Questions 2 & 3 are based on the following structures

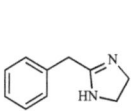

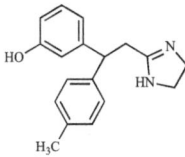

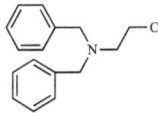

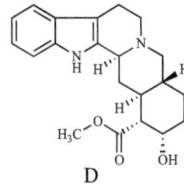

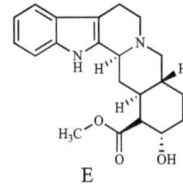

2. Which one is an irreversible α-adrenergic blocker?

3. Which one is a selective α_2-adrenergic blocker?

4. Statement 1: Both albuterol and metaproterenol are stable against COMT and MAO.

Statement 2: Both albuterol and metaproterenol are β_1 selective agonists.

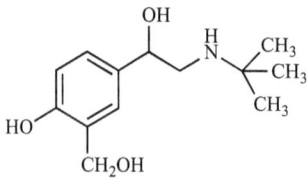

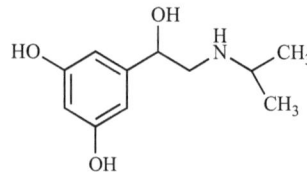

Albuterol   Metaproterenol

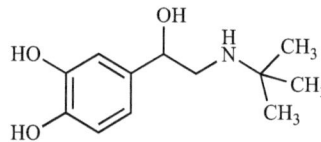

A. Statement 1 is true but statement 2 is false

B. Statement 2 is true but statement 1 is false

C. Both statements are true

D. Both statements are false

5. Statement 1: Both isoproterenol and colterol are stable against COMT and MAO.

Statement 2: Both isoproterenol and colterol are β_2 selective agonists.

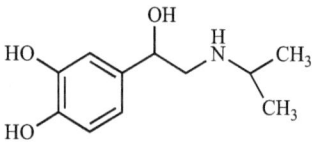

Isoproterenol   Colterol

A. Statement 1 is true but statement 2 is false

B. Statement 2 is true but statement 1 is false

C. Both statements are true

D. Both statements are false

6. Which one is a nonselective α-blocker?

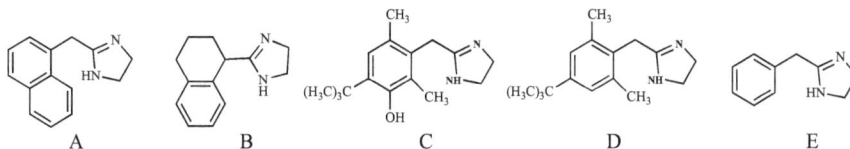

A   B   C   D   E

7. Which one is an α₁ adrenergic antagonist?

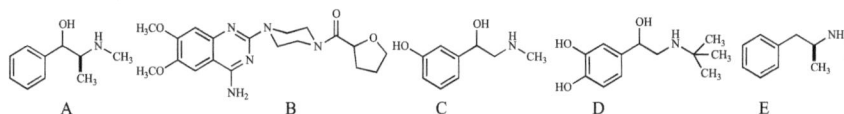

A   B   C   D   E

8. Which of the following structure is a selective β₁ blocker?

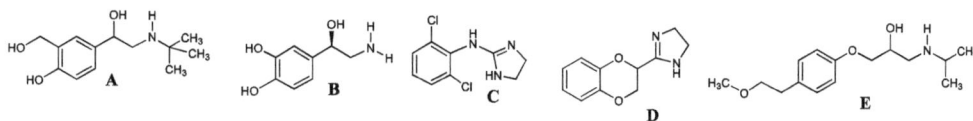

A   B   C   D   E

Part II:

Directions: Each item below contains three suggested answers of which **one or more** is correct. Chose the answer

A. if **I only** is correct

B. if **III only** is correct

C. if **I and II** are correct

D. if **II and III** are correct

E. if **I, II, and III** are correct

9. Guanethidine blocks the adrenergic activity because:

I. it inhibits the uptake of norepinephrine

II. it inhibits the release of norepinephrine

III. it stabilizes the norepinephrine storage vesicle

10. The drug structure shown:

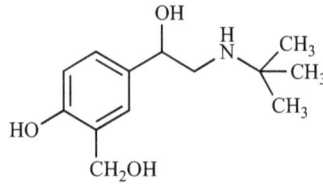

I. is a direct acting β-adrenergic agonist

I. its *R*-enantiomer is biologically more potent

II. is quickly metabolized by COMT

11. Which ones are <u>indirectly</u> acting sympathomimetic drugs?

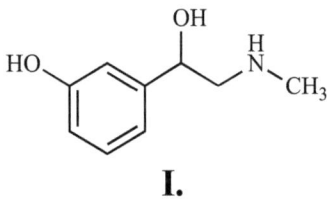

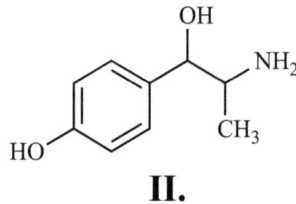

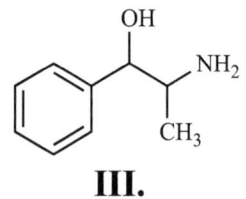

I.   **II.**   **III.**

12. Which ones are <u>irreversible</u> α-adrenergic blockers?

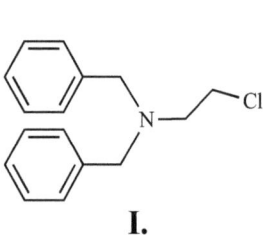

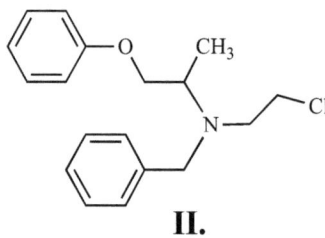

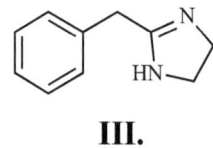

I.   **II.**   **III.**

13. The structure shown below:

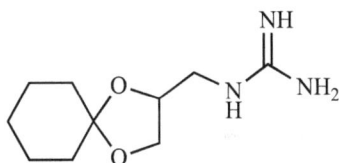

I. inhibits catecholamine release from storage vesicle

II. inhibits catecholamine uptake into the storage vesicles

III. inhibits catecholamine synthesis by blocking tyrosine hydrolase

14. The β-phenylethylamine derivatives with general structure shown may include:

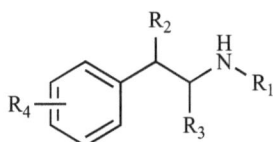

Where:
R_1 and R_2 are H, or any alkyl chain
R_3 is H or hydroxyl
R_4 is H, hydroxyl, alkloxyl, or sulfonamide group (*o*, *m*, or *p*)

I. direct acting adrenergic agonists

II. indirect acting adrenergic agonists

III. β adrenergic blockers

15. The (1*R*,2*S*)-α-methylnorepinephrine (structure shown):

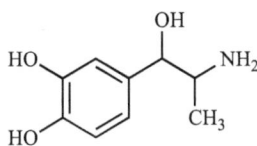

α-Methylnorepinephrine

I. if inhaled is a locally acting α agonist useful as a nasal decongestant

II. is an active metabolite of antihypertensive methyldopa works centrally as α_2 agonist

III. is not metabolized by MAO but metabolized by COMT

16. Structure shown below:

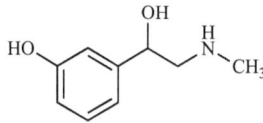

Phenylephrine

I. is a selective β_2 agonist

II. is a nasal decongestant

III. is a selective α_1 agonist

17. Structure shown below is:

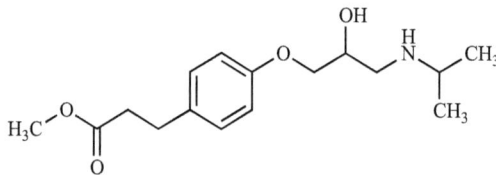

I. a nonselective β-blocker (both β_1 & β_2)

II. an antihypertensive agent

III. a short acting agent

18. Drugs acting by inhibiting synthesis, storage, or release of norepinephrine include:

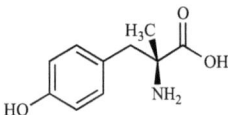

I.

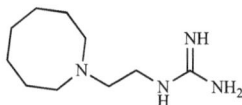

II.

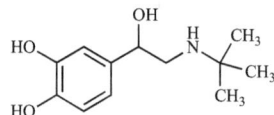

III.

19. The antihypertensive clonidine:

I. is a strong base

II. is α_2-selective agonist

III. acts centrally

Part III:

Directions: The group of items in this section consists of lettered options followed by a set of numbered items. For each item, select the **one** lettered option that is most closely associated with it. Each lettered option may be selected once, more than once, or not at all.

Match the drug structures (20-24) with the appropriate activity statements (A-E).

A. This bronchodilator is a β_2-agonist with stability against COMT

B. This α_2-agonist is used primarily in ophthalmic adrenergic preparations

C. This vasoconstrictor is an indirect acting adrenergic agonist

D. This one is a nonselective β-blocker

E. This antihypertensive drug is a selective β_1-blocker

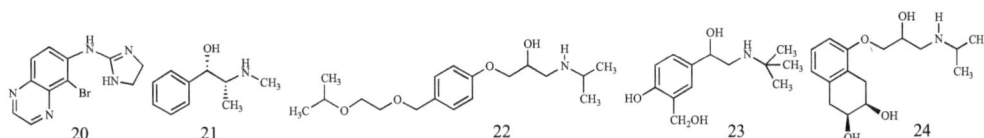

Match the drug structures (25-28) with the appropriate names (A-E).

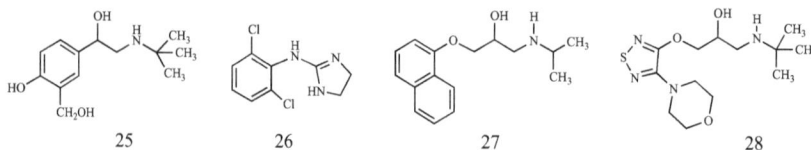

25   26   27   28

A. Clonidine

B. Terazocin

C. Propranolol

D. Timolol

E. Albuterol

Match the drug structures (29-32) with the appropriate names (A-E).

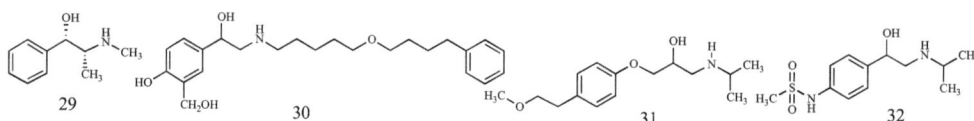

29   30   31   32

A. Clonidine

B. Metoprolol

C. Salmeterol

D. Sotalol

E. Pseudoephedrine

REFERENCES

[1]   Chen KK, Schmidt CF. The action of ephedrine, the active principle of the Chinese drug Ma Huang. J Pharmacol Exp Ther 1924; 24: 339-57.

[2]   Oliver G, Schäfer EA. On the physiological action of the extract of the suprarenal capsules. J Physiol 1894; 16: 1-4.

[3]   Moore B. On the chromogen and on the active physiological substance of the suprarenal gland. J Physiol 1897; 21(4-5): 382-9.
[http://dx.doi.org/10.1113/jphysiol.1897.sp000660] [PMID: 16992393]

[4]   Fränkel S. Physiological action of the suprarenal capsules. Wien Med Blätter 1896; 1: 14-6.

[5]   Abel JJ. On epinephrine, the active constituent of the suprarenal capsule and its compounds. Proc Am Physiol Soc 1898; 3-4: 3-5.

[6]   Takamine J. Adrenalin; the active principle of the suprarenal gland. Am J Pharm 1901; 73: 523-31.

[7]   Wilson NL. Clinical notes on adrenalin. Laryngoscope 1901; 11: 63-6.
[http://dx.doi.org/10.1288/00005537-190107000-00008]

[8]   Hartung WH. Epinephrine and related compounds: influence of structure on physiologic activity. Chem Rev 1931; 9: 389-465.
[http://dx.doi.org/10.1021/cr60034a002]

[9]   Euler USV. A specific sympathomimetic ergone in adrenergic nerve fibres (sympathin) and its relations to adrenaline and noradrenaline. Acta Physiol Scand 1946; 12: 73-97.
[http://dx.doi.org/10.1111/j.1748-1716.1946.tb00368.x]

[10]   Ahlquist RP. A study of the adrenotropic receptors. Am J Physiol 1948; 153(3): 586-600.
[http://dx.doi.org/10.1152/ajplegacy.1948.153.3.586] [PMID: 18882199]

[11]   Lands AM, Arnold A, McAuliff JP, Luduena FP, Brown TG Jr. Differentiation of receptor systems activated by sympathomimetic amines. Nature 1967; 214(5088): 597-8.
[http://dx.doi.org/10.1038/214597a0] [PMID: 6036174]

[12]   Johnson M. The β-adrenoceptor. Am J Respir Crit Care Med 1998; 158(5 Pt 3): S146-53.
[http://dx.doi.org/10.1164/ajrccm.158.supplement_2.13tac110] [PMID: 9817738]

[13]   Langer SZ. Presynaptic regulation of catecholamine release. Br J Pharmacol 1974; 60: 481-97.
[http://dx.doi.org/10.1111/j.1476-5381.1977.tb07526.x] [PMID: 20190]

[14]   Starke K, Montel H, Gayk W, Merker R. Comparison of the effects of clonidine on pre- and post-synaptic adrenoceptors in the rabbit pulmonary artery. Naunyn Schmiedebergs Arch Pharmacol 1974; 285: 133-50.
[http://dx.doi.org/10.1007/BF00501149] [PMID: 4155791]

[15]   Berthelsen S, Pettinger WA. A functional basis for classification of α-adrenergic receptors. Life Sci 1977; 21(5): 595-606.
[http://dx.doi.org/10.1016/0024-3205(77)90066-2] [PMID: 20542]

[16]   Rau JL. Inhaled adrenergic bronchodilators: historical development and clinical application. Respir Care 2000; 45(7): 854-63.
[PMID: 10926383]

[17]   Stapleton MP. Sir James Black and propranolol. The role of the basic sciences in the history of cardiovascular pharmacology. Tex Heart Inst J 1997; 24(4): 336-42.
[PMID: 9456487]

[18]   Sneader W. Hormone analogues.Drug Discovery: A History. West Sussex, England: John Wiley & Sons Ltd. 2005.
[http://dx.doi.org/10.1002/0470015535]

[19]   Ruffolo RRJr, Hieble JP. The adrenoceptors: historical perspectives, current status and future directions.Adrenoceptors: Structure, Function and Pharmacology. PA, USA: Harwood Academic Publishers 1995.

[20]   Griffith RK. Adrenergic and adrenergic blocking agents.Burger's Medicinal Chemistry and Drug Discovery. 6th ed. Hoboken, NJ: John Wiley & Sons Inc 2003; Vol. 6.
[http://dx.doi.org/10.1002/0471266949.bmc093]

[21]   Weis WI, Kobilka BK. The Molecular Basis of G Protein-Coupled Receptor Activation. Annu Rev Biochem 2018; 87: 897-919.
[http://dx.doi.org/10.1146/annurev-biochem-060614-033910] [PMID: 29925258]

[22]   Li Y-O, Hieble JP, Bergsma DJ, Swift AM, Ganguly S. Ruffolfo RRJr. The β-hydroxyl group of

catecholamines may interact with Ser90 of the second transmembrane helix of the α_{2A}-adrenoceptor.Adrenoceptors: Structure, Function and Pharmacology. PA, USA: Harwood Academic Publishers 1995.

[23]   Brogden RN, Heel RC, Speight TM, Avery GS. α-Methyl-p-tyrosine: a review of its pharmacology and clinical use. Drugs 1981; 21(2): 81-9.
       [http://dx.doi.org/10.2165/00003495-198121020-00001] [PMID: 7009139]

[24]   Facts & Comparisons® eAnswers. http://online.factsandcomparisons.com. February 16, 2018

[25]   Ruffolo RR Jr, Bondinell W, Hieble JP. Ruffolfo RRJr. α- and β-adrenoceptors: from the gene to the clinic. 2. Structure-activity relationships and therapeutic applications. J Med Chem 1995; 38(19): 3681-716.
       [http://dx.doi.org/10.1021/jm00019a001] [PMID: 7562902]

[26]   Tuttle RR, Mills J. Dobutamine: development of a new catecholamine to selectively increase cardiac contractility. Circ Res 1975; 36(1): 185-96.
       [http://dx.doi.org/10.1161/01.RES.36.1.185] [PMID: 234805]

[27]   Bergman J, Persson H, Wetterlin K. 2 new groups of selective stimulants of adrenergic beta-receptors. Experientia 1969; 25(9): 899-901.
       [http://dx.doi.org/10.1007/BF01898049] [PMID: 4391906]

[28]   Johnson M. Salmeterol. Med Res Rev 1995; 15: 225-57.
       [http://dx.doi.org/10.1002/med.2610150303] [PMID: 7658751]

[29]   Green SA, Spasoff AP, Coleman RA, Johnson M, Liggett SB. Sustained activation of a G protein-coupled receptor *via.* "anchored" agonist binding. Molecular localization of the salmeterol exosite within the 2-adrenergic receptor. J Biol Chem 1996; 271(39): 24029-35.
       [http://dx.doi.org/10.1074/jbc.271.39.24029] [PMID: 8798639]

[30]   FDA Drug Safety Communication. Drug labels now contain updated recommendations on the appropriate use of long-acting inhaled asthma medications called Long-Acting Beta-Agonists (LABAs).   http://www.fda.gov/Drugs/DrugSafety/PostmarketDrugSafetyInformationfor PatientsandProviders/ucm213836.htm Accessed February 07, 2018

[31]   Casarosa P, Kollak I, Kiechle T, *et al.* Functional and biochemical rationales for the 24-hour-long duration of action of olodaterol. J Pharmacol Exp Ther 2011; 337(3): 600-9.
       [http://dx.doi.org/10.1124/jpet.111.179259] [PMID: 21357659]

[32]   Bouyssou T, Hoenke C, Rudolf K, *et al.* Discovery of olodaterol, a novel inhaled β2-adrenoceptor agonist with a 24 h bronchodilatory efficacy. Bioorg Med Chem Lett 2010; 20(4): 1410-4.
       [http://dx.doi.org/10.1016/j.bmcl.2009.12.087] [PMID: 20096576]

[33]   van Noord JA, Smeets JJ, Drenth BM, *et al.* 24-hour bronchodilation following a single dose of the novel β(2)-agonist olodaterol in COPD. Pulm Pharmacol Ther 2011; 24(6): 666-72.
       [http://dx.doi.org/10.1016/j.pupt.2011.07.006] [PMID: 21839850]

[34]   Myrbetriq. Northbrook, IL: Astellas Pharma US Inc 2012.

[35]   Acheampong AA, Chien DS, Lam S, *et al.* Characterization of brimonidine metabolism with rat, rabbit, dog, monkey and human liver fractions and rabbit liver aldehyde oxidase. Xenobiotica 1996; 26(10): 1035-55.
       [http://dx.doi.org/10.3109/00498259609167421] [PMID: 8905918]

[36]   Bowen JS, Davis GB, Kearney TE, Bardin J. Diffuse vascular spasm associated with 4-bromo-2-5-dimethoxyamphetamine ingestion. JAMA 1983; 249(11): 1477-9.
       [http://dx.doi.org/10.1001/jama.1983.03330350053028] [PMID: 6827726]

[37]   https://pubchem.ncbi.nlm.nih.gov/compound/Lofexidine#section=Top Accessed August 20, 2018

[38]   Malamed S. What's new in local anaesthesia? SAAD Dig 2009; 25: 4-14.
       [PMID: 19267135]

[39]   Frang H, Cockcroft V, Karskela T, Scheinin M, Marjamäki A. Phenoxybenzamine binding reveals the helical orientation of the third transmembrane domain of adrenergic receptors. J Biol Chem 2001; 276(33): 31279-84.
[http://dx.doi.org/10.1074/jbc.M104167200] [PMID: 11395517]

[40]   Caine M, Perlberg S, Meretyk S. A placebo-controlled double-blind study of the effect of phenoxybenzamine in benign prostatic obstruction. Br J Urol 1978; 50(7): 551-4.
[http://dx.doi.org/10.1111/j.1464-410X.1978.tb06210.x] [PMID: 88984]

[41]   Condon ME, Cimarusti CM, Fox R, *et al.* Nondepressant beta-adrenergic blocking agents. 1. Substituted 3-amino-1-(5,6,7,8-tetrahydro-1-naphthoxy)-2-propanols. J Med Chem 1978; 21(9): 913-22.
[http://dx.doi.org/10.1021/jm00207a014] [PMID: 31485]

[42]   Boriani G, Lubinski A, Capucci A, *et al.* Ventricular Arrhythmias Dofetilide Investigators. A multicentre, double-blind randomized crossover comparative study on the efficacy and safety of dofetilide vs sotalol in patients with inducible sustained ventricular tachycardia and ischaemic heart disease. Eur Heart J 2001; 22(23): 2180-91.
[http://dx.doi.org/10.1053/euhj.2001.2679] [PMID: 11913480]

[43]   Singh BN, Singh SN, Reda DJ, *et al.* Sotalol Amiodarone Atrial Fibrillation Efficacy Trial (SAFE-T) Investigators. Amiodarone versus sotalol for atrial fibrillation. N Engl J Med 2005; 352(18): 1861-72.
[http://dx.doi.org/10.1056/NEJMoa041705] [PMID: 15872201]

[44]   Wasson BK, Gibson WK, Stuart RS, Williams HW, Yates CH. -adrenergic blocking agents. 3-(--Substituted-amino-2-hydroxypropoxy)-4-substituted-1,2,5-thiadiazoles. J Med Chem 1972; 15(6): 651-5.
[http://dx.doi.org/10.1021/jm00276a022] [PMID: 4402289]

[45]   Fahed S, Grum DF, Papadimos TJ. Labetalol infusion for refractory hypertension causing severe hypotension and bradycardia: an issue of patient safety. Patient Saf Surg 2008; 2: 13.
[http://dx.doi.org/10.1186/1754-9493-2-13] [PMID: 18505576]

[46]   Schlanz KD, Thomas RL. Penbutolol: a new beta-adrenergic blocking agent. DICP 1990; 24(4): 403-8.
[http://dx.doi.org/10.1177/106002809002400412] [PMID: 2183495]

[47]   Harting J, Becker KH, Bergmann R, *et al.* Pharmacodynamic profile of the selective beta 1-adrenoceptor antagonist bisoprolol. Arzneimittelforschung 1986; 36(2): 200-8.
[PMID: 2870720]

[48]   Schnabel P, Maack C, Mies F, Tyroller S, Scheer A, Böhm M. Binding properties of beta-blockers at recombinant beta1-, beta2-, and beta3-adrenoceptors. J Cardiovasc Pharmacol 2000; 36(4): 466-71.
[http://dx.doi.org/10.1097/00005344-200010000-00008] [PMID: 11026647]

[49]   Agon P, Goethals P, Van Haver D, Kaufman JM. Permeability of the blood-brain barrier for atenolol studied by positron emission tomography. J Pharm Pharmacol 1991; 43(8): 597-600.
[http://dx.doi.org/10.1111/j.2042-7158.1991.tb03545.x] [PMID: 1681079]

[50]   Deng CY, Lin SG, Zhang WC, *et al.* Esmolol inhibits Na^+ current in rat ventricular myocytes. Methods Find Exp Clin Pharmacol 2006; 28(10): 697-702.
[http://dx.doi.org/10.1358/mf.2006.28.10.1037498] [PMID: 17235414]

[51]   Jaillon P, Drici M. Recent antiarrhythmic drugs. Am J Cardiol 1989; 64(20): 65J-9J.
[http://dx.doi.org/10.1016/0002-9149(89)91203-4] [PMID: 2688391]

[52]   Cuthbert MF, Owusu-Ankomah K. Effect of M & B 17803A, a new -adrenoceptor blocking agent, on the cardiovascular responses to tilting and to isoprenaline in man. Br J Pharmacol 1971; 43(3): 639-48.
[http://dx.doi.org/10.1111/j.1476-5381.1971.tb07193.x] [PMID: 4400530]

[53]   Sneader W. Hormone Analogues. Drug Discovery A History. West Sussex, England: John Wiley & Sons Ltd 2005.

[http://dx.doi.org/10.1002/0470015535]

[54]   Barger G, Dale HH. Chemical structure and sympathomimetic action of amines. J Physiol 1910; 41(1-2): 19-59.
[http://dx.doi.org/10.1113/jphysiol.1910.sp001392] [PMID: 16993040]

[55]   Powell CE, Slater IH. Blocking of inhibitory adrenergic receptors by a dichloro analog of isoproterenol. J Pharmacol Exp Ther 1958; 122(4): 480-8.
[PMID: 13539775]

[56]   Moran NC, Perkins ME. Adrenergic blockade of the mammalian heart by a dichloro analogue of isoproterenol. J Pharmacol Exp Ther 1958; 124(3): 223-37.
[PMID: 13588535]

[57]   Black JW, Stephenson JS. Pharmacology of a new adrenergic beta-receptor antagonist. Lancet 1962; 2: 311-4.
[http://dx.doi.org/10.1016/S0140-6736(62)90103-4] [PMID: 13869657]

CHAPTER 3

Phenothiazines and Related Antipsychotic Drugs

Mamoon Rashid[1], Mehbuba Rahman[1] and M. O. Faruk Khan[2,*]

[1] *Department of Pharmaceutical Sciences, Appalachian College of Pharmacy, VA 24631, USA*

[2] *School of Pharmacy, University of Charleston, Charleston, WV 25304, USA*

Abstract: This chapter is a comprehensive account of the medicinal chemistry of antipsychotic drugs. It provides the mechanism of drug action and detail structure-activity relationships of the first- and second-generation antipsychotic and related drugs to give the knowledge base for pharmacists. Upon completion of this chapter, students will be able to:

• Describe the historical background about the development of antipsychotic therapeutics.

• Apply the principles of fundamental pathophysiology of schizophrenia and other psychotic disorders and receptors associated with it to their pharmacological action.

• Recognize the dopamine and its chemical analogues and identify the essential structural features to become an antipsychotic agent.

• Differentiate between the positive and negative symptoms and extrapyramidal side effects and distinguish between the typical and atypical classes of antipsychotics.

• Apply the principles of structure-activity relationships to the antipsychotic drugs.

• Delineate the clinical significance of all classes of antipsychotic drugs and their therapeutic indications.

• Identify the therapeutic use, side effects and metabolic pathways of selected first- and second-generation antipsychotic agents.

Keywords: Antipsychotic Drugs, Antianxiety Drugs, Drug-Receptor Interaction, Dopamine, First-Generation Antipsychotics, Structure-Activity Relationship, Second-Generation Antipsychotics, Typical And Atypical Antipsychotic Agents.

* **Corresponding author M. O. Faruk Khan:** School of Pharmacy, University of Charleston. Charleston, WV 25304, USA; Tel: 304-357-4860; E-mail: mdomarkhan@ucwv.edu

HISTORICAL BACKGROUNDS

The first antipsychotic drug chlorpromazine was introduced to the medical world in 1952 [1] and was considered highly significant to open a new era of treating mental illness. In 1891, German Bacteriologist Paul Erlich noted the therapeutic potency of methylene blue, a phenothiazine derivative, against malarial symptoms [2]. The chains of the central nitrogen atom were substituted to synthesize different derivatives of phenothiazine, which lost the antimalarial property but appeared to gain a potent antihistaminic effect [3, 4]. The search for better antihistaminic agents by Rhone-Poulenc lab led to the discovery of promethazine [5], an aminoalkyl phenothiazine, bearing pronounced sedative property. A French navy surgeon Henri Laborit (1949) observed this sedative property while researching various synthetic antihistamines as a means of potentiating surgical anesthetics [6]. He also noted that the application of promethazine resulted in abated anxiety in the patient. Using this as an anxiolytic lead, scientists of Rhone-Poulenc continued the research to develop derivatives of superior anxiolytic properties that led to the synthesis of chlorpromazine [6], a drug that (a) prolongs barbiturate-induced sedation, (b) prevents apomorphine-induced emesis, and (c) inhibits conditioned avoidance-escape response. Moreover, the drug was found to keep the patients relaxed and anxiety-free when applied as a part of surgery. Based on this observation, the drug was applied to a small group of psychotic patients in a military hospital with a successful outcome. Psychiatrists Jean Delay and Pierre Denikar documented this and were the first to present the antipsychotic effect of chlorpromazine to the scientific world in 1952 [7]. The drug was approved in the USA by the FDA in 1954. However, the search for safer anxiolytics continued due to their serious side effects, especially the Parkinson's-like involuntary muscle movement referred to as Extrapyramidal Side Effect (EPS) [3, 4].

Many other derivatives that were structurally different from phenothiazine were synthesized as effective antipsychotic agents (*e.g.*, haloperidol, thiothixene), but were not free of EPS demanding the need to develop atypical antipsychotics with no or minimal EPS [8]. Clozapine, a dibenzodiazepine, is credited as the progenitor (1959) of atypical antipsychotic drug [9] which was first marketed in 1972 but was quickly withdrawn after three years due to reports of serious side effects of agranulocytosis [10]. It was, however, re-introduced to the market in 1975 and ultimately to the US market in 1990, with mandatory monitoring of leukocyte count [10]. Over time, many other atypical antipsychotics including risperidone, olanzapine, sertindole, quetiapine, and ziprasidone have been introduced that steadily replaced the market of conventional antipsychotics [11]. Currently, a more precise receptor targeting strategy is used to develop new antipsychotic drugs although the newer drugs are not as efficacious as the "gold standard" drug clozapine [12]. Instead of developing pure dopamine receptor antagonists, researchers are now also targeting serotonin, glutamate (including NMDA), cholinergic, or even neuropeptide receptors in developing highly effective antischizophrenic drugs free from side effects including EPS [4]. Today, both phenothiazine derivatives and atypical, or second-generation antipsychotic agents are frequently appearing in the top 200 drug list (Fig. **1**) [13].

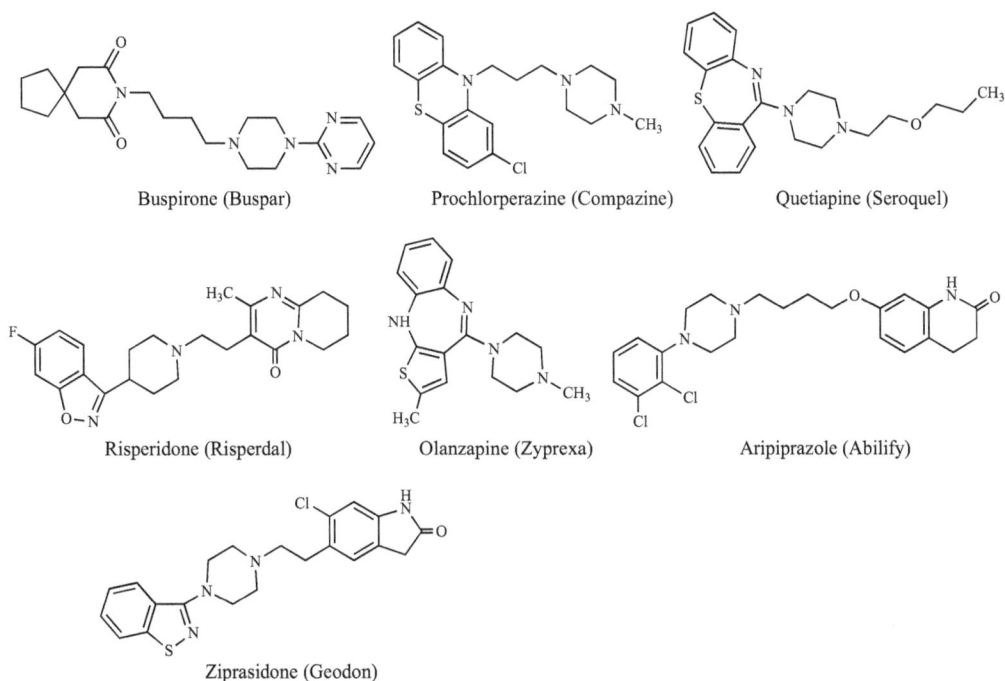

Buspirone (Buspar)　　　Prochlorperazine (Compazine)　　　Quetiapine (Seroquel)

Risperidone (Risperdal)　　　Olanzapine (Zyprexa)　　　Aripiprazole (Abilify)

Ziprasidone (Geodon)

Fig. (1). Antipsychotics frequently occurring in the top 200 drug list.

INTRODUCTORY CONCEPTS

Psychotic Disorders and Relevant Terminologies

The word psychosis is made up of two parts: Greek 'psyche' meaning mind or soul and '-osis', a suffix used to represent any abnormal pathophysiological condition. Though etymologically psychosis should be used to define an abnormal condition of a person's mind [14], it includes conditions where a person communicates imaginary objects and loses contact with the surrounding reality. In fact, the broader definition of psychosis embraces mental disorders from relatively normal aberrant experience to severe symptoms of schizophrenia and bipolar disorder [15, 16]. Mental disorders are usually more complicated to diagnose and conditions like hallucinations, delusions, occasional violence and disturbed cognitive behavior are sometimes described by the broad generic term *psychosis*

[17, 18]. These abnormalities sometimes stem from altered expression or metabolism of neurotransmitters or biochemical components of the brain and nervous system. However, in many cases, the etiology remains elusive [19].

The terms positive and negative symptoms are frequently used to describe the nature of psychosis [18]. *Positive symptoms* are additive to a normal healthy person's mental condition. This means these are symptoms that a non-psychotic person does not experience but have been added to a mentally ill person's way of functioning. Hallucinations, delusions, bizarre behavior are common positive symptoms. *Negative symptoms* are those that a healthy non-psychotic person usually exhibits but absent in a psychotic person's normal nature of behavior. Some examples are social withdrawal, apathy, and inability to experience pleasure [20].

Delusion is a type of strong belief in things that are either impossible or based on incomplete information [21]. An unshakable firm belief that FBI personnel is hiding in the attic to spy on the reporting person is a classic example of delusion. *Hallucination* is a false perception of objects or events [22]. The reporting person experiences the presence of objects or events through visual, auditory, gustatory, tactile, or other senses despite the objects or events that do not exist.

Schizophrenia is a mental abnormality manifested by unusual social behavior and inability to realize and respond to the real world [23]. The Greek root *skhizein* (to split) and *phren* (mind) give schizophrenia a literal meaning of a pathological condition where the patient shows abnormal or contrasting mental condition. The common symptoms of schizophrenia include delusion, auditory hallucination, impaired cognition, social isolation, inactivation, and unusual emotional expression [17].

Psychoactive medication refers to psychoactive substances prescribed and administered to create an effect on the biochemical environment of the cells of the brain and the nervous system as a whole [24]. Their general purpose is to treat the mental illness of various kinds. Antipsychotics, antidepressants, mood stabilizers, anxiolytic-hypnotics, and stimulants are common members of psychoactive medication family [25].

Dopamine Hypothesis of Psychosis and Site of Action of Antipsychotics

The unique brain regions are believed to be contributing to various symptom domains of schizophrenia [26]. The brain is extremely complex in its anatomy and function, and the same emotional response may be originated from more than one region of the brain. According to the current hypothesis, the malfunctioning mesolimbic circuits are responsible for positive symptoms of schizophrenia, while the negative symptoms of schizophrenia are related to mesocortical circuits as well as some mesolimbic areas such as the nucleus accumbens [27]. Nucleus accumbens is a part of the reward pathway of the brain and therefore plays a direct role in the motivational response of the individual [28]. Various schizophrenia-related symptoms and their associated regions in the brain are summarized in Table **1**.

Table 1. Localization of the schizophrenia symptom domains.

Positive symptoms	Mesolimbic
Affective symptoms	Ventromedial prefrontal cortex
Aggressive symptoms	Orbitofrontal cortex
	Amygdala
Cognitive symptoms	Dorsolateral prefrontal cortex
Negative symptoms	Mesocortical/prefrontal cortex
	Nucleus accumbens reward circuits

Different regions of the brain crosstalk and produce complex cognitive and emotional perception, indicating an overlap in their function [26]. A thorough understanding of which region of the brain is principally involved in a precise symptom is pivotal to develop drugs associated with the symptom. The major dopamine pathways in the brain are shown in Fig. (**2**).

Schizophrenia-associated Neurotransmitters and Circuitry in the Brain

The dopamine hypothesis stemmed from the observation that a large number of antipsychotic drugs function as dopamine receptor antagonists [29]. Also, symptoms of psychoses including schizophrenia may be attributed to hyperactivation of dopamine receptors in the brain. However, neither the hyperactivation of the receptor nor the excessive expression of dopamine ligand exclusively appears as the etiology of schizophrenia [30]. There are four main dopaminergic pathways in the brain which transmit neurotransmitter dopamine from one region of the brain to another [31, 32]. The mesolimbic dopaminergic pathway originates from the ventral tegmental area (sitting in the midbrain) and reaches the limbic system *via* nucleus accumbens. The mesocortical pathway begins from the ventral tegmental area and transmits towards the frontal cortex. Dopamine is transmitted from the area of substantia nigra to the striatum through the nigrostriatal pathway, which is related to locomotion and motor control. The tuberoinfundibular pathway is the fourth pathway and transmits dopamine from the hypothalamus to the pituitary gland region. The secretion of prolactin and other hormones may be induced by this pathway (Fig. **2**) [27].

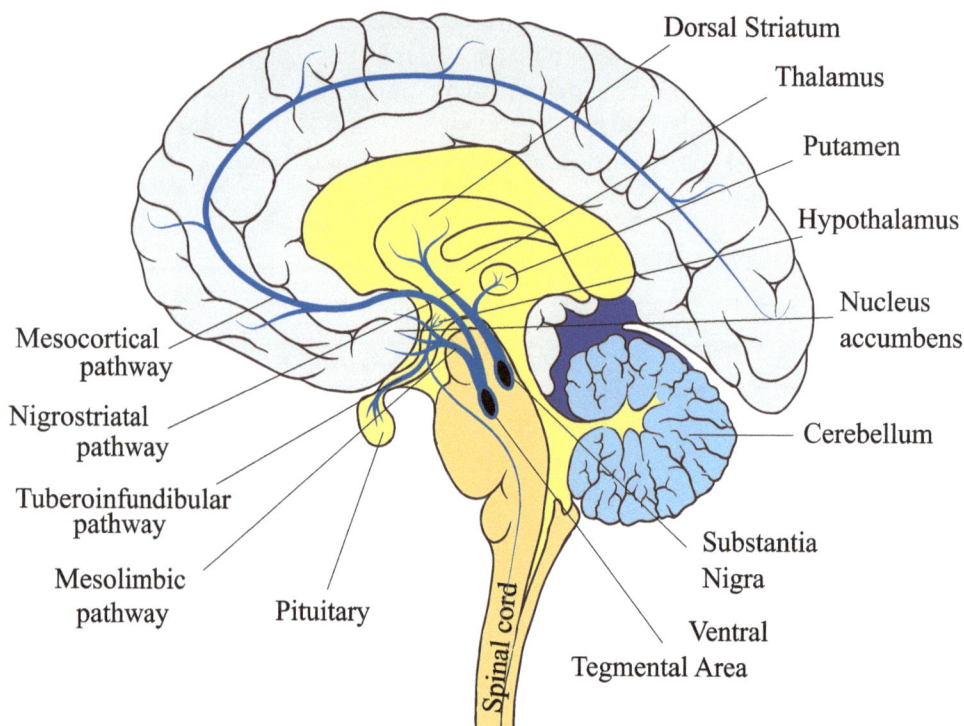

Fig. (2). Some dopamine pathways in the mammalian brain: 1. Nigro-striatal pathway – between substantial nigra and basal ganglia involved in movement causing EPS; 2. Meso-limbic pathway ("reward" pathway) – between VTA and nucleus accumbens involved in positive symptoms of schizophrenia; 3. Meso-cortical pathway – between VTA and cortex involved in motivation and emotional response causing the negative symptoms of schizophrenia; 4. Tuberoinfundibular pathway – between the hypothalamus and posterior pituitary. By Slashme, Patrick J. Lynch, and Fvasconcellos. The permission to reproduce is obtained under the creative commons.

Antipsychotics such as the phenothiazines and butyrophenones function as dopamine receptor (particularly D_2) antagonists with a therapeutic dose that is inversely proportional to the binding affinity to the D_2 receptor [33, 34].

Prolonged exposure to amphetamine and cocaine elevate dopamine level in the brain and induces psychosis-like symptoms, a phenomenon commonly known as 'amphetamine/cocaine psychosis'. Likewise, when Parkinson's patients are treated with levodopa to increase the dopamine level, they show symptoms similar to the patients with schizophrenia. The level of dopamine is found to be higher in schizophrenic patients than non-schizophrenic group upon administering amphetamine [35]. Dopamine-like compounds such as methylphenidate and amphetamine exacerbate psychotic symptoms up to 75% of schizophrenic patients at a dose that does not create any effect in healthy non-psychotic humans [25, 36].

Evidence Against the Hypothesis

Newer technologies such as positron emission tomography (PET) on living patients revealed that even after 90% blockade of D_2 receptor with antipsychotic drugs, some patients showed little improvement of psychoses. This occurs mainly in patients with a psychotic history of 10-30 years. A psychotic patient usually takes several days to show improved symptoms after the onset of the treatment whereas dopamine-inhibiting drugs lower the level of dopamine within minutes. This observation concludes that dopamine may be connected to psychosis only passively [37]. The new generation of antipsychotics (atypical antipsychotics) have similar efficacy to control psychosis but higher effectiveness to control negative symptoms. These atypical antipsychotics have a lower affinity for dopamine receptors [38].

The Dopaminergic Neurons, Synthesis, and Degradation of Dopamine

The most established hypothesis for schizophrenia is founded on the anomaly of biochemical pathways involving dopamine (DA) neurotransmitter (Figs. **3a** & **3b**) [39]. How dopamine plays a role in schizophrenia pathology and how various antipsychotic drugs serve to abate them requires a clear understanding of the synthesis, receptor-interaction, metabolism, and regulation of dopamine neurotransmitters.

Amino acid tyrosine is pumped in *via* the tyrosine transporter and served as the precursor at the dopaminergic nerve terminals for the dopamine biosynthesis (Fig. **3a**). Synthesized dopamine molecules are stored in the synaptic vesicles and released during the process of neurotransmission. The synaptic action of dopamine may be paddled back by the action of a presynaptic transporter (DAT). DAT is specific for dopamine and terminates the action of dopamine in the synapse by pulling it back to the vesicles. Different neurons have a varying density of DAT on their membranes, resulting in the diverse extent of vesicular uptake. Monoamine oxidase (MAO) A or B degrade dopamine within the cells, and catechol-O-methyl-transferase (COMT), as well as aldehyde dehydrogenase (AD), destroy it when in the synaptic cleft. Also, norepinephrine transferases (NETs) contribute to diminishing the dopamine action by binding them as a secondary substrate [40].

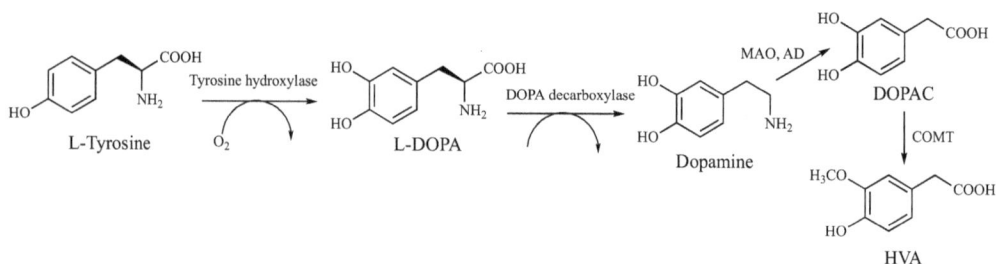

Fig. (3A). Biosynthesis and degradation of dopamine. L-DOPA, L-dihydroxy methyl alanine; DOPAC, dihydroxy phenyl acetic acid; HVA, homovanillic acid.

Receptors of Dopamine

Dopaminergic neurotransmission is critically regulated by dopamine receptors. A wide variety of transports (DAT and VMAT2) and receptors are there to transport or bind dopamine. There are at least five pharmacological subtypes as well as isoform variations of dopamine receptors exist [41]. Dopamine receptor 2 (D_2) has been the most expansively probed member of this family, mainly because of its stimulation by dopamine agonists (as in the case of Parkinson's disease) and blockade by antagonists (as in the case of psychotic disorders) [42]. D_1, D_2, D_3, and D_4 receptors are all blocked by some atypical antipsychotics. However, to what extent the D_1, D_3, and D_4 receptors contribute to the clinical properties of the antipsychotic drugs is not fully elucidated [41].

The D_2 receptor may function as an autoreceptor in the presynaptic membrane and thus plays the role of "gatekeeper" by two fashions — enabling vesicular DA to be released when they are not bound to DA, and preventing vesicular DA to be released when they are prevalent in the synapse (which results in their own binding) [43]. The occupancy of the D_2 receptor, therefore, sends negative feedback to the presynaptic dopaminergic neurons (Fig. **3b**).

The Interaction of Dopamine Receptor and Antipsychotic Agents

The dopamine D_2 receptor (D2R) has only one site favorable for binding with the dopamine and related antipsychotic agents [30]. D2R is a G-Protein Coupled Receptor (GPCR), and the ligands bind at the top third part of the domains 3, 4, 5, and 6 of the heptahelical transmembrane barrels (Fig. **4**). It is the primary target for antipsychotic drugs. Recently the structure of dopamine receptor bound to risperidone (an atypical antipsychotic agent) has been established, which provides a template for the development of safer and more effective medications [44].

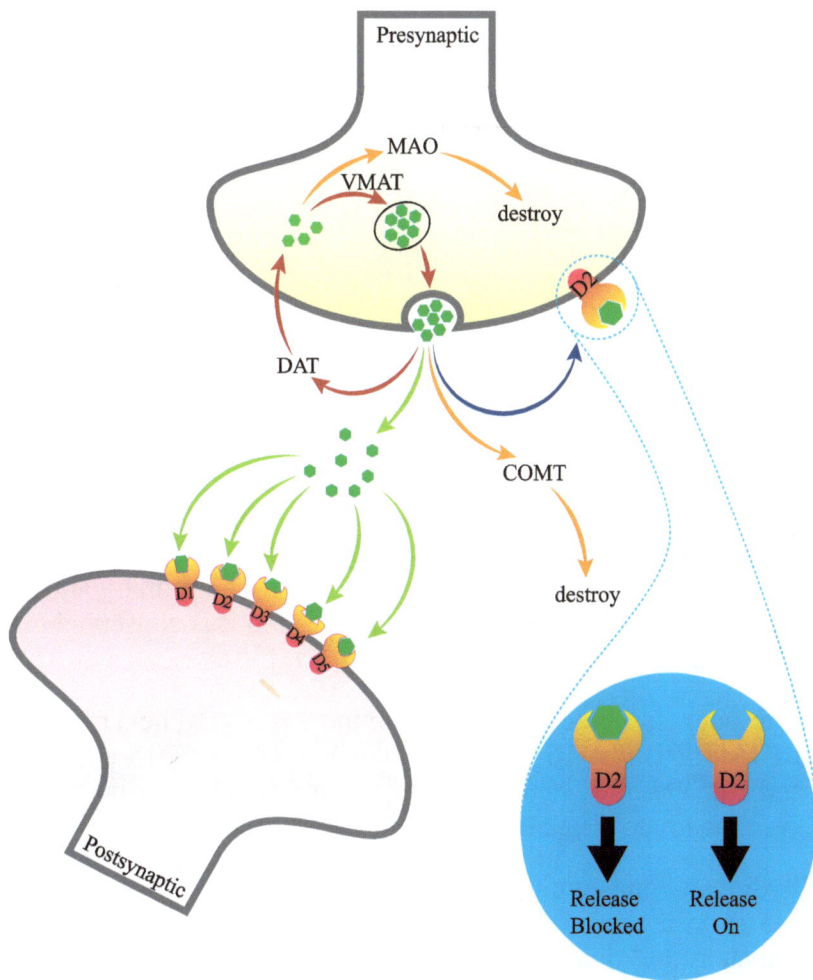

Fig. (3B). Production, release, binding and destruction of dopamine in synaptic membranes. Vesicle-contained dopamine is released to the synaptic cleft, which may bind various DA receptors (D_1, D_2, D_3, D_4, and D_5 receptors) and exert subsequent signal transduction. Catechol-O-Methyl-Transferase (COMT) metabolizes and inactivates free dopamine at this site. Also, dopamine transferase (DAT) capture these free neurotransmitter and pump back to the presynaptic cytosol where the mitochondria-provided enzymes monoamine oxidases A and B (MAO-A and MAO-B) process dopamine into an inactive metabolite. Cytosolic dopamine molecules are again packed into vesicles with the help of vesicular monoamine transporter (VMAT) until they are released. The presynaptic membrane also contains the D_2 receptor, which, upon binding with dopamine prevents the release of more dopamine into the synapse. Thereby it serves as the "gatekeeper" of dopamine from the presynaptic vesicles.

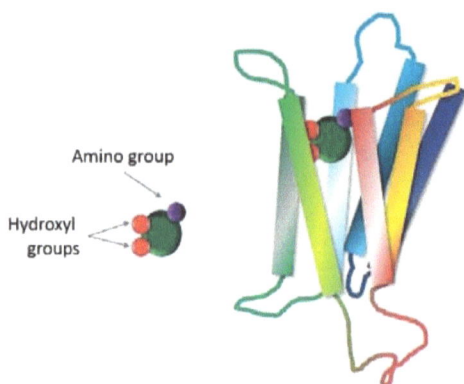

Fig. (4). The dopamine molecule and its bound state inside the heptahelical D_2 receptor.

The amino acids essential for proper binding of the ligands to the D2R are broadly classified into three groups. Conserved ASP-114 in TM3: Dopamine and antipsychotic analogues directly interact with the carboxylic group of this aspartate moiety through a tight salt bridge (2.6 Å). The primary amino group of dopamine interacts with the acid tail of aspartate, and it is conserved over all five subtypes of the human dopamine receptor (Fig. **5a**) [30].

Hydrophobic pocket: Three clusters of amino acids (i) Phe-110, Met-117 and Cys-118 of TM3; (ii) Phe-164, Phe-189 and Val-190 of TM5 and (iii) Trp-386, Phe-390 and His-394 of TM6 shape a hydrophobic pocket for housing dopamine and antipsychotic drugs (Fig. **5a**) [30].

Multiple hydrogen bonds with p- and m- hydroxyl groups: The Ser-193 and Ser-197 of TM5 form hydrogen bonds with meta and para hydroxyl groups of the dopamine nucleus and therefore play a crucial role in ligand recognition. These two residues along with the adjacent Ser-194 are conserved in all five types of dopamine receptors in humans. The Ser-194 also forms a hydrogen bond with the ligand, although the nitrogen residue of moiety 192 has been found to be linked to the Ser-194 through hydrogen bonding (Fig. **5a**) [30].

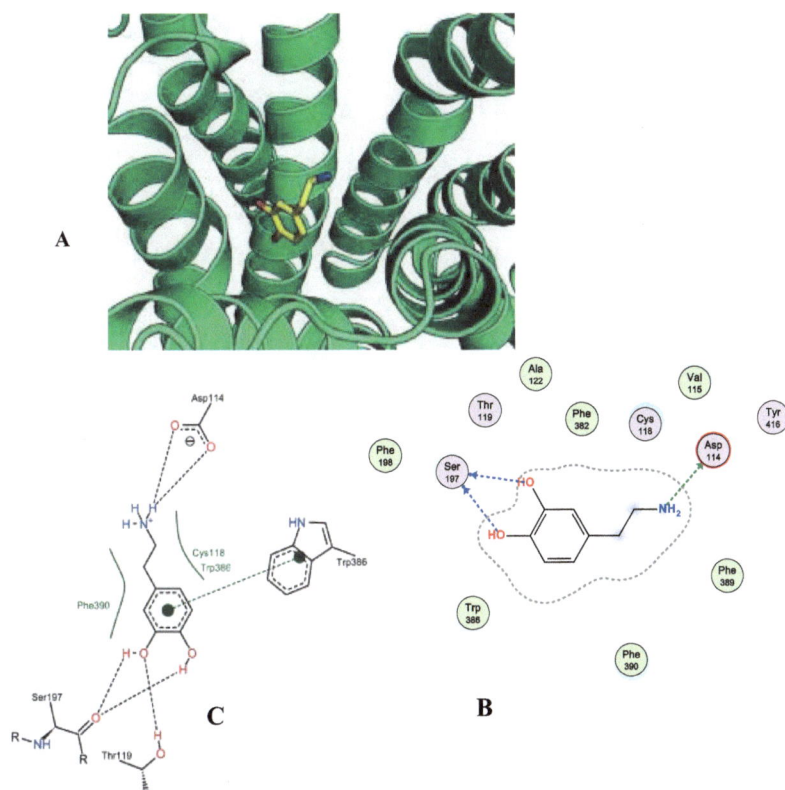

Fig. (5A). Predicted binding mode of dopamine at the human D$_2$ receptor (hD2R). A) Cartoon representation of haloperidol docked to the hD2R at its orthosteric ligand-binding cavity. Docking was performed using GOLD5.3 (CCDC, Cambridge, UK) in its default mode and PyMOL (www.pymol.org) was used to generate the Fig. B & C) 2D ligand-interaction diagrams for the dopamine-hD2R complex shown above. The diagrams were generated using POSEVIEW (C) (https://proteins.plus/) and MOE 2015 (B) (https://www.chemcomp.com/). Courtesy of Dr. Taufiq Rahman, University of Cambridge, UK.

Class-I antagonists of D2R (clozapine is a representative example; Fig. **5B**) occupy the region enclosed by transmembrane helices 3, 4, 5, and 6 — the location where the agonist binds. Therefore, clozapine will perform the following set of interactions:

a. Helix 3: a 2.8 Å salt bridge with Asp-114
b. Helix 5: a 3.2 Å hydrogen bond to Ser-193; no hydrogen bond with Ser-194 or Ser-197
c. Helix 6: 3.1 Å spaced heteroatomic interactions with Trp-386
d. Multiple helices: enclosure of the multi-barrel hydrophobic pocket formed by specific amino acid residues from helices 2, 3, 4, 5, 6 and 7.

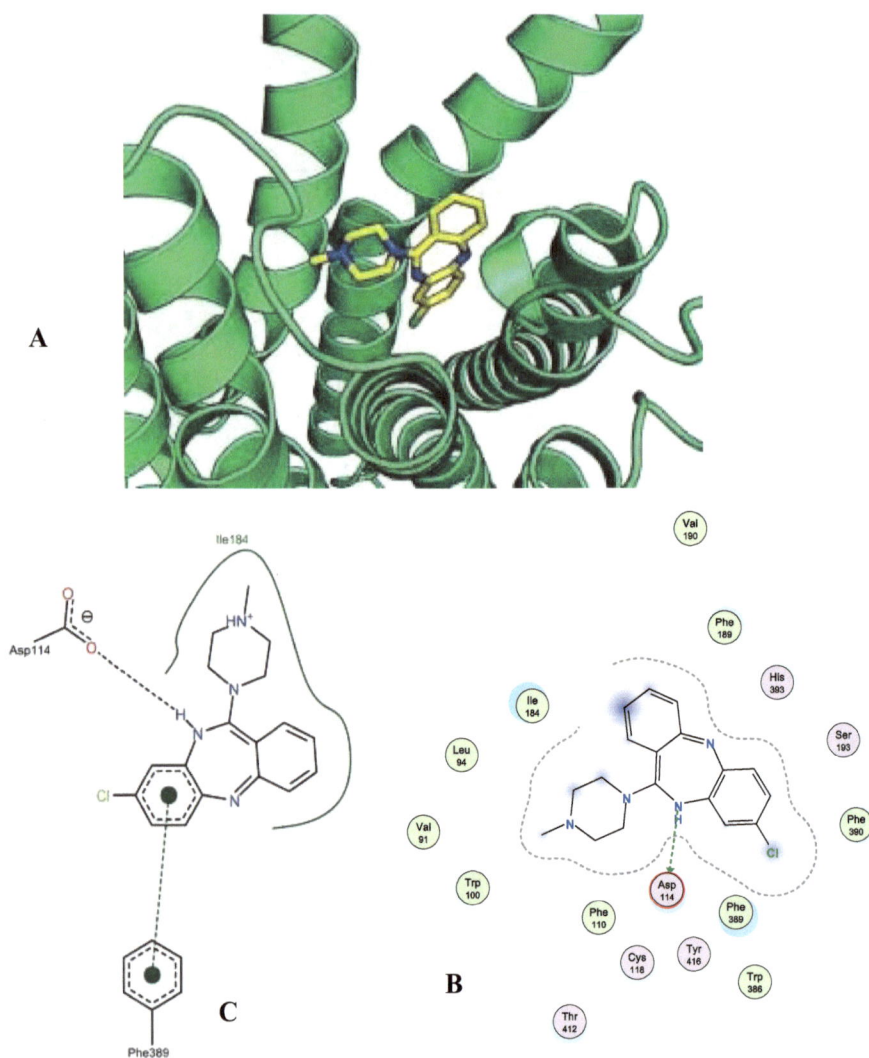

Fig. (5B). Predicted binding mode of haloperidol at human D_2 receptor (hD2R). A) Cartoon representation of clozapine docked to the hD2R at its orthosteric ligand-binding cavity. Docking was performed using GOLD5.3 (CCDC, Cambridge, UK) in its default mode and PyMOL (www.pymol.org) was used to generate the Fig. B & C) 2D ligand-interaction diagrams for the clozapine-hD2R complex shown above. The diagrams were generated using POSEVIEW (C) (https://proteins.plus/) and MOE 2015 (B) (https://www.chemcomp.com/). Courtesy of Dr. Taufiq Rahman, University of Cambridge, UK.

Class-II antagonists of D2R (haloperidol is a representative example; Fig. **5C**) contact the helices 4 and 5 only minimally and occupy the region surrounded by helices 2, 3, 6, and 7 [30]. Therefore, haloperidol molecule demonstrates the following interactions:

a. Helix 3: a 2.8 Å salt bridge with Asp-114
b. Helix 5: a 3.2 Å hydrogen bond to Ser-193, however, there is no hydrogen bond with Ser-194 or Ser-197
c. Heteroatomic interaction with Trp-386 at helix 6 (3.8 Å) and Trp-90 at helix 2 at 3.0 Å.
d. The hydrophobic pocket formed by various residue groups at the helices 2, 3, 4, 5, 6, and 7.

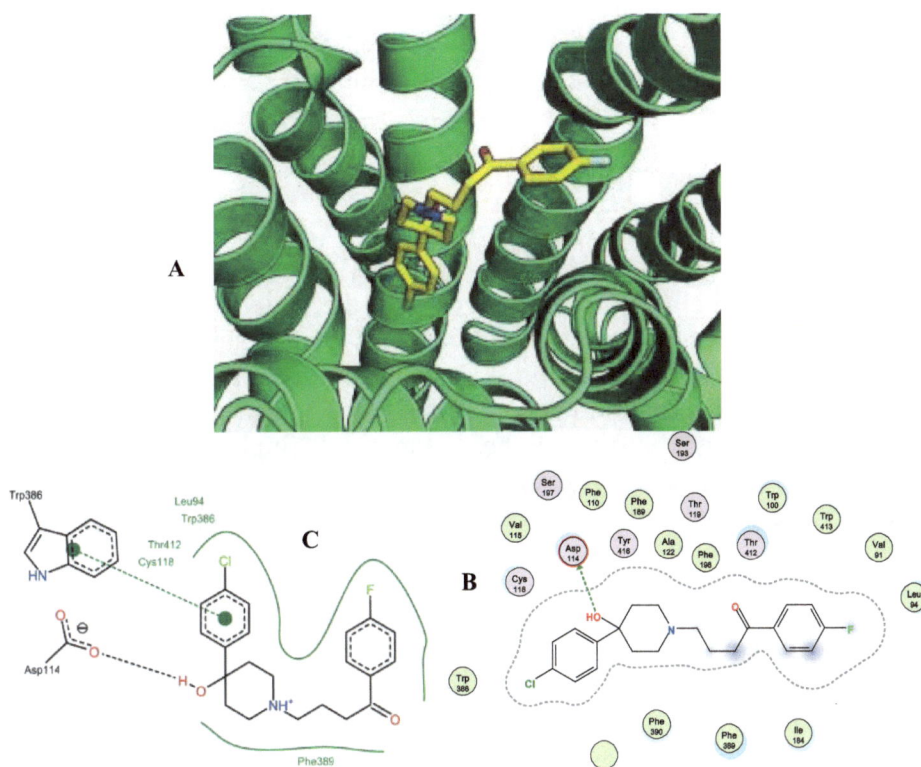

Fig. (5C). Predicted binding mode of haloperidol at human D$_2$ receptor (hD2R). A) Cartoon representation of haloperidol docked to the hD2R at its orthosteric ligand-binding cavity. Docking was performed using GOLD5.3 (CCDC, Cambridge, UK) in its default mode and PyMOL (www.pymol.org) was used to generate the Fig. B & C) 2D ligand-interaction diagrams for the haloperidol-hD2R complex shown above. The diagrams were generated using POSEVIEW (C) (https://proteins.plus/) and MOE 2015 (B) (https://www.chemcomp.com/). Courtesy of Dr. Taufiq Rahman, University of Cambridge, UK.

Other Receptors Involved in Antipsychotic Drug Action

Receptors other than classical dopamine types have also been identified as the contributor in psychotic pathogenesis and the design of associated therapeutics. The positive and negative psychotic symptoms have associations with the activation of α_1 and α_2 adrenergic receptors [45]. Histamine H_1 Receptor is also an off-target of the antipsychotics, binding of which results in sedation and subsequent alleviation of the psychotic symptoms [46]. The regulation of synaptic plasticity of the prefrontal cortex is contributed by muscarinic receptors [47]. The disturbance of cholinergic neurotransmission has an association with schizophrenia [48]. The NMDA receptor functioning, cortical microcircuitry and synaptic plasticity may be affected by aberrant glutamatergic neurotransmission [49]. NMDA receptor antagonists such as phencyclidine and ketamine cause psychosis in experimental animals and healthy subjects [50, 51], which serves as evidence that these receptors are also important in psychotic pathogenesis.

THE ANTIPSYCHOTIC DRUGS

Classes of Antipsychotic Drugs

Depending on the type of receptor antagonized, the incidence of extrapyramidal side effects (EPS), efficacy on the treatment-resistant groups and freedom from untoward side effects, antipsychotic drugs are broadly divided into two classes [52]: (a) the first-generation antipsychotic drugs also called the 'typical' antipsychotics such as chlorpromazine, haloperidol, fluphenazine, flupenthixol, clopenthixol; and (b) second-generation or 'atypical' antipsychotics, such as clozapine, risperidone, sertindole, quetiapine, amisulpride, aripiprazole, and zotepine.

Based on the mechanism of action, antipsychotics are grouped into three different categories: (a) typical antipsychotics causing high D_2 antagonism and low serotonin-2 receptor [5-HT$_{2A}$] antagonism; (b) atypical antipsychotics causing moderate to high D_2 antagonism and high 5-HT$_{2A}$ antagonism; and (c) atypical clozapine-like antipsychotics causing low D_2 antagonism and high 5-HT$_{2A}$ antagonism [53].

First Generation (Typical) Antipsychotic Drugs

SAR of the Phenothiazine Ring

The SAR of phenothiazine antipsychotics depends on four aspects as shown in the color-mapped pharmacophoric illustration (Fig. **6**) and discussed in this section [54 - 56].

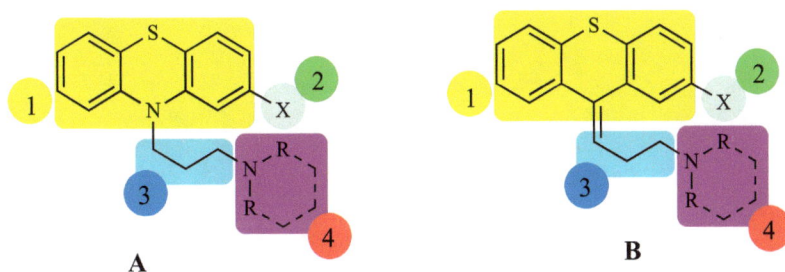

Fig. (6). Structures of phenothiazine (A) and related thioxanthene (B) antipsychotics pharmacophores 1) Phenothiazene/thioxanthene nucleus, 2) ring substituent, 3) 3-carbon side chain, 4) side chain N-substituents.

Key features of the SAR are as follows:

1. The phenothiazine or isosteric thioxanthene ring system (the Ring binding site).
2. Substitution at position no. 2 with the desired electronic effect.
3. Presence of a spacer group between the phenothiazine and amine group with the optimum length of three carbons.
4. Presence of a protonated amine moiety to interact with the electron-rich groove of the receptor.

   SAR 1: The phenothiazine nucleus with N at 10 or isosteric thioxanthene with a double bond at C-10 possesses the optimal structural conformation to bind the dopamine receptors. For the case of thioxanthene, it is an unsymmetrical alkene, which requires a Z -(cis) conformation for optimal receptor-ligand interaction.

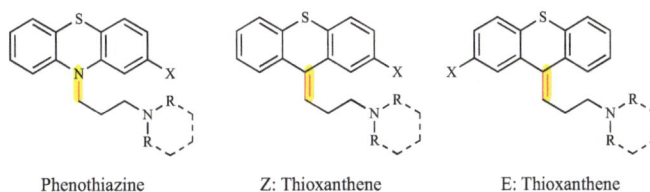

Phenothiazine   Z: Thioxanthene   E: Thioxanthene

   SAR 2: The substituent at position 2 should be an electron-withdrawing moiety to exert optimum receptor-ligand affinity.

Electron withdrawing groups (X) enhance activity through two effects:

1. Pulls the electrons away from ring "A" resulting in a $\delta+$ charge on the ring increasing binding of the ring to an electron-rich area on the receptor which is another aromatic ring (induced dipole-induced dipole interaction)
2. Pulls the protonated nitrogen toward the phenyl ring providing the proper spacing between the nitrogen and the ring (two-carbon distance)

   SAR 2.1: Substitution at positions 1, 3, and 4 diminishes or decreases the activity.

SAR 2.2: Commonly occurring various groups at position 2 are as follows.

$$
\begin{array}{cccccccccccc}
& CH_3 & & & & & & & & H_3C\diagdown{}_N\diagup CH_3 & & \\
& | & & & & & & & & | & & \\
& CH_2 & CH_3 & & & & & & & & CF_3 & \\
& | & | & & & & & & & & | & \\
& CH_2 & CH_2 & CH_3 & CH_3 & CH_3 & CH_3 & CF_3 & & & CF_3 & \\
& | & | & | & | & | & | & | & & | & | & \\
OH\ \ H\ \ CH_3 & O=C & O=C & O=C & O=S=O & Cl\ \ S & O=S & S & & O=S=O & O=S=O & CF_3 \\
|\ \ \ \ |\ \ \ \ | & & & & & & & & & | & | & | \\
\end{array}
$$

Least Potent   Most Potent

•

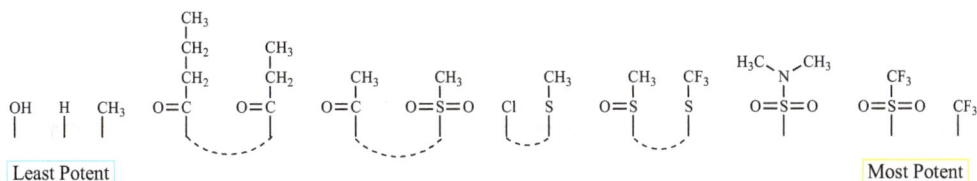

The Chlorpromazine Index (CI) may be compared (Table **2**) to evaluate the best-fitting position of X on the phenyl ring. The CI is the ratio of the potency of the compound to that of chlorpromazine. Hence, CI values higher than 1 indicates a compound more potent than chlorpromazine [57].

Table 2. The Chlorpromazine Index (CI) of various chemical groups as substituents at various positions in ring A [57].

Substituent	Ring A Position	CI
–H	2	0.4
–Cl	2	1.0
	3	0.18
	4	<0.08
–CF_3	2	2.4
	3	0.43
	4	<0.06
–S–CF_3	2	1.0
–OH	1	0.02
	2	0.025
	3	0.13
	4	~0.4
–CH_3	2	0.28
–$(CH_2)_2CH_3$	2	0.18
–CHO	2	0.5
–$COCH_3$	2	0.6
– $COCH_2CH_3$	2	2.0
– $CO(CH2)_2CH_3$	2	2.0
–SO_2CH_3	2	0.6

Few points are clearly evident from Table **2**:

SAR 2.2.1: The dopamine-shaped conformation of the ligand is achieved when the side chain is bent due to the affinity between the 2-substituent and nitrogen moiety. Therefore, the presence of an electron-withdrawing group at C2 facilitates the antipsychotic effect.

SAR 2.2.2: The rank order of potency is position 2>3>4>1

SAR 2.2.3: The bending of the nitrogen-bearing arm is blocked if C1 has a substitution. Therefore, substitution at this point may result in the depletion of drug action. Likewise, the substitution at C4 may interfere with substrate binding to the receptor as the p-OH of the dopamine molecule does.

SAR 2.2.4: With exceptions, stronger electron withdrawers are usually more potent.

SAR 2.2.5: More than one substitution on the ring system decreases the potency

SAR 2.2.6: Oxidizing the ring-sulfur to sulfoxide or sulfone reduces the potency

SAR 3: Increasing or decreasing the length from 3 carbons decreases the potency. The further from 3 the less potent. Two carbon side chains increase H_1 antagonism (Fenethazine)

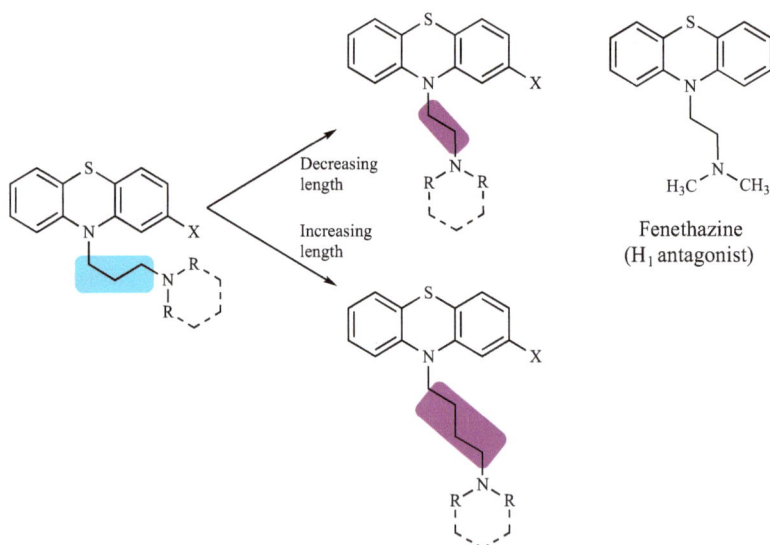

SAR 3.2: Substitution on the α, β- or γ-carbon alters the potency and induces side effects.

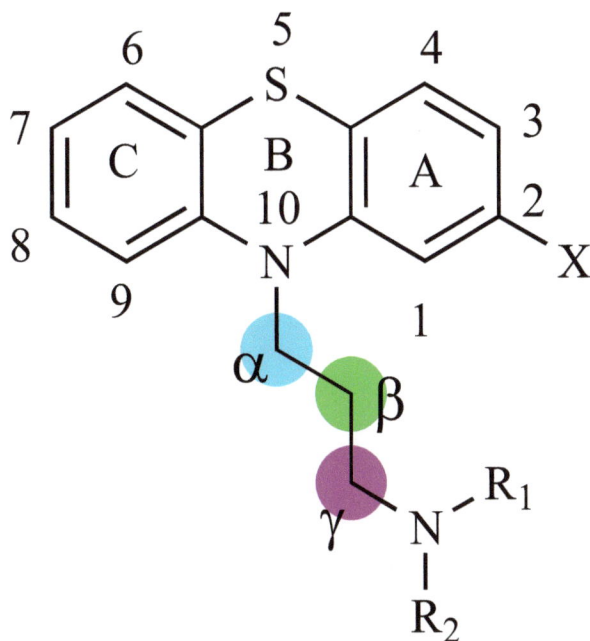

SAR 3.2.1: The dopamine antagonism effect of the ligand may increase or decrease if a methyl group is substituted on the β- carbon.

SAR 3.2.2: A methyl substituent on the β- carbon increases H1 antagonism. However, substituents that are larger than the methyl group decrease antihistaminic activity unless they are part of a heterocycle (Methdilazine).

SAR 3.2.3: The dopamine antagonism effect is reduced but simultaneously the anticholinergic effect is increased if a substitution is made on the γ- carbon. All the piperidines fit this category.

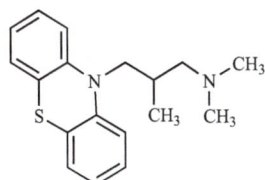

Trimeprazine   Thioridazine   Methdilazine

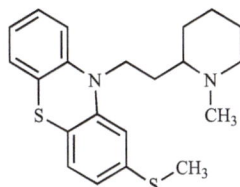

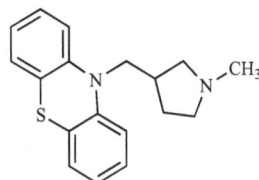

SAR 4: The optimal affinity for the dopamine receptors relies on the terminal amine moiety. The substitution on γ-nitrogen may lead to three classes of phenothiazines:

1. N,N-Dimethyl (aliphatic);
2. Piperazine;
3. Piperidine   derivatives.

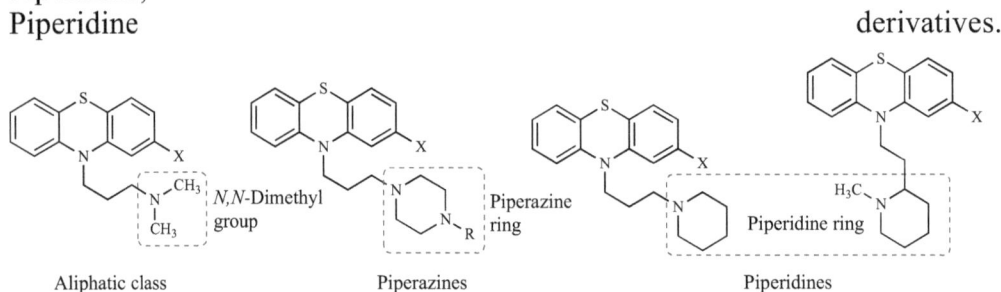

Aliphatic class   Piperazines   Piperidines

SAR 4.1: Two methyl groups may substitute the hydrogens at the γ-nitrogen to produce an *N,N*-dimethyl derivative. The compounds usually have *-promazine* at the suffix, and the C-2 substitution determines the prefix.

SAR 4.1.1: No substitution (*i.e.*, primary amines) exerts low potency.

SAR 4.1.2: Monomethyl compounds are better but still very weak.

SAR 4.1.3: Highest potency is exerted by dimethyl substitution.

SAR 4.1.4: Potency is decreased if the carbon length of the substituted group is increased. However, if the increased carbon-length forms a heterocyclic shape, then the potency is increased (as observed in the cases of piperazines and piperidines).

SAR 4.1.5: The γ- N substitution renders potency based on the following order: piperazine > aliphatic > piperidine.

SAR 4.2: In the piperazines class of antipsychotics, the γ- nitrogen becomes a part of the piperazine ring. In general, if the para nitrogen has a methyl attached, the suffix becomes '-perazine'; and if the para nitrogen has a hydroxyethyl group attached the suffix becomes '-phenazine'. The prefix of the name depends on the C2 substituent. For example, Fluphenazine has a trifluoromethyl substituent at the C2 position of the phenothiazine ring.

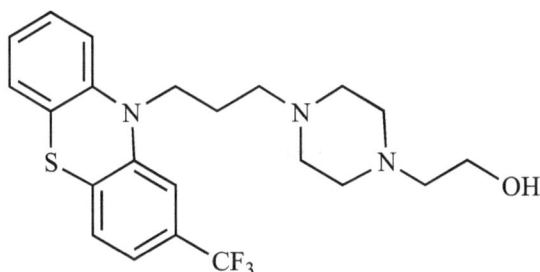

Fluphenazine

SAR 4.2.1: 5-membered rings show higher potency than 6 membered rings. However, at present, there are no 5 membered ring drugs available in the market.

SAR 4.2.2: The presence of para nitrogen enhances receptor binding than the absence. Therefore, piperazine is better than piperidine (attached at nitrogen or N1).

SAR 4.2.3: Substitution at the ring increases potency. Therefore, hydroxyethyl substitution is more potent than methyl substitution, which is more potent than the unsubstituted analogue.

SAR 4.2.4: Piperazine bearing phenothiazines possess the highest degree of D_2 antagonism.

SAR 4.3: Piperidine compounds have the γ- nitrogen incorporated into a piperidine ring. The phenothiazines using this derivative are 2-piperidines. A 1-piperidine behaves more like piperazine. Their names commonly end with the "–ridazine" and the nature of C2 substituent determines the prefix of the name. For example, thioridazine has a thiomethyl group at the C2 position.

SAR 4.3.1: Since the branching on γ-carbon adversely affects D_2 affinity, these compounds have the lowest potency of the three classes of phenothiazines. However, they exert the most potent anticholinergic effect.

SAR 4.3.2: Thioridazine is a thioether, oxidation of the sulfur gives mesoridazine that retains activity.

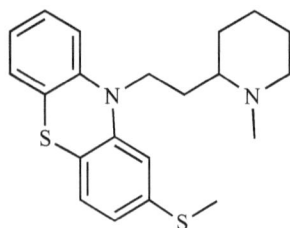

Thioridazine   Mesoridazine

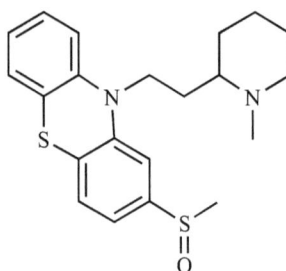

Potency Comparison of Piperazine, Aliphatic and Piperidine Type Antipsychotic Agents

Potency at the D_2 Receptors [58]

If the C2 substitution remains unchanged, then the order of potency is: Piperazine > Aliphatic > Piperidine. Some major pharmacologic and therapeutic effects are summarized in Table 3. The abbreviated "Zin", "Din", and "Phatic" forms are used for the sake of simplicity.

Table 3. Potency comparison of various antipsychotic drug groups in specific therapeutic applications.

Property or Effect	Order
DA receptor affinity	Zin > Din > Phatic
mACh receptor affinity	Din = Phatic > Zin
Alpha-1 receptor affinity	Din = Phatic > Zin
H1 receptor affinity	Din = Phatic > Zin
Antipsychotic potency	Zin > Din > Phatic
EPS frequency	Zin > Phatic > Din
Sedation	Din = Phatic > Zin
Orthostatic Hypotension	Phatic > Din > Zin
Ejaculatory Disturbance	Phatic = Din > Zin

Butyrophenone Antipsychotics and Related SAR

Butyrophenone Pharmacophore and SAR

Butyrophenone (*but-* for four carbons, *phen-* for benzene and *-one* for the presence of a ketone group) compounds are a potent group of neuroleptics possessing a general structure and the pharmacophore as shown in Fig. 7.

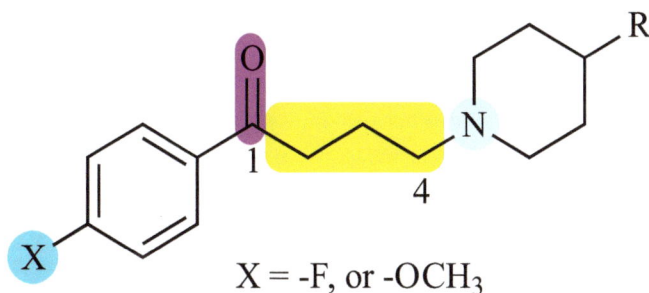

Fig. (7). General structure of butyrophenone derivatives showing the pharmacophore.

SAR 1: The nitrogen attached to the C4 should be tertiary for optimum neuroleptic function.

SAR 2: The space between nitrogen and carbonyl carbon should be three-carbon long; shortening or elongating decreases the potency.

SAR 3: Alteration of the keto moiety decreases potency. This includes:
- Replacing with thioketone (as in butyrothienones).
- Replacing with olefinic or phenoxy groups.
- Reduction of the carbonyl functional group.

SAR 4: Most potent butyrophenone compounds bear a fluorine substitution in the para position of the benzene ring (such as haloperidol).

SAR 5: Potency may be retained if a variation is introduced into the tertiary amino group. For instance, the nitrogen may be a part of a six-membered ring (*e.g.*, piperidine, tetrahydropyridine, or piperazine) in which a substitution is made at the para position.

SAR 6: The haloperidol butyrophenone side chain may be modified by replacing the keto group with a di-4flurophenylmethane, which results in diphenylbutyl piperidine neuroleptics (*e.g.*, pimozide) possessing a longer duration of action.

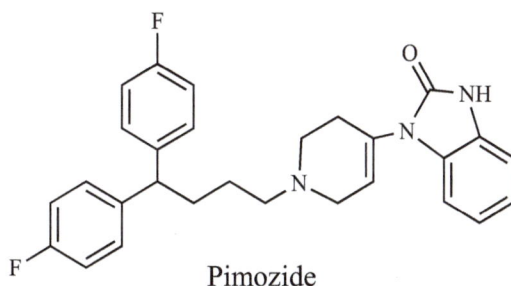

Pimozide

Selected Clinically Used First-Generation Antipsychotic Drugs

The structures of a few selected first-generation antipsychotic agents that are discussed in detail in this section are shown in Fig. (**8**).

Chlorpromazine

Discovered in 1950, chlorpromazine (Thorazine®) is the first phenothiazine drug categorized as a first-generation (typical) antipsychotic (FGA), containing an aliphatic amine side chain. It is used primarily to treat schizophrenia and also to treat bipolar disorder, attention deficit hyperactivity disorder, nausea, vomiting and anxiety. It is a low-potency antipsychotic, which works by blocking different dopamine receptors with a high affinity for the D_2 receptor. Chlorpromazine exhibits a high incidence of sedative, EPS, and anticholinergic side effects and orthostatic hypotension. It causes the most weight gain among all FGAs. Due to the presence of the phenothiazine ring system, it exhibits mild urticarial-type rash or photosensitivity.

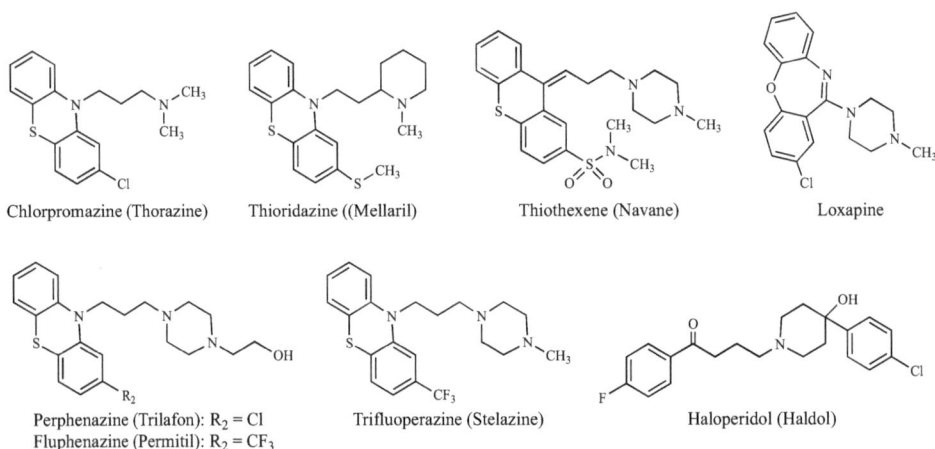

Fig. (8). Structures of selected first-generation antipsychotic agents.

It is highly lipophilic, thus is easily absorbed after oral administration. The drug and its metabolites are widely distributed throughout the tissues including breast milk and placenta with a very high volume of distribution. It is recommended not to use in pediatric patients younger than 6 months old. However, due to high protein binding (92-97%), and metabolic transformation the bioavailability is 10-30%. The metabolism is mediated through cytochrome P450 isozymes CYP3A4 (major pathway), flavin mono-oxidase 3 as well as glucuronide conjugation to active and inactive metabolites. Hydroxylation, N-oxidation, sulphoxidation, demethylation, deamination and conjugation reactions are common metabolic pathways and 7-hydroxychlorpromazine is its major active metabolite (Fig. **9**). The metabolites are mostly excreted *via* urine, only less than 1% is excreted unchanged.

Thioridazine

Thioridazine (Mellaril®) is an FGA with a phenothiazine ring system containing a piperidine amine side chain. It is a low-potency antipsychotic, which works by blocking dopamine receptors with a high affinity for the D_2 receptor. It is used primarily to treat schizophrenia when all other treatments are failed. It exhibits a high incidence of sedative, EPS and anticholinergic side effects and low incidence of orthostatic hypotension and weight gain. Thioridazine may cause life-threatening *torsades de pointes*-type arrhythmias and sudden death due to prolongation of QTc interval in a dose-related manner. This is why it is used in the treatment of schizophrenic patients only if they fail to show an acceptable response to other antipsychotic drugs. Like all other phenothiazines, it also causes photosensitivity. It is well absorbed with a bioavailability of 25-33% due to high protein binding (96-99.3%. The metabolism is mediated through hepatic enzymes *via* sulphoxidation (primarily), demethylation (2%), and hydroxylation (limited) [59].

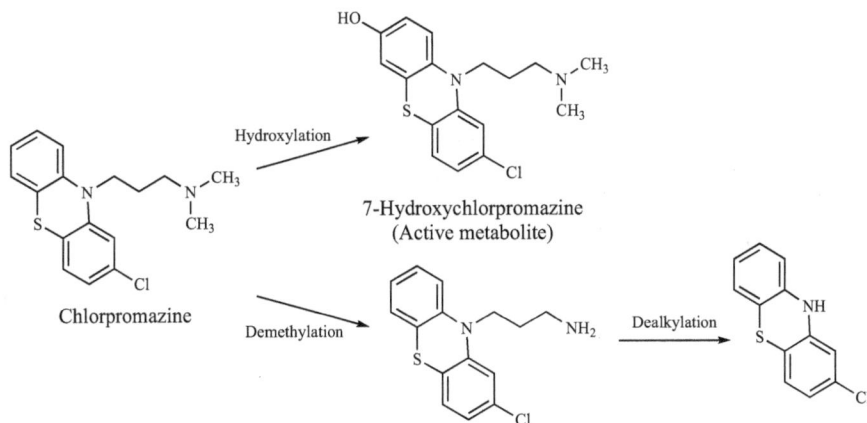

Fig. (9). Major metabolites of chlorpromazine.

Fluphenazine

Fluphenazine (Prolixin®) is a piperazine side containing phenothiazine class of FGA. It is a high-potency antipsychotic, which works by blocking dopamine receptors with a high affinity for the D_2 receptor. It is used primarily to treat schizophrenia. It exhibits a high incidence of sedative, EPS and anticholinergic side effects and low incidence of orthostatic hypotension and weight gain. It is contraindicated in liver impaired patients as well as in patients less than 12 years old (decanoate salt only). The hydrochloride salt absorbs quicker than the decanoate salt with peak plasma concentration reaching within 2.8 and 8-10 hrs., respectively. The half-life of the former is 14-16 hrs., while that of the later is about 14 days [60]. It is primarily metabolized by CYP2D6, which is susceptible to polymorphism.

Perphenazine

Perphenazine (Trilafon®) is a medium-potency (five times more potent than chlorpromazine) FGA of the phenothiazine group with a piperazine side chain [61]. It is effectively used to treat psychosis (schizophrenia), and in low doses may be used to treat agitated depression. However, it is rarely used at present. It exhibits moderate sedative, and anticholinergic side effects, high EPS and low incidence of orthostatic hypotension and weight gain It is readily absorbed after oral administration with a bioavailability of 20-25%. It is metabolized extensively in the liver to active and inactive metabolites by CYP2D6 and glucuronidase *via* sulfoxidation, hydroxylation, dealkylation, and glucuronidation. Because of CYP2D6 mediated metabolism, this drug may show polymorphism requiring dose adjustments. Its major active metabolite is 7-hydroxyperphenazine. The metabolites are excreted in urine and feces.

Trifluoperazine

Trifluoperazine (Stelazine®) is a high-potency FGA of phenothiazine group with a piperazine side chain. It is primarily used to treat schizophrenia and non-psychotic anxiety. It exhibits moderate sedative, and anticholinergic side effects, high EPS, and low incidence of orthostatic hypotension and weight gain. It is readily absorbed after oral administration and undergoes hepatic metabolism with a half-life of 3 to 12 hrs.

Thiothixene

Thiothixene (Navane®) is a high-potency FGA of the thioxanthene group that acts by blocking dopamine receptors, especially the D_2 receptor. It is primarily used to treat schizophrenia exhibiting low incidence of sedative, anticholinergic side effects, orthostatic hypotension and weight gain and high EPS. It is readily absorbed, widely distributed including in breast milk, highly protein-bound (90%), and has a half-life of 34 hrs. It undergoes hepatic metabolism mainly by CYP1A2.

Haloperidol

Haloperidol (Haldol®) is a high-potency FGA of butyrophenone group that acts primarily through the blockade of dopamine receptors, with a high affinity for D_2. It is used to treat schizophrenia, nausea, vomiting, delirium, OCD and other psychotic diseases. It exhibits a low incidence of sedative, anticholinergic side effects, orthostatic hypotension and weight gain and high EPS. It also causes significant hematological disturbances. Unlike the phenothiazine and thiothixene groups, it does not show photosensitivity. It is well absorbed with about 40-70% oral bioavailability. It is widely distributed throughout the body tissues including breast milk and placenta. It undergoes hepatic metabolism *via* glucuronidation (50% to 60%; inactive), CYP3A4-mediated reduction to an active metabolite (23%; some back-oxidation to haloperidol); and CYP3A4-mediated N-dealkylation (20% to 30%), including minor CYP1A2- and CYP2D6-mediated oxidation pathways to *N*-oxides and toxic pyridinium derivative (Fig **10**).

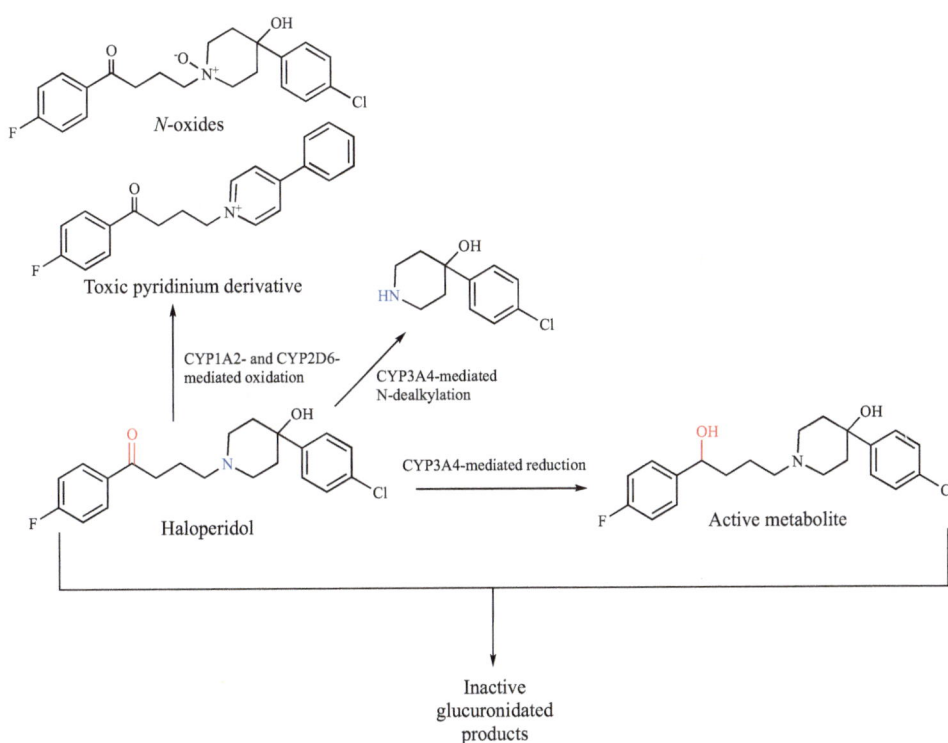

Fig. (10). Major metabolic pathways of haloperidol.

Loxapine

Structurally dibenzoxazepine, loxapine is an FGA drug of dibenzoxazepine group available for oral (Loxitane®), injectable (Loxitane®), and inhalation (Adasuve®) routes. It is indicated for schizophrenia and other psychotic agitations. It causes side effects typical for FGAs in addition to a series of cardiovascular and gastrointestinal events. It may also cause bronchospasm so recommended to administer in an enrolled health care facility with advanced airways management. Be especially cautious of patients' history of asthma and COPD. Loxapine REMS (risk evaluation and mitigation strategy) is a specialized program for loxapine therapy to overcome the bronchial risk [62]. Loxapine is metabolized mainly through CYP1A2, CYP3A4, and CYP2D6 and glucuronide conjugation and the metabolites are excreted in urine and feces.

SECOND GENERATION (ATYPICAL) ANTIPSYCHOTICS

General Mechanisms of Action and Side Effects

The atypical antipsychotics have an affinity to not only the dopamine D_2-type receptors but also other receptors including serotonin 5-HT_{2A} G-protein coupled receptors (GPCRs) at varying degrees (Fig. **11**). The higher affinity for the serotonin receptor is the cause of their fewer extrapyramidal side effects. The overall psychotherapeutic effect or tapering off the "negative" symptoms of the first-generation antipsychotic is believed to be associated with interaction with a range of non-dopamine receptors such as [63 - 65]:

- Serotonin GPCRs, such as 5-HT_{2A}, 5-HT_6, and/or 5-HT_7.
- Adrenergic GPCRs — α_1 and/or α_2 receptors.
- Acetylcholine muscarinic (mACh) GPCRs, such as M_1 and M_5
- Histamine H_1 receptors.

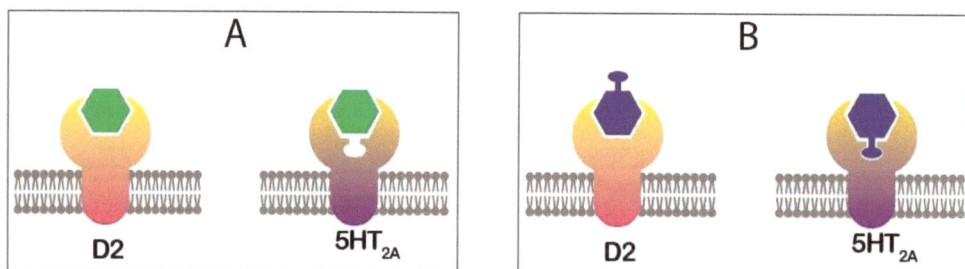

Fig. (11). Schematic representation of the conventional antipsychotics (A) and atypical antipsychotics (B) with their ability to bind different receptors.

Binding to various receptors has been linked to antipsychotic-associated weight gain and general metabolic dysregulation leading to cardiovascular and diabetic disorders [66]. Clozapine and olanzapine cause the highest weight gain, followed by the group of quetiapine, risperidone and chlorpromazine for moderate and the group of haloperidol, ziprasidone and aripiprazole for smallest weight gain [66, 67]. While the exact mechanism behind these side effects is not clearly elucidated, the pathways are believed to be linked to the serotonin $5HT_{2C}$ and/or antagonism or inverse agonism of the histamine H_1 receptors [67 - 69]. According to the most recent studies including meta-analyses, the SGAs differ in their mechanisms of action and in the manner in which they produce an atypical therapeutic profile. There hasn't been enough evidence to declare a therapeutic superiority of one atypical antipsychotic drug over others [70 - 73]. The recent solution of risperidone binding mode to the D2R will shed some light on their mechanism of antipsychotic action and the development of new safer, more efficacious drugs (Fig. **5**) [34].

Selected Clinically Used Second-Generation Antipsychotics

The dibenzodiazepine group member clozapine is the prototype of second-generation antipsychotic drugs and beneficial to the patients not responding well to phenothiazines or butyrophenone antipsychotics. Its receptor interaction is well characterized but the functional relationship with the chemical structure is not fully understood [71]. According to the majority of the studies [70, 74 - 76], the molecule behaves to be an antagonist at various GPCRs, which has been refuted by hypothesis related to functional selectivity [77 - 79]. Newer second-generation antipsychotics have been developed over recent years and are in clinical practice. Structures of a few selected second-generation antipsychotic (SGA) drugs in clinical practice are shown in Fig. (**12**).

Clozapine and Olanzapine

The dibenzodiazepine, clozapine (Clozaril®), and isosteric thienobenzodiazepine, olanzapine (Zyprexa®), are new generation atypical antipsychotics that have greatly reduced or minimal extrapyramidal side effects and do not produce tardive dyskinesia. They are beneficial in schizophrenic patients showing no response to classical neuroleptics (phenothiazines or butyrophenones). Clozapine has a relatively low affinity for brain dopamine D_1 and D_2 receptors (moderate affinity for D_4) in comparison to its affinity at adrenergic α_1 and α_2, histamine H_1, muscarinic M_1 and serotonin $5\text{-}HT_{2A}$ receptors. Olanzapine has somewhat different neurological profiles in that it is a more potent antagonist at dopamine D_2 and serotonin $5\text{-}HT_{2A}$ receptors. The use of clozapine is limited due to its potential side effect of agranulocytosis [80]. Both of these drugs cause very high weight gain and hyperglycemia. Clozapine causes high sedation, anticholinergic and orthostatic side effects and olanzapine causes these in moderation.

Both of these drugs are orally active with rapid and almost complete absorption and are metabolized by CYP3A4 (clozapine) or CYP1A2 (olanzapine) to inactive metabolites. Desmethylclozapine (active) and clozapine N-oxide (inactive) are the major metabolites of clozapine. Olanzapine-10-*N*-glucuronide, 2-hydroxymethyl olanzapine and olanzapine-4-*N*-oxide are the major metabolites of olanzapine (Fig. **13**) [81, 82]. Clozapine has a half-life of 12 hours while olanzapine has a variable half-life of 20 to 50 hours. Polymorphisms in CYP1A2 may lead to polymorphism in clozapine and olanzapine metabolism and thus requiring dose adjustments. Clozapine's efficacy is associated with its plasma concentration greater than 350 ng/mL and its serum concentration should be monitored before exceeding 600 mg daily in high-risk patients or in patients with potential drug interactions [83].

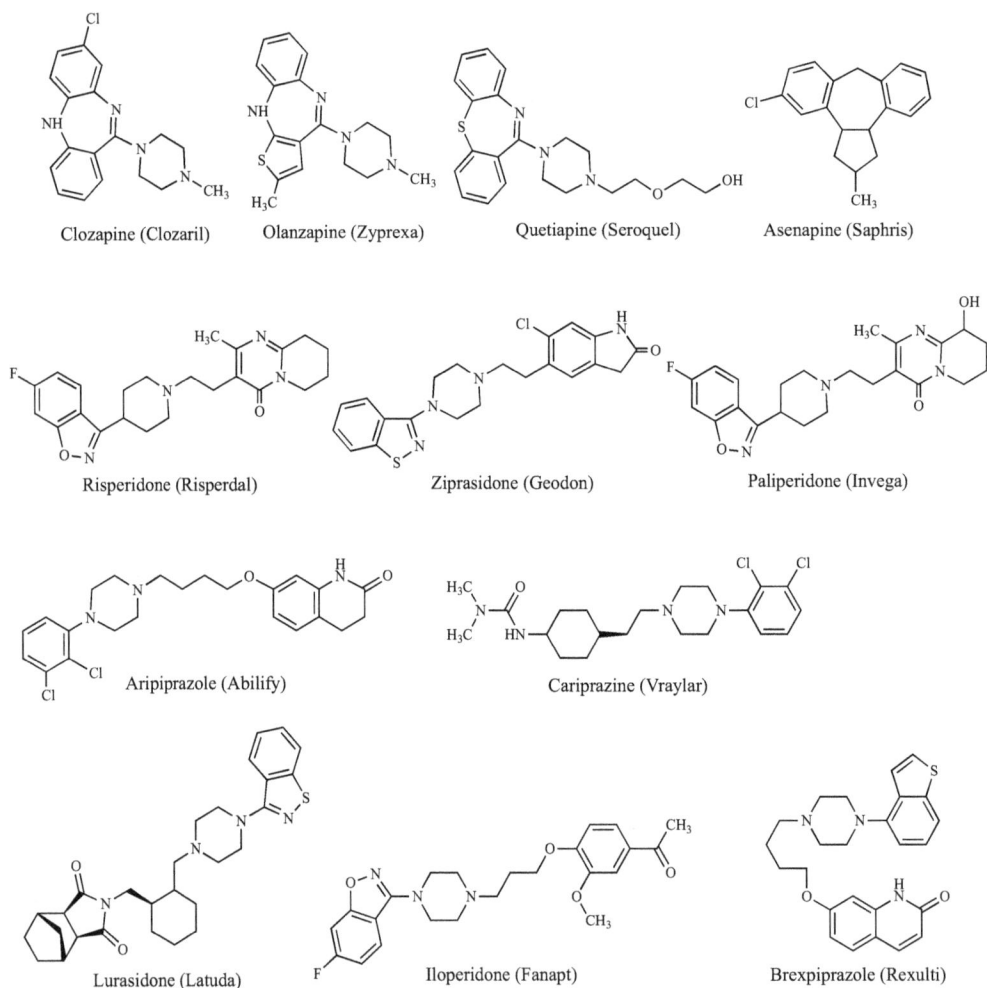

Fig. (12). Structures of selected second-generation antipsychotic (SGA) drugs in clinical practice.

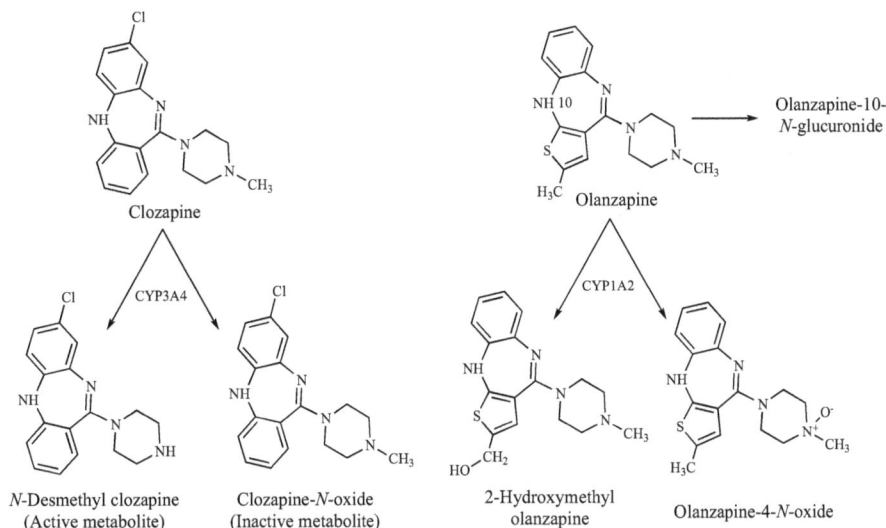

Fig. (13). Metabolic routes of clozapine and olanzapine.

Quetiapine

Quetiapine (Seroquel®), a dibenzo-thiazepine derivative with a piperazine side chain, has a similar brain receptor binding profile as clozapine, except that it has the lowest D_2 binding among all SGAs. It is approved for acute and maintenance treatment of multiple symptoms associated with bipolar as well as major depressive disorders and schizophrenia, in addition to off-label use for many other psychological disorders including OCD, PTSD and psychosis in Parkinson's disease, to name a few. As an atypical (SGA) drug, it exhibits moderate sedation, orthostatic hypotension and weight gain and minimal EPS and anticholinergic side effects. In order to minimize the withdrawal symptoms, the drug should be discontinued gradually with close monitoring of the patient.

This atypical antipsychotic drug is absorbed completely from the gastrointestinal tract after oral administration but is about 83% protein-bound and extensively metabolized that reduces the bioavailability of the active free drug. The drug is primarily metabolized by CYP3A4 isozyme to form active and inactive metabolites. The major active metabolite is *N*-desalkylquetiapine, which is further metabolized by CYP3A4 to sulfoxide metabolite (inactive) and by CYP2D6 to 7-hydroxy-N-desalkylquetiapine (active) (Fig. **14**) [84]. About 70% of the metabolites are excreted in the urine and 20% in the feces [85].

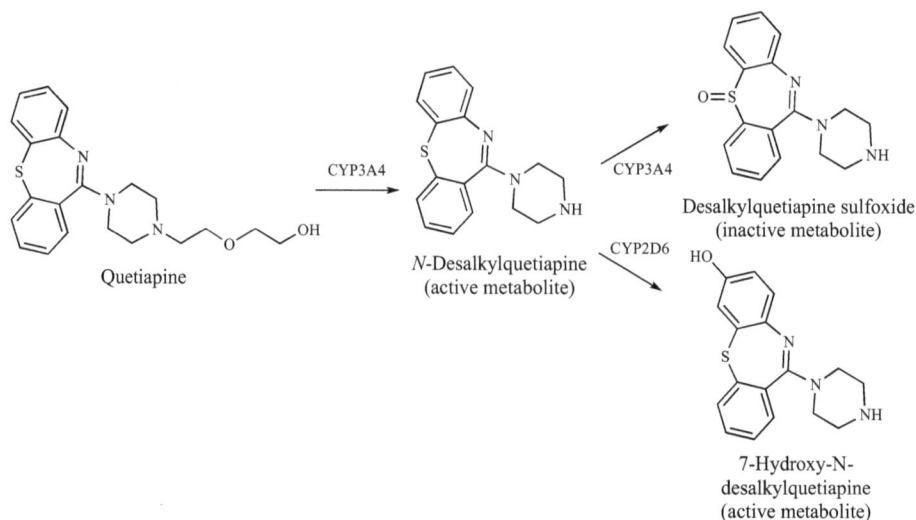

Fig. (14). Metabolism of quetiapine.

Asenapine

Asenapine (Saphris®), a benzoxepine, is an atypical antipsychotic agent approved for the acute treatment of adults with schizophrenia and acute treatment of manic or mixed episodes associated with bipolar I disorder with or without psychotic features in adults. It shows high affinity (antagonistic) for numerous receptors, including the serotonin receptors (5-HT$_{2A}$), the adrenergic receptors (α_1), the dopamine receptors (D$_2$), and the histamine (H$_1$) receptors and much lower affinity for the muscarinic acetylcholine receptors. It causes little or no anticholinergic side effects with low sedation and weight gain and moderate EPS. Asenapine is reasonably absorbed with an absolute bioavailability of 35% from sublingual dosing, which is the FDA approved route of administration with the recommendation of no food or drink within 10 minutes of administration that reduces bioavailability. If administered orally, its bioavailability is only about 2%. It has high plasma protein binding (~95%), It is primarily metabolized by oxidative metabolism by CYP1A2 and also by direct glucuronidation by UGT1A4. It is excreted by both renal and hepatic routes in approximately similar proportions.

Cariprazine

Cariprazine (Vraylar®) is an atypical antipsychotic which is used in the treatment of schizophrenia, manic disorders and mixed episodes associated with bipolar disorder. It is unique in that it is a partial agonist of D$_3$ and D$_2$ receptors with high selectivity for the D_3 receptor; it antagonizes overstimulated dopamine receptors but stimulates these receptors at a low endogenous dopamine level [86]. Its major side effects include akathisia, insomnia, and weight gain. EPS, sedation, nausea, vomiting, anxiety, and constipation were minimally observed.

Like all other antipsychotics, cariprazine is lipophilic that allows it to have high oral bioavailability and easy access through the blood-brain barrier. It is metabolized by CYP3A4 (major) and CYP2D6 (minor) *via* hydroxylation and demethylation. Desmethyl cariprazine (DCAR) and didesmethyl cariprazine (DDCAR) are its active metabolites. DCAR is metabolized to DDCAR by CYP3A4 and CYP2D6, and DDCAR is then metabolized by CYP3A4 to a hydroxylated metabolite (Fig. **15**).

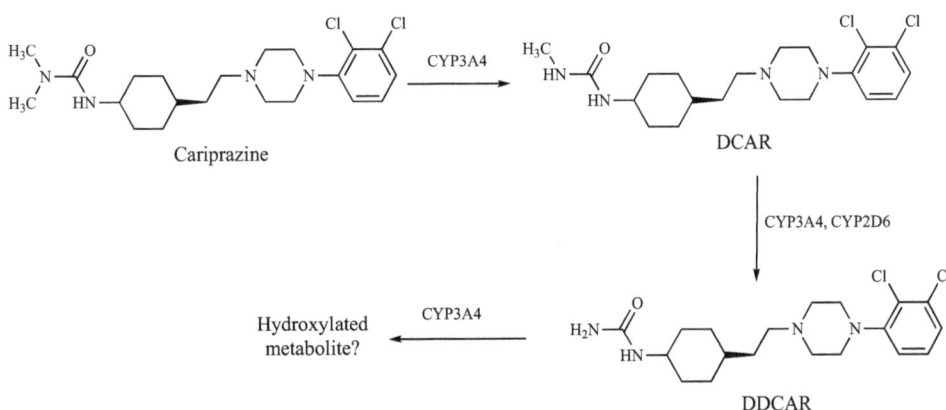

Fig. (15). Active metabolites of cariprazine.

Risperidone Paliperidone and Ziprasidone

Risperidone (Risperdal®) is a benzisoxazole and ziprasidone (Geodon®) is a benzisothiazole containing SGA. Risperidone is a $5\text{-HT}_{2A}/D_2$ antagonist with relatively high affinity at histamine H_1 and adrenergic α_1 and α_2 receptors. It has less extrapyramidal side effects due to no dopamine inhibitory effect in the striatum and cortex. Ziprasidone is also a $5\text{-HT}_{2A/C}/D_2$ antagonist with relatively high affinity at histamine H_1 and adrenergic α_1 and α_2 receptors. It can also activate 5-HT_{1A} in the brain and partial D_2 agonist activity in some selective cells which are important for these atypical antipsychotics for little or no extrapyramidal effects. Risperidone at a low dose (2-5 mg/day), binds the D_2 receptor in the ranges of 60% to 79%, but at a higher dose (>6 mg/day) leads to higher binding exceeding the 77% threshold associated with the development of EPS. Among all the currently available SGAs, ziprasidone has the highest

5-HT$_{2A}$-to-D$_2$ affinity ratio. Risperidone has low sedation and anticholinergic side effects and moderate EPS, orthostasis and weight gain. Ziprasidone leads to low anticholinergic side effects, orthostasis, and weight gain and moderate EPS and sedation.

Risperidone is well absorbed orally (bioavailability ~68%) and metabolized by hepatic CYP2D6 to 9-hydroxy-risperidone (also known as paliperidone) active metabolite with a half-life of 22 hours (Fig. **16**).

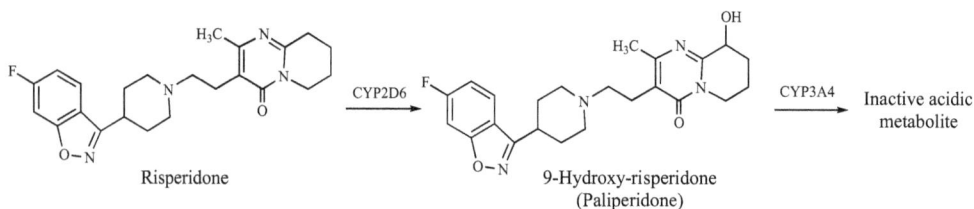

Fig. (16). Major metabolic pathways for risperidone and paliperidone.

As mentioned above, paliperidone (Invega®) is chemically 9-hydroxyrisperidone, the major hepatic metabolite of risperidone with similar pharmacological and toxicological profiles. It exerts its antipsychotic action by blocking dopamine D$_2$ and 5HT$_{2A}$ receptors. It also works as an antagonist of α_1, α_2, and H$_1$ receptors. This drug is available as both oral and injectable dosage forms. It is absorbed orally with a bioavailability of about 28%, which may increase if taken with food. It is metabolized through CYP2D6 and CYP3A4 isozymes to inactive metabolites.

Ziprasidone is also well absorbed orally. It has a half-life of 6 hours with oral bioavailability ~60%. It is unique in that it is largely (about two-thirds) metabolized by aldehyde oxidase (reductive cleavage of benzisothiazole ring), unlike all other antipsychotics which are mostly metabolized by CYP isozymes. About one-third of ziprasidone is also metabolized by CYP3A4 (oxidation). The reductive cleavage coupled with N-dearylation of the benzisothiazole ring results in S-methyl-dihydroziprasidone, S-methyl-dihydro-ziprasidone sulfoxide, and 6-chloro-5-(2-piperazin-1-yl-ethyl)-1,3-dihydro-indol-2-one, respectively. Ziprasidone sulfoxide and sulfone are the major metabolites in the human serum (Fig. **17**) [87]. The metabolites are excreted *via* urine (~20%) and feces (~66%).

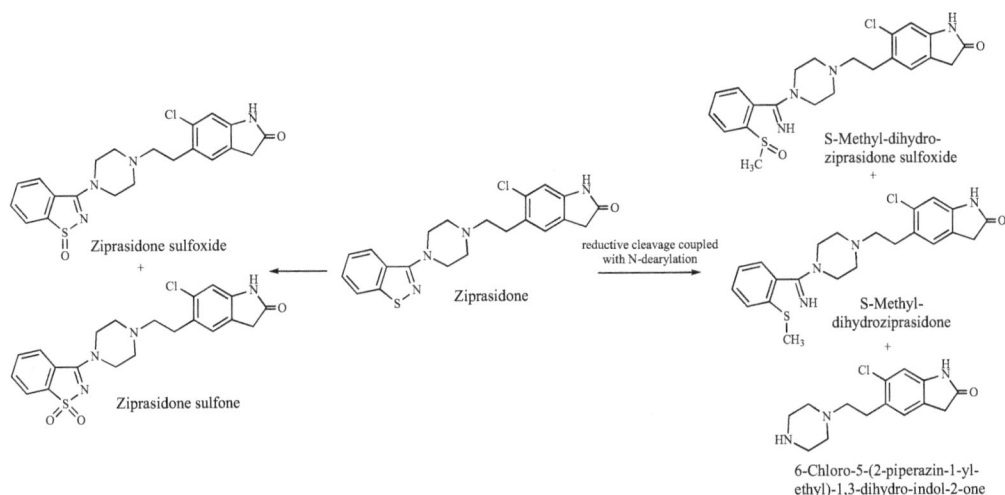

Fig. (17). Major metabolic pathways of ziprasidone.

Lurasidone

Lurasidone (Latuda®) is also a benzisothiazole derivative like ziprasidone, but also contains a norbornane ring on the other half of the molecule. It is available as film-coated tablets only. It is indicated for the treatment of schizophrenia, depressive episodes in adults with bipolar I disorder and major depressive disorder. Like the other SGAs, lurasidone acts as an antagonist of dopamine D_2 and serotonin $5HT_{2A}$ receptors. As an antagonist, it possesses a moderate affinity for adrenergic α_2 receptors. It works as a partial agonist for serotonin $5\text{-}HT_{1A}$ receptors. Lurasidone is as effective as iloperidone and less effective than ziprasidone, chlorpromazine, and asenapine. It is relatively well-tolerated with a low propensity for weight gain, EPS, anticholinergic side effects, and sedation [88].

Lurasidone is taken orally with ~10-20% bioavailability. It is recommended to take with food for better absorption. It is highly protein-bound (~99%) [89]. The drug is metabolized mainly in the liver by CYP3A4 *via* oxidative *N*-dealkylation between the piperazine and cyclohexane rings, hydroxylation of the norbornane ring, and S-oxidation. The hydroxylation of the cyclohexane ring and reductive cleavage of the isothiazole ring followed by S-methylation are also minor metabolic routes. ID-14283 and ID-14326 are two major active metabolites resulting from norbornane hydroxylation; and ID-20219 (carboxylic acid), ID-11614 (piperazine) and ID-20220 (a norbornane hydroxylated derivative of ID-20219) are major inactive metabolites resulting from *N*-dealkylation and hydroxylation (Fig. **18**) [90]. The drug and/or metabolites are excreted in feces and urine with a biological half-life of 18 hours [89].

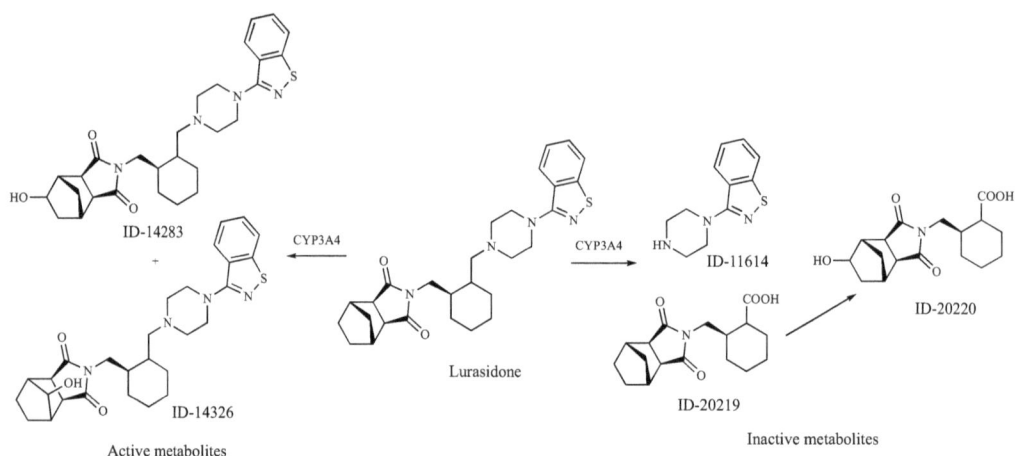

Fig. (18). Major active and inactive metabolites of lurasidone.

Iloperidone

Iloperidone (Fanapt®) is a piperidinyl-benzisoxazole derivative atypical antipsychotic for the treatment of schizophrenia. The tertiary amine makes the molecule basic, but otherwise, the molecule is largely lipophilic in character. It blocks the sites of noradrenaline, dopamine, and serotonin receptors. It has a high affinity for D_2, D_3, and 5-HT$_{2A}$ receptors, and moderate affinity for D_4, 5-HT$_6$, 5-HT$_7$, and α_1-receptors. It causes high orthostatic hypotension, moderate weight gain and anticholinergic side effects and low sedation and EPS.

Iloperidone is well absorbed orally and has high bioavailability (96%). It is metabolized primarily by CYP2D6 and CYP3A4 forming two predominant metabolites, P95 (~48%, 5) and P88 (~20%, 2), which is pharmacologically active (Fig. **19**). It is excreted primarily through urine and to some extent through feces. Due to CYP2D6-mediated metabolism, metabolic polymorphism is identified. The poor metabolizers of CYP2D6 show enhanced response to iloperidone during acute treatment of schizophrenia and thus special care with dosing in such patients should be taken.

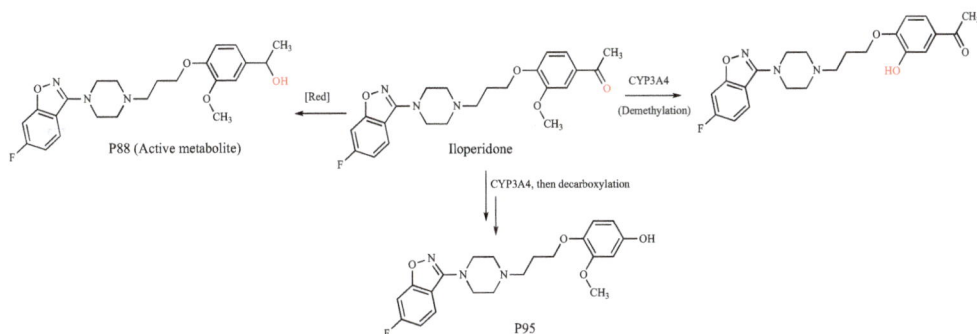

Fig. (19). Major metabolic routes of iloperidone.

Aripiprazole

Aripiprazole (Abilify®) is an arylpiperazine quinoline derivative with complex pharmacology. Dopamine (D_2) and serotonin (5-HT_{1A} & 5-$HT_{2A/C}$) receptor inhibitions are believed to be involved in its antischizophrenic activity. It has a high affinity partial agonist effect to some D_2 receptors depending on cell type, which explains its low EPS. It also has low anticholinergic side effects as well as low sedation, orthostatic hypotension and weight gain.

Aripiprazole is well absorbed after oral administration with high bioavailability (~90%). It is extensively metabolized in the liver principally by CYP2D6 and CYP3A4 through dehydrogenation, hydroxylation, and N-dealkylation. Dehydroaripiprazole is its only known active metabolite (Fig. **20**). The metabolites are excreted *via* feces and urine.

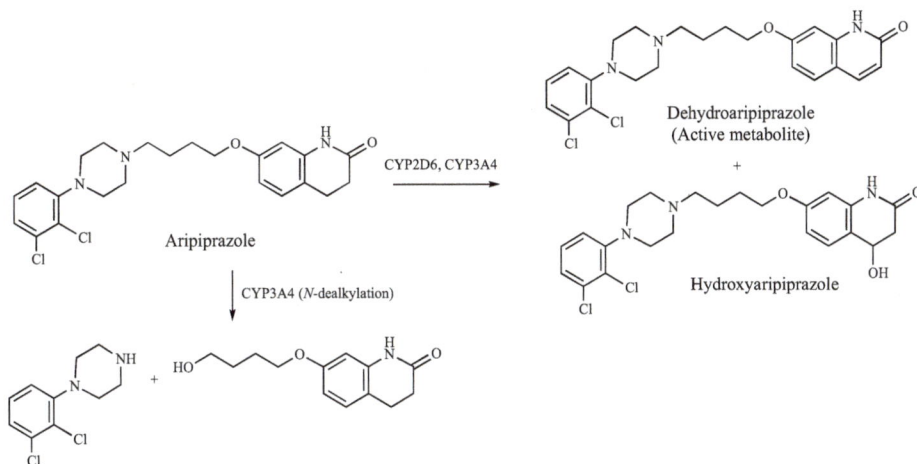

Fig. (20). Aripiprazole metabolism.

Brexpiprazole

Brexpiprazole (Rexulti®) is a successor of aripiprazole containing the same quinoline ring system of its active metabolite dehydroaripiprazole, and a thiophene ring system replaced the dichlorobenzene ring. It is developed by the same pharmaceuticals (Otsuka and Lundbeck) to provide improved efficacy and tolerability. It is a partial agonist at D_2, D_3, and 5-HT$_{1A}$ receptors and considered as a modulator of serotonin-dopamine activity. It has lower dopamine receptor affinity, but higher serotonin receptor affinity than aripiprazole. It is used for the treatment of schizophrenia with less akathisia, restlessness and/or insomnia compared to other established antipsychotic agents. It is well absorbed after oral administration with a bioavailability of 95% and a long half-life (~90 hrs). It is extensively metabolized by CYP2D6 and CYP3A4 *via* sulfoxidation forming the major metabolite DM-3411 (brexpiprazole sulfoxide).

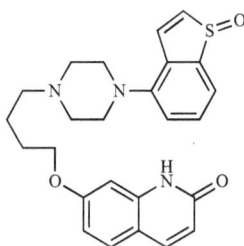

DM-3411

Selected Antipsychotic Drugs and Their Interaction with Dopamine and other Receptors

Table **4** summarizes various antipsychotics' interaction with pertinent receptors. As it is evident, the typical antipsychotics have pronounced antagonizing effect on the dopamine receptors, which is absent or irregular among the atypical members (PA indicates partial antagonism in the case of aripiprazole).

CASE STUDIES

Clinically Relevant Case Studies

SS is a 35-year-old woman with chronic schizophrenia, which is now well controlled. After taking **A** for several years, she has switched to **B** 10 months ago due to the development of tardive dyskinesia. Her current medicines are: olanzapine and 15 mg daily omeprazole 20 mg daily (due to gastric acidity). She is overweight and her physician recently diagnosed her as prediabetic. She is now concerned that her weight is getting uncontrolled even though she has been in regular diet like usual over the last few months when she is on this medication. She takes her medicines from the pharmacy where you intern, and she was asking the attending pharmacist about her being overweight and prediabetic and if there is anything to do with these medications she is taking. You learn that she has a family history of Parkinsonism and that you are also worried about her getting EPS with many of the antipsychotic agents. You have the following first- and second-generation antipsychotic agents in your stock.

Table 4. Comparative interaction profile of selected typical and atypical antipsychotics with various receptors. The presence and absence of the blocking effects are represented with + and — signs respectively.

	Drug	D1	D$_2$	α-Adr	H1	mACh	5-HT$_2$
Typical	Chlorpromazine	++	+++	+++	++	++	++
	Thioridazine	+	++	+++	+	++	++
	Haloperidol	+	+++	++	–	±	+
	Flupenthixol	++	+++	++	++	–	+++
Atypical	Sulpiride	–	+++	–	–	–	–
	Clozapine	++	++	++	++	++	+++
	Risperidone	–	++	++	++	++	+++
	Sertindole	–	++	++	–	–	+++
	Quetiapine	–	+	+++	–	+	+
	Aripiprazole	–	+++ (PA)	+	+	-	++
	Zotepine	++	++	+	+	+	+

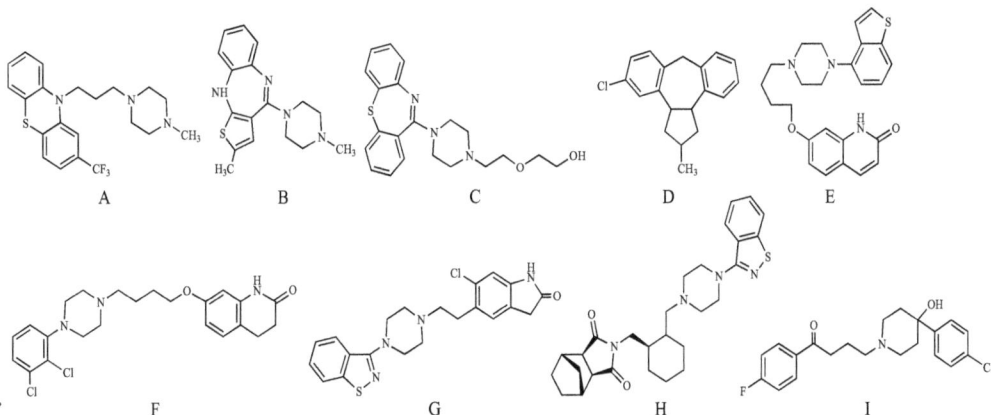

- Classify each of the drug structure chemically as well as pharmacologically.
- Do you think Structure B is the reason for her weight gain? What other drugs

may cause high weight gain.

- Are there any of these drug(s) that will have the lowest risk of diabetes and weight gain and diabetes and is thus advantageous for this patient to control her weight while also controlling her schizophrenia?
- Which antipsychotic drug(s) are least likely to cause extrapyramidal side effects?
- Which drug would be a more appropriate choice for this patient and what monitoring might be necessary if any?

DRUG DISCOVERY CASE STUDIES

Discovery of Haloperidol

The successful discovery of dextromoramide as a potent narcotic analgesic in the mid-1950s, Paul Janssen chemically modified pethidine to a new potent analgesic, R951, by replacing the methyl group attached to its nitrogen atom. He then lengthened the chain to a butyrophenone to yield R1187, another analgesic that progressively calmed and sedated the mice similar to chlorpromazine (Fig. **21**).

Intrigued by this chlorpromazine-like sedative and calming effects of R1187, Janssen then synthesized its analogues by replacing the ester function with a hydroxyl group to find tranquillizer devoid of analgesic activity. He then prepared hundreds of analogues with different substituents in the benzene rings, an effort led to the development of haloperidol (Fig. **21**) in 1958 as a highly potent tranquillizer, 50–100 times more potent than chlorpromazine with fewer side effects [91].

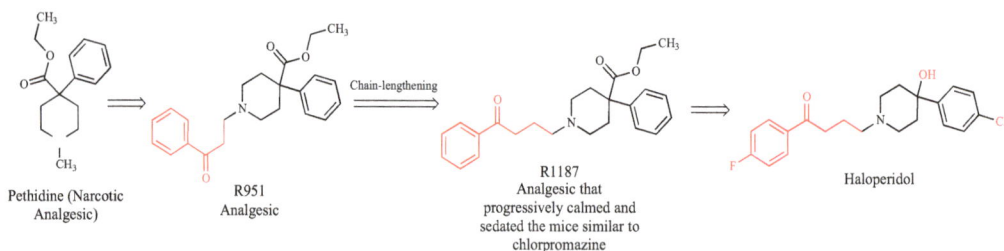

Fig. (21). Discovery of haloperidol from pethidine.

Discovery of Ziprasidone

The accidental discovery of chlorpromazine in the 1950s for the treatment of schizophrenia led Paul Janssen in 1953 to develop animal models to predict clinical activity relying on the ability of chlorpromazine to block the locomotor effects of stimulants such as amphetamine and apomorphine, with the subsequent discovery of the antipsychotic, haloperidol. Later, *in vitro* receptor-based pharmacology emerged in the 1980s and 1990s based on the finding that haloperidol and related drugs' antipsychotic activity is the result of the blockade of dopamine type 2 (D_2) receptors. The first atypical antipsychotic drug clozapine that lacks the undesirable extra-pyramidal symptoms (EPS) of haloperidol and chlorpromazine, binds to both D_2 and 5-hydroxytryptamine type 2 (5-HT$_2$) receptors.

Dopamine

5-Hydroxytryptamine
(5-HT, serotonin)

EPSs, caused by excessive D_2-receptor blockade, are hypothesized to be protected by the binding to 5-HT$_2$ receptor possibly with a D_2/5-HT$_2$-receptor blockade ratio of 10. Medicinal chemists with the drug discovery group used this background scientific information along with animal and receptor models to discover the new therapeutic agent Ziprasidone (Fig. **22**). Naphthylpiperazine was known to strongly bind serotonin receptors including 5-HT$_2$, which was used to target this receptor for finding an agent without EPS effects. However, since binding to the dopamine receptor is important for the antipsychotic effects, naphthylpiperazine was combined with the dopamine to yield structure **I**. The substitution of catechol moiety for oxindole in this structure furnished the compound **II**, which has both D_2 and 5-HT$_2$ antagonist activity (Fig. **22**).

Fig. (22). Development of ziprasidone.

Although compound **II** showed perfect antipsychotic effects in rats, disappointing results were obtained in monkeys. The naphthalene group was then replaced with the 1,2-benzisothiazole groups, which afforded the desired D_2/5-HT_2 blockade ratio of 25 to yield the prototype compound **III** and further modifications based on the SAR studies in this new series led to the new effective anti-schizophrenic drug, ziprasidone, without EPS liability and thus validated the D_2/5-HT_2 hypothesis. A total of 17 years (5 years of discovery phase + 9 years of clinical testing + 3 years to address regulatory requirements) were needed to receive final approval by the United States Food & Drug Administration (FDA) to market this drug in 2001 [92].

STUDENT SELF-STUDY GUIDE

- Learn detail about dopamine hypothesis and dopamine pathways.
- What are the different types of dopamine and serotonin receptors and what are their roles in antipsychotics and other actions?
- Discuss the binding mode of dopamine, haloperidol and clozapine in the dopamine receptor site.
- Why phenothiazines are antagonists to dopamine receptors? Explain the binding modes.
- What is the effect of ring substitution on antipsychotic potency of phenothiazines? Know about both types and positions of substitution.
- What type of side-chain favors antipsychotic activity? What is the effect of branching the side chain on both antihistaminic and antipsychotic effects?
- What are the different types of amine functions on the side chain? Compare their antipsychotic and other effects of all three types of amines – the aliphatic, piperidine and piperazine.
- What are thiothexenes and their activities?
- What are atypical antipsychotics? Why do they not possess extrapyramidal side effects?
- What are the different chemical classes of atypical antipsychotics?
- Identify the atypical drugs from a group of structures. How were haloperidol and ziprasidone developed?
- Know all about individual FGAs and SGAs in detail including indications, toxicities, pharmacokinetics, and metabolic routes.

STUDENTS SELF-ASSESSMENT QUESTIONS

1. Chlorpromazine is an antagonist to: I) Cholinergic receptor; II) Histamine receptor; III) Adrenergic receptor.

A. I only

B. III only

C. I and II only

D. II and III only

E. All of the above

2. Phenothiazine ring substitution that significantly increases antipsychotic activity include: I) 4-Substitution with -CF$_3$; II) 1-Substitution with -SCH$_3$; III) 2-Substitution with –Cl.

A. I only

B. III only

C. I and II only

D. II and III only

E. All of the above

3. Which statement(s) is/are true regarding the activity of piperazine, aliphatic, and piperidine analogs of antipsychotic phenothiazines? I) Piperazine side-chain exhibits the highest inhibitory potency on D$_2$ receptor; II) Aliphatic side-chain exhibits the highest inhibitory effect on α-adrenergic receptor; III) Piperidine side-chain exhibits highest extrapyramidal side effects.

A. I only

B. III only

C. I and II only

D. II and III only

E. All of the above

4. Antipsychotics with little or no extrapyramidal side effects include:

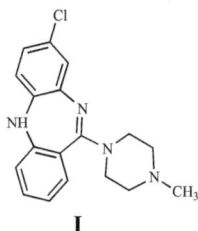

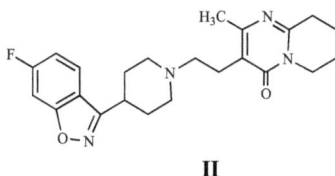

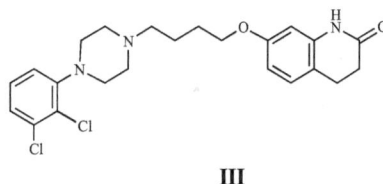

I   II   III

A. I only

B. III only

C. I and II only

D. II and III only

E. All of the above

5. Asenapine (Structure shown):

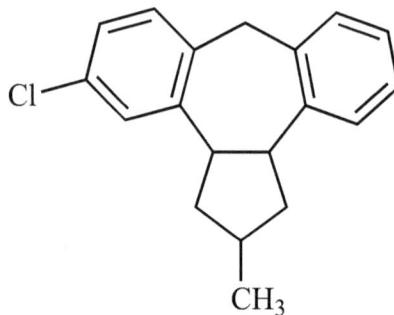

Asenapine (Saphris)

I) is a second-generation antipsychotic used in schizophrenia and manic episodes for adult

II) is only orally used that have high bioavailability

III) has low plasma protein binding and is minimally metabolized by CYP enzymes.

A. I only

B. III only

C. I and II only

D. II and III only

E. All of the above

6. Match the drug structures (I-V) with appropriate statements (A-E).

A. This arylpiperazine quinoline derivative with low EPS has low anticholinergic side effects as well as low sedation, orthostatic hypotension and weight gain.

B. This first-generation antipsychotic agent may cause life-threatening *torsades de pointes*-type arrhythmias and sudden death due to prolongation of QTc interval in a dose-related manner.

C. The use of this SGA is limited due to its potential side effect of agranulocytosis.

D. It is unique in that it is a partial agonist of D3 and D_2 receptors with high selectivity for the D_3 receptor; it antagonizes overstimulated dopamine receptors but stimulates these receptors at a low endogenous dopamine level.

E. This classic typical antipsychotic agent with an aliphatic side chain causes the most weight gain among all FGAs.

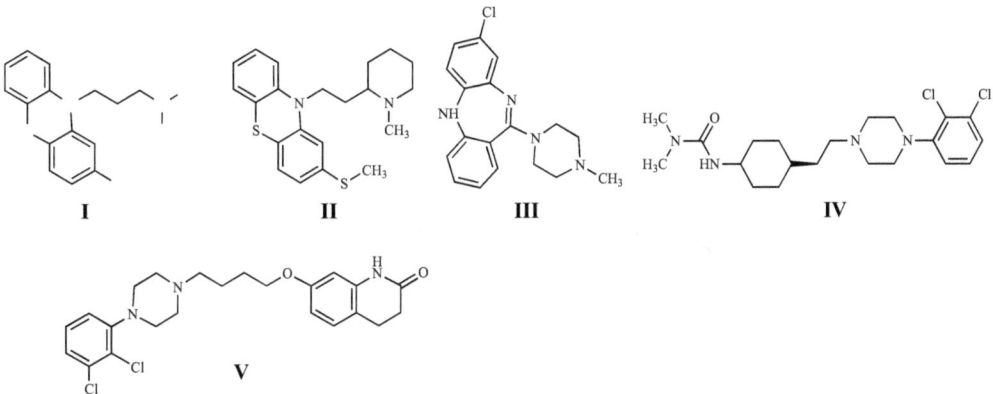

7. Which receptor is responsible for the antipsychotic activity of phenothiazines?

A. α-Adrenergic

B. D_2

C. 5-HT

D. H2

E. Uptake-1

8. Which SAR statement(s) is/are true regarding the alkyl side chain of the phenothiazine derivatives?

I) Increasing or decreasing the length of the chain from 3 carbons decreases the antipsychotic potency

II) Substitution on the alpha carbon decrease antipsychotic potency

III) A methyl or larger group substituent on the β carbon increases dopamine antagonism.

A. I only

B. III only

C. I and II only

D. II and III only

E. All of the above

9. Metabolic routes of phenothiazine antipsychotics include:

I) Ring hydroxylation followed by glucuronidation

II) S-oxidation

III) Dealkylation of the side chain amine and/or deamination.

A. I only

B. III only

C. I and II only

D. II and III only

E. All of the above

10. The antipsychotic potency of X, Y, Z is in order:

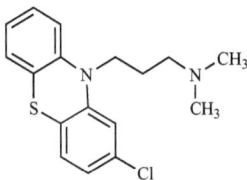 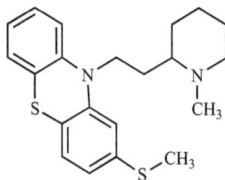 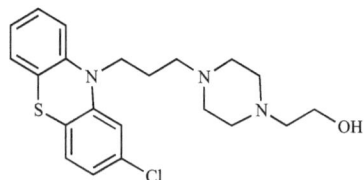

        X   **Y**   **Z**

A. X>Y>Z

B. Z>Y>Z

C. Z>X>Y

D. X>Z>Y

E. Y>X>Z

11. Which antipsychotic agent is least likely to cause extrapyramidal side effects and/or photosensitivity and skin pigmentation?

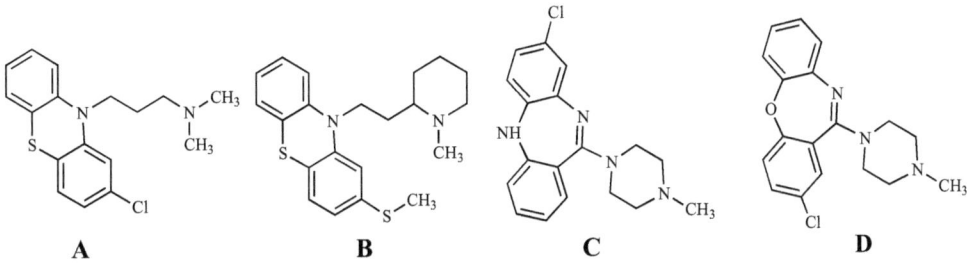

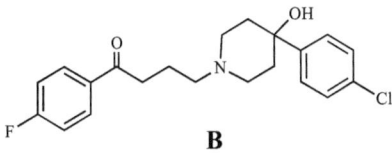

12. Which statement(s) regarding drug structure shown is/are true?

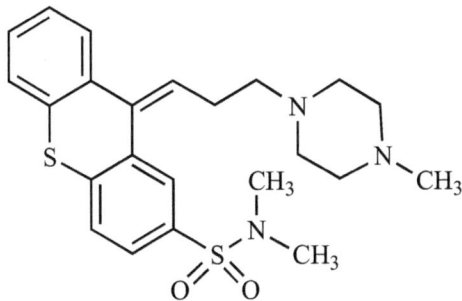

I) Its E isomer is more potent

II) It is an antipsychotic agent

III) It causes extrapyramidal side effects.

A. I only

B. III only

C. I and II only

D. II and III only

E. All of the above

13. Which statements are true about aripiprazole?

I) It is an arylpiperazine quinoline derivative with complex pharmacology

II) Dopamine D_2 and serotonin 5-HT1A & 5-HT2A/C receptor inhibitions are believed to be involved in its antischizophrenic therapy

III) It has high extrapyramidal side effects.

A. I only

B. III only

C. I and II only

D. II and III only

E. All of the above

NOTES

Databases for Accessing Drug Details and Receptor Information

[1] DrugBank: https://www.drugbank.ca/

[2] PubChem: https://pubchem.ncbi.nlm.nih.gov/

[3] IUPHAR-GPCR:
https://www.guidetopharmacology.org/GRAC/ReceptorFamiliesForward?type=GPCR

CONSENT FOR PUBLICATION

Not applicable.

CONFLICT OF INTEREST

The authors confirm that the contents of this chapter have no conflict of interest.

ACKNOWLEDGEMENTS

Declare none.

REFERENCES

[1]   Castillo R, Carlat D, Millon T, Millon C, Meagher S, Grossman S, *et al.* Diagnostic and statistical manual of mental disorders. Washington, DC: American Psychiatric Association Press 2007.

[2]   Bosch F, Rosich L. The contributions of Paul Ehrlich to pharmacology: a tribute on the occasion of the centenary of his Nobel Prize. Pharmacology 2008; 82(3): 171-9.
[http://dx.doi.org/10.1159/000149583] [PMID: 18679046]

[3]   López-Muñoz F, Alamo C, Cuenca E, Shen WW, Clervoy P, Rubio G. History of the discovery and clinical introduction of chlorpromazine. Ann Clin Psychiatry 2005; 17(3): 113-35.
[http://dx.doi.org/10.1080/10401230591002002] [PMID: 16433053]

[4]   Shen WW. A history of antipsychotic drug development. Compr Psychiatry 1999; 40(6): 407-14.
[http://dx.doi.org/10.1016/S0010-440X(99)90082-2] [PMID: 10579370]

[5]   Rocha E, Silva M, Antonio A. Bioassay of antihistaminic action Histamines II and antihistamines: chemistry, metabolism and physiologic and pharmacologic actions. Berlin: Springer-Verlag 1978; pp. 381-438.
[http://dx.doi.org/10.1007/978-3-642-66445-8_10]

[6]   Maxwell RA, Eckhardt SB. Chlorpromazine. In: Drug Discovery. Totowa, NJ: Humana Press 1990; pp. 111-22.
[http://dx.doi.org/10.1007/978-1-4612-0469-5_8]

[7]   Delay J, Deniker P. Neuroleptic effects of chlorpromazine in therapeutics of neuropsychiatry. Int Rec Med Gen Pract Clin 1955; 168(5): 318-26.
[PMID: 14381100]

[8]   Peek BM, Ross GT, Edwards SW, Meyer GJ, Meyer TJ, Erickson BW. Synthesis of redox derivatives of lysine and related peptides containing phenothiazine or tris(2,2'-bipyridine)ruthenium(II). Int J Pept Protein Res 1991; 38(2): 114-23.
[http://dx.doi.org/10.1111/j.1399-3011.1991.tb01418.x] [PMID: 1783487]

[9]   Hippius H. A historical perspective of clozapine. J Clin Psych 1999; 60: 22-3.

[10]   Hippius H. The history of clozapine. Psychopharmacology (Berl) 1989; 99 (Suppl.): S3-5.
[http://dx.doi.org/10.1007/BF00442551] [PMID: 2682730]

[11]   Leucht S, Wahlbeck K, Hamann J, Kissling W. New generation antipsychotics versus low-potency conventional antipsychotics: a systematic review and meta-analysis. Lancet 2003; 361(9369): 1581-9.
[http://dx.doi.org/10.1016/S0140-6736(03)13306-5] [PMID: 12747876]

[12]   Alphs LD, Anand R. Clozapine: The commitment to patient safety. J Clin Psych 1999; 60: 39-42.

[13]   Fuentes AV, Pineda MD, Venkata KCN. Comprehension of Top 200 Prescribed Drugs in the US as a Resource for Pharmacy Teaching, Training and Practice. Pharmacy (Basel) 2018; 6(2): 43.

[http://dx.doi.org/10.3390/pharmacy6020043] [PMID: 29757930]

[14]   Bougousslavsky JBF. Neurological disorders in Famous Artists. 1st ed., Karger Medical and Scientific Publishers 2005.
[http://dx.doi.org/10.1159/isbn.978-3-318-01206-4]

[15]   https://www.nimh.nih.gov/health/topics/schizophrenia/raise/raise-questions-and-answers.shtml

[16]   National Health Service U. Psychosis 2016; 23(December) [Available from: https://www.nhs.uk/conditions/psychosis/.].

[17]   2016. https://www.nhs.uk/conditions/psychosis/symptoms/

[18]   2016. https://www.nhs.uk/conditions/psychosis/causes/

[19]   Stegmayer K, Walther S, van Harten P. Tardive dyskinesia associated with atypical antipsychotics: prevalence, mechanisms and management strategies. CNS Drugs 2018; 32(2): 135-47.
[http://dx.doi.org/10.1007/s40263-018-0494-8] [PMID: 29427000]

[20]   Griswold KS, Del Regno PA, Berger RC. Recognition and Differential Diagnosis of Psychosis in Primary Care. Am Fam Physician 2015; 91(12): 856-63.
[PMID: 26131945]

[21]   Moutoussis M, Eldar E, Dolan RJ. Building a new field of computational psychiatry. Biol Psychiatry 2017; 82(6): 388-90.
[http://dx.doi.org/10.1016/j.biopsych.2016.10.007] [PMID: 27876357]

[22]   Unterrainer H-F. Functional and Dysfunctional Religious/Spiritual Beliefs in Psychotic Disorders Processes of Believing: The Acquisition, Maintenance, and Change in Creditions. Springer 2017; pp. 167-80.

[23]   Organization WH. Schizophrenia—fact sheet no. 397. Retrieved 3 February. 2016.

[24]   Daiello LA, Cizginer S, Pelosi MA, Ott BR. Psychoactive medication and memory impairment among members of an Alzheimer prevention registry. Alzheimer's & Dementia. J Alzh Assoc 2015; 11(7): 734.

[25]   Curran C, Byrappa N, McBride A. Stimulant psychosis: systematic review. Br J Psychiatry 2004; 185: 196-204.
[http://dx.doi.org/10.1192/bjp.185.3.196] [PMID: 15339823]

[26]   Uhrig S, Hirth N, Broccoli L, *et al.* Reduced oxytocin receptor gene expression and binding sites in different brain regions in schizophrenia: A post-mortem study. Schizophr Res 2016; 177(1-3): 59-66.
[http://dx.doi.org/10.1016/j.schres.2016.04.019] [PMID: 27132494]

[27]   Gründer G, Cumming P. The dopamine hypothesis of schizophrenia: Current status Neurobiology of Schizophrenia. Elsevier 2016; pp. 109-24.
[http://dx.doi.org/10.1016/B978-0-12-801829-3.00015-X]

[28]   Hikida T, Morita M, Macpherson T. Neural mechanisms of the nucleus accumbens circuit in reward and aversive learning. Neurosci Res 2016; 108: 1-5.
[http://dx.doi.org/10.1016/j.neures.2016.01.004] [PMID: 26827817]

[29]   Lau CI, Wang HC, Hsu JL, Liu ME. Does the dopamine hypothesis explain schizophrenia? Rev Neurosci 2013; 24(4): 389-400.
[http://dx.doi.org/10.1515/revneuro-2013-0011] [PMID: 23843581]

[30]   Kalani MY, Vaidehi N, Hall SE, *et al.* The predicted 3D structure of the human D_2 dopamine receptor and the binding site and binding affinities for agonists and antagonists. Proc Natl Acad Sci USA 2004; 101(11): 3815-20.
[http://dx.doi.org/10.1073/pnas.0400100101] [PMID: 14999101]

[31]   Center GSL. Beyond the Reward Pathway 2013. https://learn.genetics.utah.edu/ content/ addiction/beyond/

[32] Kenneth L, Davis DC, Joseph T Coyle. Charles Nemeroff Neuropsychopharmacology – 5th Generation of Progress. Philadelphia, Pennsylvania: Lippincott, Williams, & Wilkins 2002.

[33] Creese I, Burt DR, Snyder SH. Dopamine receptor binding predicts clinical and pharmacological potencies of antischizophrenic drugs. Science 1976; 192(4238): 481-3.
[http://dx.doi.org/10.1126/science.3854] [PMID: 3854]

[34] Seeman P, Lee T, Chau-Wong M, Wong K. Antipsychotic drug doses and neuroleptic/dopamine receptors. Nature 1976; 261(5562): 717-9.
[http://dx.doi.org/10.1038/261717a0] [PMID: 945467]

[35] Jacobs D, Silverstone T. Dextroamphetamine-induced arousal in human subjects as a model for mania. Psychol Med 1986; 16(2): 323-9.
[http://dx.doi.org/10.1017/S0033291700009132] [PMID: 3726006]

[36] Lieberman JA, Kane JM, Alvir J. Provocative tests with psychostimulant drugs in schizophrenia. Psychopharmacology (Berl) 1987; 91(4): 415-33.
[http://dx.doi.org/10.1007/BF00216006] [PMID: 2884687]

[37] Thompson RF. The brain: A neuroscience primer. New York: Worth Publishers 2000.

[38] Diaz J, Diaz J. How drugs influence behavior: A neuro-behavioral approach. New jersey: Prentice Hall 1997.

[39] Schulz SC, Green MF, Nelson KJ. Schizophrenia and Psychotic Spectrum Disorders. Oxford: Oxford University Press 2016.
[http://dx.doi.org/10.1093/med/9780199378067.001.0001]

[40] Howes OD, Kambeitz J, Kim E, *et al.* The nature of dopamine dysfunction in schizophrenia and what this means for treatment. Arch Gen Psychiatry 2012; 69(8): 776-86.
[http://dx.doi.org/10.1001/archgenpsychiatry.2012.169] [PMID: 22474070]

[41] Beaulieu JM, Espinoza S, Gainetdinov RR. Dopamine receptors - IUPHAR Review 13. Br J Pharmacol 2015; 172(1): 1-23.
[http://dx.doi.org/10.1111/bph.12906] [PMID: 25671228]

[42] Segura-Aguilar J, Paris I, Muñoz P, Ferrari E, Zecca L, Zucca FA. Protective and toxic roles of dopamine in Parkinson's disease. J Neurochem 2014; 129(6): 898-915.
[http://dx.doi.org/10.1111/jnc.12686] [PMID: 24548101]

[43] Ford CP. The role of D_2-autoreceptors in regulating dopamine neuron activity and transmission. Neuroscience 2014; 282: 13-22.
[http://dx.doi.org/10.1016/j.neuroscience.2014.01.025] [PMID: 24463000]

[44] Wang S, Che T, Levit A, Shoichet BK, Wacker D, Roth BL. Structure of the D_2 dopamine receptor bound to the atypical antipsychotic drug risperidone. Nature 2018; 555(7695): 269-73.
[http://dx.doi.org/10.1038/nature25758] [PMID: 29466326]

[45] Svensson TH. Alpha-adrenoceptor modulation hypothesis of antipsychotic atypicality. Prog Neuropsychopharmacol Biol Psychiatry 2003; 27(7): 1145-58.
[http://dx.doi.org/10.1016/j.pnpbp.2003.09.009] [PMID: 14642973]

[46] He M, Deng C, Huang XF. The role of hypothalamic H1 receptor antagonism in antipsychotic-induced weight gain. CNS Drugs 2013; 27(6): 423-34.
[http://dx.doi.org/10.1007/s40263-013-0062-1] [PMID: 23640535]

[47] Ghoshal A, Rook JM, Dickerson JW, *et al.* Potentiation of M1 Muscarinic Receptor Reverses Plasticity Deficits and Negative and Cognitive Symptoms in a Schizophrenia Mouse Model. Neuropsychopharmacology 2016; 41(2): 598-610.
[http://dx.doi.org/10.1038/npp.2015.189] [PMID: 26108886]

[48] Dean B, Scarr E. Possible involvement of muscarinic receptors in psychiatric disorders: a focus on schizophrenia and mood disorders. Curr Mol Med 2015; 15(3): 253-64.

[http://dx.doi.org/10.2174/1566524015666150330144821] [PMID: 25817858]

[49]   Harrison PJ, Weinberger DR. Schizophrenia genes, gene expression, and neuropathology: on the matter of their convergence. Mol Psychiatry 2005; 10(1): 40-68.
[http://dx.doi.org/10.1038/sj.mp.4001558]

[50]   Paoletti P, Neyton J. NMDA receptor subunits: function and pharmacology. Curr Opin Pharmacol 2007; 7(1): 39-47.
[http://dx.doi.org/10.1016/j.coph.2006.08.011] [PMID: 17088105]

[51]   Cull-Candy S, Brickley S, Farrant M. NMDA receptor subunits: diversity, development and disease. Curr Opin Neurobiol 2001; 11(3): 327-35.
[http://dx.doi.org/10.1016/S0959-4388(00)00215-4] [PMID: 11399431]

[52]   Meltzer HY, Matsubara S, Lee JC. Classification of typical and atypical antipsychotic drugs on the basis of dopamine D-1, D-2 and serotonin2 pKi values. J Pharmacol Exp Ther 1989; 251(1): 238-46.
[PMID: 2571717]

[53]   Miyamoto S, Miyake N, Jarskog LF, Fleischhacker WW, Lieberman JA. Pharmacological treatment of schizophrenia: a critical review of the pharmacology and clinical effects of current and future therapeutic agents. Mol Psychiatry 2012; 17(12): 1206-27.
[http://dx.doi.org/10.1038/mp.2012.47] [PMID: 22584864]

[54]   Jaszczyszyn A, Gąsiorowski K, Świątek P, et al. Chemical structure of phenothiazines and their biological activity. Pharmacol Rep 2012; 64(1): 16-23.
[http://dx.doi.org/10.1016/S1734-1140(12)70726-0] [PMID: 22580516]

[55]   Foye WO. Foye's principles of medicinal chemistry. Pennsylvania: Lippincott Williams & Wilkins 2008.

[56]   Stahl SM, Stahl SM. Stahl's essential psychopharmacology: neuroscientific basis and practical applications. Cambridge: Cambridge University Press 2013.

[57]   Lieberman JA, Phillips M, Gu H, et al. Atypical and conventional antipsychotic drugs in treatment-naive first-episode schizophrenia: a 52-week randomized trial of clozapine vs chlorpromazine. Neuropsychopharmacology 2003; 28(5): 995-1003.
[http://dx.doi.org/10.1038/sj.npp.1300157] [PMID: 12700715]

[58]   Singh MM, Kay SR. A comparative study of haloperidol and chlorpromazine in terms of clinical effects and therapeutic reversal with benztropine in schizophrenia. Theoretical implications for potency differences among neuroleptics. Psychopharmacology (Berl) 1975; 43(2): 103-13.
[http://dx.doi.org/10.1007/BF00421012] [PMID: 1103205]

[59]   2018. https://www.drugs.com/mtm/thioridazine.html

[60]   2018. https://www.drugs.com/mtm/fluphenazine.html

[61]   Rees L. Chlorpromazine and allied phenothiazine derivatives. BMJ 1960; 2(5197): 522-5.
[http://dx.doi.org/10.1136/bmj.2.5197.522] [PMID: 14436902]

[62]   2019. https://www.drugs.com/mtm/loxapine.html

[63]   Miller R. Mechanisms of action of antipsychotic drugs of different classes, refractoriness to therapeutic effects of classical neuroleptics, and individual variation in sensitivity to their actions: Part I. Curr Neuropharmacol 2009; 7(4): 302-14.
[http://dx.doi.org/10.2174/157015909790031229] [PMID: 20514210]

[64]   Tarsy D, Baldessarini RJ, Tarazi FI. Effects of newer antipsychotics on extrapyramidal function. CNS Drugs 2002; 16(1): 23-45.
[http://dx.doi.org/10.2165/00023210-200216010-00003] [PMID: 11772117]

[65]   Wong EH, Tarazi FI, Shahid M. The effectiveness of multi-target agents in schizophrenia and mood disorders: Relevance of receptor signature to clinical action. Pharmacol Ther 2010; 126(2): 173-85.
[http://dx.doi.org/10.1016/j.pharmthera.2010.02.001] [PMID: 20171983]

[66]   Kirk SL, Glazebrook J, Grayson B, Neill JC, Reynolds GP. Olanzapine-induced weight gain in the rat: role of 5-HT2C and histamine H1 receptors. Psychopharmacology (Berl) 2009; 207(1): 119-25.
[http://dx.doi.org/10.1007/s00213-009-1639-8] [PMID: 19688201]

[67]   Rowland NE, Crump EM, Nguyen N, Robertson K, Sun Z, Booth RG. Effect of (-)-trans-PAT, a novel 5-HT2C receptor agonist, on intake of palatable food in mice. Pharmacol Biochem Behav 2008; 91(1): 176-80.
[http://dx.doi.org/10.1016/j.pbb.2008.07.004] [PMID: 18692085]

[68]   Reynolds GP, Kirk SL. Metabolic side effects of antipsychotic drug treatment--pharmacological mechanisms. Pharmacol Ther 2010; 125(1): 169-79.
[http://dx.doi.org/10.1016/j.pharmthera.2009.10.010] [PMID: 19931306]

[69]   Kroeze WK, Hufeisen SJ, Popadak BA, et al. H1-histamine receptor affinity predicts short-term weight gain for typical and atypical antipsychotic drugs. Neuropsychopharmacology 2003; 28(3): 519-26.
[http://dx.doi.org/10.1038/sj.npp.1300027] [PMID: 12629531]

[70]   Asenjo Lobos C, Komossa K, Rummel-Kluge C, et al. Clozapine versus other atypical antipsychotics for schizophrenia. Cochrane Database Syst Rev 2010; (11): CD006633.
[http://dx.doi.org/10.1002/14651858.CD006633.pub2] [PMID: 21069690]

[71]   Bhattacharjee J, El-Sayeh HG. Aripiprazole versus typical antipsychotic drugs for schizophrenia. Cochrane Database Syst Rev 2008; (3): CD006617.
[http://dx.doi.org/10.1002/14651858.CD006617.pub3] [PMID: 18646161]

[72]   Crossley NA, Constante M, McGuire P, Power P. Efficacy of atypical v. typical antipsychotics in the treatment of early psychosis: meta-analysis. Br J Psychiatry 2010; 196(6): 434-9.
[http://dx.doi.org/10.1192/bjp.bp.109.066217] [PMID: 20513851]

[73]   Leucht S, Corves C, Arbter D, Engel RR, Li C, Davis JM. Second-generation versus first-generation antipsychotic drugs for schizophrenia: a meta-analysis. Lancet 2009; 373(9657): 31-41.
[http://dx.doi.org/10.1016/S0140-6736(08)61764-X] [PMID: 19058842]

[74]   Leucht S, Komossa K, Rummel-Kluge C, et al. A meta-analysis of head-to-head comparisons of second-generation antipsychotics in the treatment of schizophrenia. Am J Psychiatry 2009; 166(2): 152-63.
[http://dx.doi.org/10.1176/appi.ajp.2008.08030368] [PMID: 19015230]

[75]   Komossa K, Rummel-Kluge C, Schmid F, et al. Aripiprazole versus other atypical antipsychotics for schizophrenia. Cochrane Database Syst Rev 2009; (4): CD006569.
[http://dx.doi.org/10.1002/14651858.CD006569.pub3] [PMID: 19821375]

[76]   Komossa K, Rummel-Kluge C, Schwarz S, et al. Risperidone versus other atypical antipsychotics for schizophrenia. Cochrane Database Syst Rev 2011; (1): CD006626.
[http://dx.doi.org/10.1002/14651858.CD006626.pub2] [PMID: 21249678]

[77]   Milligan G. Mechanisms of multifunctional signalling by G protein-linked receptors. Trends Pharmacol Sci 1993; 14(6): 239-44.
[http://dx.doi.org/10.1016/0165-6147(93)90019-G] [PMID: 8396793]

[78]   Raymond JR. Multiple mechanisms of receptor-G protein signaling specificity. Am J Physiol 1995; 269(2 Pt 2): F141-58.
[PMID: 7653589]

[79]   Urban JD, Clarke WP, von Zastrow M, et al. Functional selectivity and classical concepts of quantitative pharmacology. J Pharmacol Exp Ther 2007; 320(1): 1-13.
[http://dx.doi.org/10.1124/jpet.106.104463] [PMID: 16803859]

[80]   Kane J, Honigfeld G, Singer J, Meltzer H. Clozapine for the treatment-resistant schizophrenic. A double-blind comparison with chlorpromazine. Arch Gen Psychiatry 1988; 45(9): 789-96.
[http://dx.doi.org/10.1001/archpsyc.1988.01800330013001] [PMID: 3046553]

[81]   Kassahun K, Mattiuz E, Franklin R, Gillespie T. Olanzapine 10-nglucuronide: A tertiary n-glucuronide humans. Drug Metab Dispos 1998; 26(9): 848-55.

[82]   Schaber G, Stevens I, Gaertner HJ, Dietz K, Breyer-Pfaff U. Pharmacokinetics of clozapine and its metabolites in psychiatric patients: plasma protein binding and renal clearance. Br J Clin Pharmacol 1998; 46(5): 453-9.
[http://dx.doi.org/10.1046/j.1365-2125.1998.00822.x] [PMID: 9833598]

[83]   2019. https://www.drugs.com/clozapine.html

[84]   Bakken GV, Molden E, Knutsen K, Lunder N, Hermann M. Metabolism of the active metabolite of quetiapine, N-desalkylquetiapine *in vitro*. Drug Metab Dispos 2012; 40(9): 1778-84.
[http://dx.doi.org/10.1124/dmd.112.045237] [PMID: 22688609]

[85]   2019.https://www.drugs.com/mtm/quetiapine.html

[86]   Caccia S, Invernizzi RW, Nobili A, Pasina L. A new generation of antipsychotics: pharmacology and clinical utility of cariprazine in schizophrenia. Ther Clin Risk Manag 2013; 9: 319-28.
[http://dx.doi.org/10.2147/TCRM.S35137] [PMID: 23966785]

[87]   Prakash C, Kamel A, Gummerus J, Wilner K. Metabolism and excretion of a new antipsychotic drug, ziprasidone, in humans. Drug Metab Dispos 1997; 25(7): 863-72.
[PMID: 9224781]

[88]   Leucht S, Cipriani A, Spineli L, *et al.* Comparative efficacy and tolerability of 15 antipsychotic drugs in schizophrenia: a multiple-treatments meta-analysis. Lancet 2013; 382(9896): 951-62.
[http://dx.doi.org/10.1016/S0140-6736(13)60733-3] [PMID: 23810019]

[89]   2018. https://www.drugs.com/mtm/lurasidone.html

[90]   Caccia S, Pasina L, Nobili A. Critical appraisal of lurasidone in the management of schizophrenia. Neuropsychiatr Dis Treat 2012; 8: 155-68.
[http://dx.doi.org/10.2147/NDT.S18059] [PMID: 22570547]

[91]   Sneader W. Drug discovery: a history. New Jersey: John Wiley & Sons 2005.
[http://dx.doi.org/10.1002/0470015535]

[92]   Lombardino JG, Lowe JA III. The role of the medicinal chemist in drug discovery--then and now. Nat Rev Drug Discov 2004; 3(10): 853-62.
[http://dx.doi.org/10.1038/nrd1523] [PMID: 15459676]

CHAPTER 4

Antidepressant Drugs

Horrick Sharma[1], Michaela Leffler[2] and M. O. Faruk Khan[3,*]

[1] Department of Pharmaceutical Sciences, College of Pharmacy, Southwestern Oklahoma State University, Weatherford, OK 73096

[2] Department of Pharmacy Practice, University Charleston School of Pharmacy, Charleston, WV 25304, USA; University of Charleston School of Pharmacy, Charleston, WV 25304, USA

[3] School of Pharmacy, University of Charleston, Charleston, WV 25304, USA

Abstract: This chapter is a comprehensive account of the medicinal chemistry of the antidepressant drugs. It provides the mechanism of drug action and details of the structure-activity relationships (SAR) of the antidepressant and related drugs to give the knowledge base for pharmacists. After a study of this chapter, students will be able to:

• Relate principles of affective disorders including the biogenic amine hypothesis and depression.

• Describe the roles of dopamine, serotonin and norepinephrine in depression and how these roles relate to the mechanism of action of antidepressant drugs.

• Describe different classes of antidepressant drugs with examples.

• Compare the chemical structures of all the classes of antidepressant drugs and relate their action with structures.

• Illustrate the mechanism of action, SAR, metabolites, and clinical considerations of:

▪ Serotonin and norepinephrine reuptake inhibitors

  o Tricyclic antidepressants (TCAs)

  o Phenylalkylamines

▪ Selective serotonin reuptake inhibitors (SSRIs)

  o Phenoxyphenylalkyl amines

* **Corresponding author M. O. Faruk Khan:** School of Pharmacy, University of Charleston, Charleston, WV 25304, USA; Tel: 304-357-4860; E-mail:mdomarkhan@ucwv.edu

M. O. Faruk Khan & Ashok E. Philip (Eds.)

o Phenylalkylamine

• Monoamine oxidase inhibitors (MAOIs)

• Miscellaneous antidepressant drugs

Keywords: Antidepressant drugs, Clinical use of antidepressant Drugs, Drug receptor interaction, Major Depressive Disorder (MDD), Selective Norepinephrine Reuptake Inhibitors (NRIs), Serotonin and Norepinephrine Reuptake Inhibitors (SNRIs) Selective Serotonin Reuptake Inhibitors (SSRIs), Structure-Activity Relationship (SAR).

HISTORICAL PERSPECTIVE

Imipramine was the first TCA discovered in the late 1950s, an era that also saw iproniazid, lithium, meprobamate, and chlordiazepoxide introduced for psychiatric disorders. The history of imipramine and the TCAs is tied to the synthesis of first phenothiazines in 1883 by a German scientist who was working on chemical dyes at a chemical company, Badische Anilin und Soda Fabrik (BASF) [1]. In 1948, phenothiazines were modified to give iminodibenzylic derivatives, such as the compound named **G-22355**. Most of these compounds were found to possess some antihistaminergic and sedative effects with no significant adverse effects in toxicological studies performed on mice. Subsequently, in 1952, chlorpromazine, a phenothiazine derivative, was discovered as an antipsychotic. **G-22355** was tested in clinical research and, being a phenothiazine derivative, was expected to exert a potential antipsychotic effect. However, when tested, **G-22355** lacked any appreciable neuroleptic activity but instead showed marked improvements in patients with depressive psychosis. Structurally, replacing the sulfur of chlorpromazine, a D_2 antagonist, with an ethylene bridge (Fig. **1**) resulted in a compound that demonstrated activity at inhibiting serotonin and norepinephrine reuptake, with little or no dopamine receptor antagonist activity. These changes were probably due to the changes in the ring geometry. The ethylene bridge linking the two phenyl rings in imipramine, and other TCAs, altered the ring geometry and led to less rigid and more conformationally flexible structures than phenothiazines. **G-22355** was renamed imipramine and became the first TCA medication used for the treatment of major depressive disorder (MDD) [2].

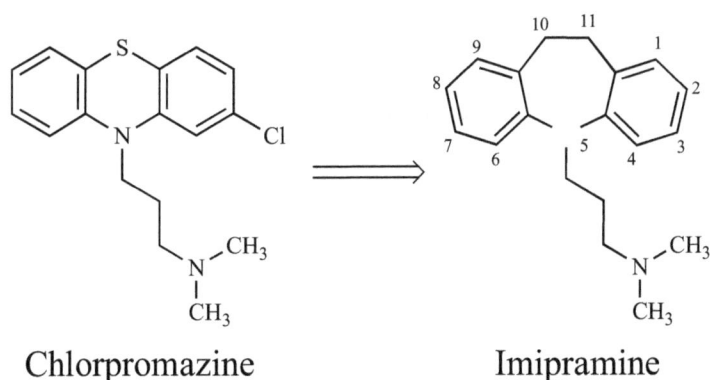

Fig. (1). Development of first-generation antidepressants.

The discovery of TCAs as antidepressants was earlier thought to be due to their ability to potentiate the effects of norepinephrine. Bernard Brodie and Julius Axelrod in studies with laboratory animals showed that imipramine interferes with the uptake of infused norepinephrine into peripheral tissues [3]. However, by the end of the 1960s, studies started to differentiate the effect of secondary and tertiary amine TCAs. Tertiary amine TCAs were found to exert a more powerful inhibition of serotonin uptake than norepinephrine uptake. This effect was even stronger with clomipramine, which possesses an electron-withdrawing chlorine atom on the TCA ring [3]. Further, the antidepressant response of iproniazid, an MAOI, is shown to result in elevated brain levels of both norepinephrine and serotonin. Subsequently, in 1965, Joseph Schildkraut proposed the catecholamine-deficit hypothesis as an explanation for the etiology of depression [4]. In 1969, Russian scientists Izyaslav Lapin and Gregory Oxenkrug of Bekhterev's Psychoneurological Research Institute associated the increased serotonergic 5-HT activity in the brain to the mood-elevation effect of antidepressants, and they suggested that the increased noradrenergic activity was responsible for the motor and energizing effects. This led to the search for selective serotonin reuptake inhibitors (SSRIs) with an aim to target specific 5-HT transporter (SERT) and avoid the undesirable sedative and anticholinergic effects of TCAs. At the Karolinska Institute, Arvid Carlsson examined the effects of antihistamines on both 5-HT and norepinephrine uptake in tissues and developed a pheniramine analog as a potent SSRI in 1971 [5]. This molecule was marketed in Europe as zimelidine in 1982, but it was withdrawn by Astra in the following year because of reports of the Guillaine–Barre´ syndrome in some patients. The second SSRI to be marketed in Europe was indalpine, which contained an indole scaffold to partially mimic the structure of serotonin. Indalpine also was withdrawn shortly after its introduction, as it resulted in agranulocytosis in a few patients. The next SSRI to be introduced was fluvoxamine which did not exhibit the above side effects and thus fueled the search for other SSRIs. In 1974, Bryan Molloy of Eli Lilly made analogs of diphenhydramine and screened them for inhibition of norepinephrine and 5-HT uptake. His research resulted in the discovery of the phenoxyphenylpropyl amine (PPA) core. About 60 PPA derivatives were synthesized, in which subtle structural changes resulted in dramatic variations in selectivity for inhibition of monoamine uptake. The *N*-methyl-phenoxyphenylpropylamine analog turned to be twice as potent at inhibiting the uptake of 5-HT as it was at inhibiting norepinephrine uptake. Further analog synthesis led to the discovery of an SSRI called fluoxetine [6]. The FDA approved fluoxetine on Dec 29th, 1987 and Eli Lilly marketed it in 1988 under the proprietary name Prozac. This medication became the most widely used antidepressant in the U.S. and worldwide. Today, a large number of SSRI antidepressants with differing structures, therapeutic efficacy, and safety are available on the market, with several being the most commonly prescribed medications (Fig. **2**).

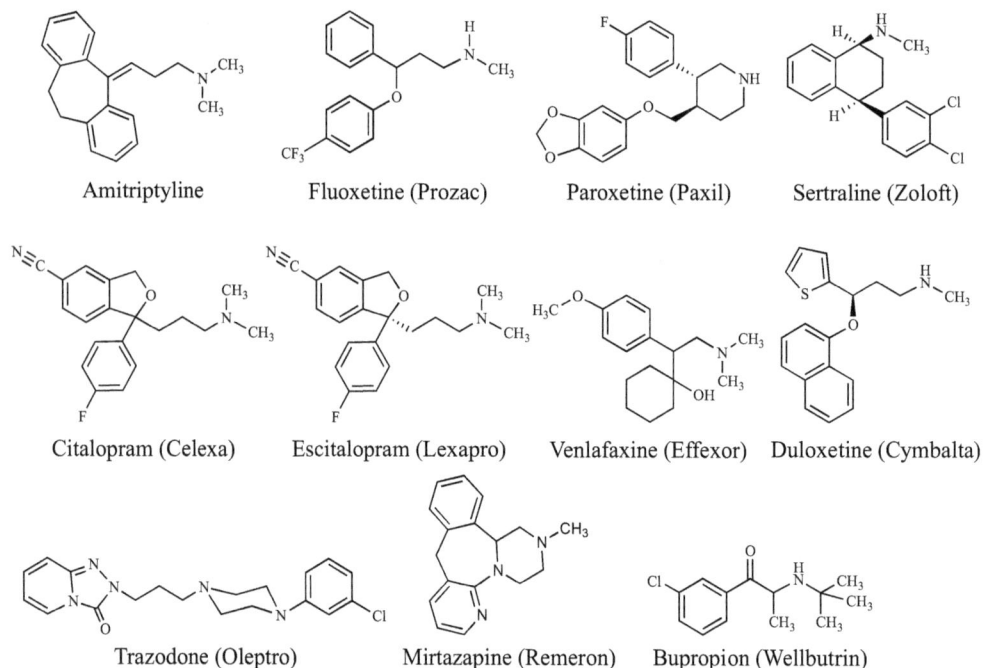

Fig. (2). Antidepressant agents frequently prescribed.

INTRODUCTORY CONCEPTS

Affective Disorders

Affective disorders are also known as mood disorders. The most common affective disorders are MDD and bipolar disorder. MDD is characterized by depressed mood, loss of interest or pleasure in life, sleep disturbances, changes in appetite, feelings of worthlessness, fatigue or less of energy, diminished ability to focus and frequent thoughts of suicide. Depressed patients can also be irritable or anxious. MDD affects over 150 million people worldwide and is associated with high rates of morbidity and mortality.

Pathophysiology - Biogenic Amine Hypothesis

The biogenic amine hypothesis (Fig. **3**) of mood postulates that brain amines, particularly norepinephrine (NE), serotonin (5-HT) and dopamine (DA), and their overlapping roles, are important in the expression of mood. According to this hypothesis, a decrease in the neurotransmission of NE, 5-HT and DA is thought to result in depression; a functional increase of these catecholamines in the brain synapses results in mood elevation [7, 8]. Prefrontal cortex, hippocampus, amygdala, and insula are regions in the brain that are involved in the pathophysiology of MDD. Serotonergic fibers in the brain project from the raphe nuclei in the midbrain to the limbic structures in the forebrain. 5-HT in the CNS is important in regulating sleep, appetite, impulsivity, sexual behavior, and aggression. It is believed that impaired 5-HT neurotransmission can decrease cortical responsiveness to emotional reactions and can lead to depression. The locus coeruleus (LC) is the major NE nucleus of the brain. Noradrenergic fibers are involved in arousal (wakefulness) and autonomic activity which results from a dense population of excitatory projections to most of the cerebral cortex. Reduction of NE is associated with a decrease in alertness, energy and interest. NE has the highest affinity for alpha-2 adrenoceptors (*i.e.* inhibitory), and therefore low-level NE release may inhibit neuronal activity, whereas increased neuronal transmission arising from NE binding to stimulatory alpha-1 and beta-adrenoceptors occurs only at higher NE concentrations [9]. As for dopaminergic fibers, the principle pathway effected is the mesolimbic pathway, sometimes referred to as motivation and the reward pathway of the brain. This pathway connects the ventral tegmental area in the midbrain to the ventral striatum of the basal ganglia in the forebrain. The ventral striatum includes the nucleus accumbens, in which DA regulates one's motivation and desire for reward. The D1 receptor is the most abundant type of DA receptor in the CNS and when activated has a stimulatory response. D1 receptors are located mostly in the basal ganglia followed by the cerebral cortex, hypothalamus and thalamus [10 - 12]. All three monoamines (Fig. **3**) regulate mood, cognition and behavior, while anxiety and depression are mostly associated with a deficit of NE and 5-HT, with a lack of dopamine too contributing to anhedonia, one of the treatment-resistant symptoms of MDD.

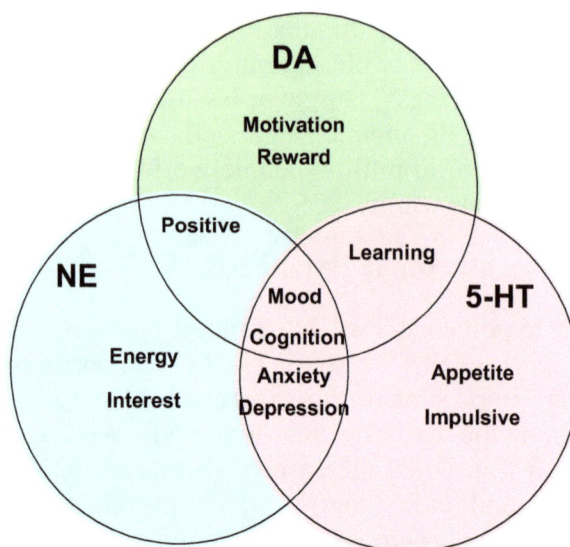

Fig. (3). Role of biogenic amines NE, 5-HT and DA in emotional control involved in depression.

The drugs used in MDD are of varied chemical structures; many have effects that enhance the CNS actions of norepinephrine, serotonin, or both. This biogenic amine hypothesis remains popular because studies have shown that antidepressant medications can alleviate symptoms of MDD by enhancing the actions of NE and 5-HT in the CNS. However, some challenges with this hypothesis include that postmortem brain tissue of patients who suffer from depression does not show evidence of decreased brain levels of NE or 5-HT. Additionally, although antidepressants may cause an increase in the levels of amines in the brain within hours, it typically takes weeks before any clinical effects are achieved. Most antidepressant drugs increase the synaptic concentration of 5-HT, and this leads to the down-regulation of presynaptic 5-HT1A autoreceptors. Evidence supports that this down-regulation of 5-HT1A autoreceptors, in turn may increase the firing rate of serotonergic fibers and thus might be responsible for the delayed therapeutic effects of antidepressant drugs [13, 14].

Classification of Antidepressants

1. Serotonin and norepinephrine reuptake inhibitors (SNRIs)
   i. Tricyclic antidepressants (TCAs).

   ii. Phenylalkylamines
2. Selective norepinephrine reuptake inhibitors (NRIs).
   i. Phenoxyphenylpropylamines
3. Selective serotonin reuptake inhibitors (SSRIs).
   i. Phenoxyphenylalkyl amines
   ii. Phenylalkylamine
4. Monoamine oxidase inhibitors (MAOIs).
5. Miscellaneous agents.

Consequence of Ring Geometry of TCA

The discovery of imipramine through structural modification of phenothiazine (Fig. **1**) resulted in changes in the ring geometry leading to several mechanistic changes [15].

- Dramatic decrease in affinity for the dopamine receptor; most TCAs do not act as dopamine antagonists, while a few have weak dopamine antagonism.
- Increased affinity for the presynaptic norepinephrine and serotonin membrane transporters, NET and SERT, respectively.
- TCAs work by competitively inhibiting the uptake of norepinephrine and serotonin. The large lipophilic ring enhanced the affinity of TCAs to exert multiple pharmacodynamic effects, both centrally and peripherally.

SEROTONIN AND NOREPINEPHRINE REUPTAKE INHIBITORS (SNRIS)

Tricyclic Antidepressants (TCAs)

This class of agents (Fig. **4**) is effective in the treatment of depression but is associated with a high incidence of adverse effects and can cause severe toxicity when taken in excess of recommended daily doses. Due to the high incidence of side effects at doses used for depression, TCA medications are more commonly used for the treatment of disordered sleep in lower doses in the modern-day medicine practice.

Tertiary Amine TCAs

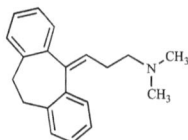

Amitriptyline   Imipramine (Tofranil)   Clomipramine (Anafranil)   Doxepin (Vivactil)

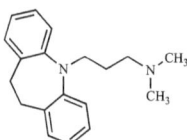

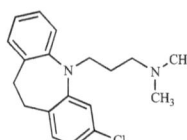

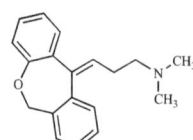

Secondary Amine TCAs

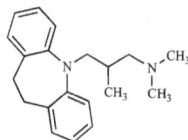

Trimepramine (Surmontil)   Prortryptyline (Vivactil)   Amoxapine (Asendin)   Maprotiline (Ludiomil)

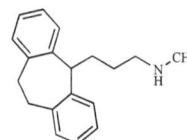

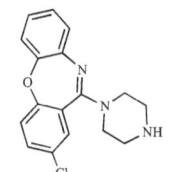

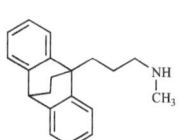

Fig. (4). Tricyclic antidepressants.

Mechanism of Action

All TCAs block the neuronal reuptake of NE and 5-HT, but to differing degrees depending on the agent. For example, tertiary amine TCAs inhibit the reuptake of 5-HT to a greater extent than they do NE reuptake. The blockade of NE and 5-HT reuptake happens as soon as drug administration begins and causes an immediate increase in the synaptic concentration of NE and 5-HT. TCAs produce an antidepressant effect that becomes evident about two weeks after therapy is initiated.

Adverse Effects

TCA medications produce autonomic side effects by blocking muscarinic and alpha-1 adrenoceptors. As a result, these medications produce significant sedation and drowsiness and thus are often administered at low doses at bedtime for the treatment of disordered sleep. Additionally, TCAs can lower the seizure threshold and thus can induce seizures at supratherapeutic concentrations. TCAs are also known to cause increased appetite and excessive weight gain in some patients. Due to the distress this causes some patients, weight gain is reported to be the most common cause for discontinuation of TCA medications [16].

General SAR of TCAs

Features common to all TCAs include: (i) A protonatable nitrogen (ii) Two aromatic rings, and (iii) approximately a 3-carbon distance between the protonatable nitrogen and the central ring of the TCA [17, 18].

Ring Substitutions

- The central ring of TCAs exhibits variations leading to a dihydrodibenzazepine ring (imipramine), its bioisosteric dibenzoxepin ring (doxepin), a dibenzocycloheptene ring (amitriptyline), and a dibenzocycloheptatriene ring (protriptyline).
- Removal of the phenyl ring from the tricyclic core results in total loss of activity.
- Substitutions on the aromatic ring are not required for activity. However, electron-withdrawing groups at position C3 of the dihydrodibenzazepine ring enhance preferential selectivity for SERT inhibition. This is exemplified by clomipramine with a 3-Cl substituent, which is five-times more selective in inhibiting SERT than imipramine. Also, the 3-CN group in 3-cyanoimipramine resulted in greater SERT inhibition. 3-cyanoimipramine was never marketed but was used as a research tool.
- Maprotiline is a tetracyclic derivative and demonstrates the highest selectivity (>100 fold) for inhibition of norepinephrine reuptake.

γ-Nitrogen Substituents

- The side chain containing γ-nitrogen may be attached to any one of the atoms in the central seven-membered ring. The side chain must have three carbons, either saturated (propyl as in imipramine) or unsaturated (as in amitriptyline or doxepin), that is connected to a γ-tertiary or secondary amine.
- The side chain may be fused into a ring system as in amoxapine, which lacks the *N*-methyl group and is related to antipsychotic loxapine. Amoxapine has side effects associated with blockade of dopamine D_2 receptors.
- TCAs inhibit the active reuptake of both norepinephrine and serotonin. However, tertiary amine TCAs have greater serotonin reuptake inhibitory activity than their secondary amine counterparts, which possess greater norepinephrine reuptake inhibition. Inhibitors of serotonin reuptake are more commonly prescribed antidepressants, including SSRIs.
- Among the secondary amine TCAs, the order of *in vitro* selectivity for NET is desipramine>protriptyline>nortriptyline>amoxapine>doxepin.
- Among the tertiary amine TCAs, the order of *in vitro* selectivity for SERT is clomipramine>imipramine>amitriptyline>doxepin.
- Tertiary amine TCAs have greater anticholinergic side effects, sedation, and orthostatic hypotension than secondary amine TCAs. This suggests that the tertiary amine TCAs exert greater effects at muscarinic receptors, H_1 receptors, and α_1 receptors than secondary amine TCAs. Tertiary amine TCAs also have a greater sodium channel blocking effect and, thus greater potential to cause cardiotoxicity.

INDIVIDUAL CLINICALLY USED TCAS

Imipramine (Tofranil™)

Imipramine was the first TCA to be discovered where the sulfur of the phenothiazine ring of antipsychotic chlorpromazine was substituted with a 10-11 ethylene bridge. Imipramine inhibits the reuptake of both serotonin and norepinephrine, but being a tertiary amine TCA, it exhibits greater serotonin reuptake inhibitory activity [19]. Imipramine is well absorbed (>95%) from the small intestine and requires 2-6 h after dosing to attain peak plasma concentrations. Food has no effect on its absorption or peak plasma concentration. In general, tertiary amine TCAs undergo rapid first-pass metabolism that includes hydroxylation on the TCA ring and *N*-demethylation reaction leading to their corresponding secondary amine metabolites. The secondary amine metabolites are more selective for NET inhibition and their plasma concentration usually exceeds their parent counterparts. Imipramine undergoes extensive CYP2C19 and CYP1A2 mediated *N*-demethylation reaction resulting in its secondary amine metabolite, desipramine (Fig. **5**). Imipramine is also metabolized by CYP2D6 catalyzed hydroxylation to its 2- and 10-hydroxylated metabolites and their glucuronide conjugates [20, 21]. The demethylated metabolite desipramine preferentially inhibits NET and exhibits less anticholinergic, antiadrenergic, and sedative side effects than the parent drug imipramine.

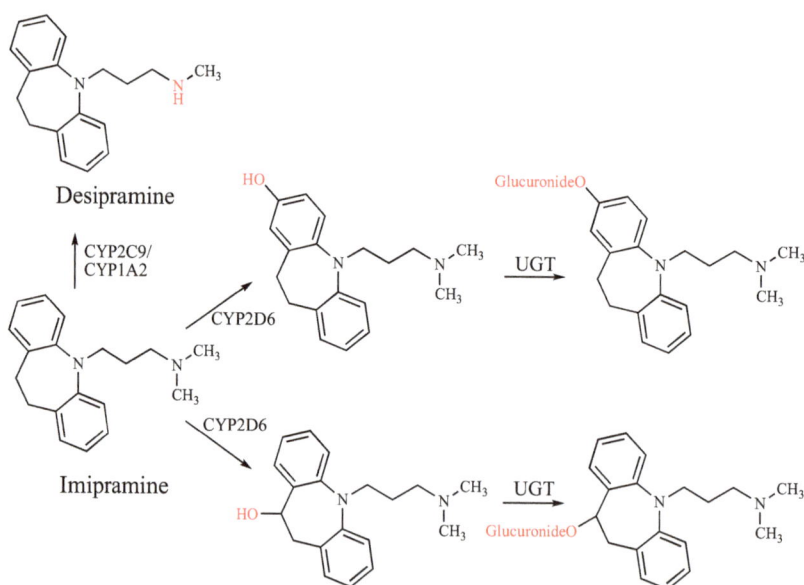

Fig. (5). Metabolic transformation of imipramine.

Clomipramine (Anafranil™)

Clomipramine is a more potent antidepressant than imipramine and exhibits greater selectivity for inhibiting SERT uptake *in vitro* [19]. Clomipramine is well absorbed from the gastrointestinal tract and, being lipophilic, undergoes extensive plasma protein binding (>97%) and has a large apparent volume of distribution (>1000 L). Clomipramine is metabolized mostly by CYP2D6 to its *N*-dealkylated and 2- and 8-hydroxylated metabolites (Fig. **6**). *N*-desmethylclomipramine, being a secondary amine TCA, exhibits greater NET inhibition. Other metabolic transformations include glucuronide conjugation of its hydroxylated metabolite and *N*-oxidation of the tertiary amine. The glucuronide conjugates are excreted in the urine. The *in vivo* antidepressant activity is a result of both the parent drug and its *N*-desmethyl metabolite, having an apparent half-life of 24 h and 96 h, respectively. Clomipramine is indicated for the treatment of patients with obsessive-compulsive disorder (OCD) [22].

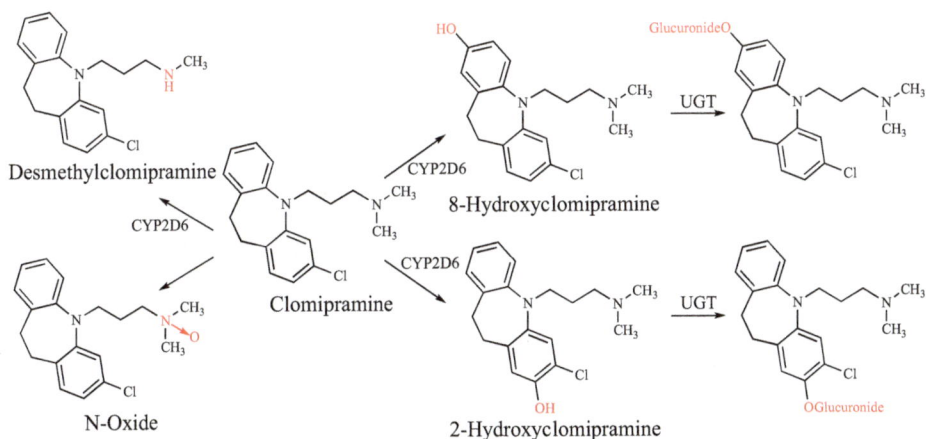

Fig. (6). Metabolic pathway of clomipramine.

Amitriptyline

Amitriptyline has an affinity for both SERT and NET and is almost twice as potent in inhibiting SERT reuptake [19]. Amitriptyline, because of its exocyclic double bond of the propylidene chain, is sensitive to photo-oxidation and should be protected from light [4]. Upon oral administration, amitriptyline is absorbed completely from the gastrointestinal tract and reaches its peak plasma concentration in 4-8 h. Due to its lipophilicity, amitriptyline shows high tissue and plasma protein binding and has large apparent volume of distribution. It is primarily metabolized (Fig. **7**) by CYP2C19/C9 to its active *N*-desmethyl metabolite nortriptyline, which has greater norepinephrine reuptake inhibitory activity. Another metabolic transformation is its CYP2D6-mediated hydroxylation to (*E*)-10 hydroxyl metabolite. The plasma half-life of amitriptyline ranges from 10-28 h, while nortriptyline's half-life is extended to 16 to 80 h [23, 24].

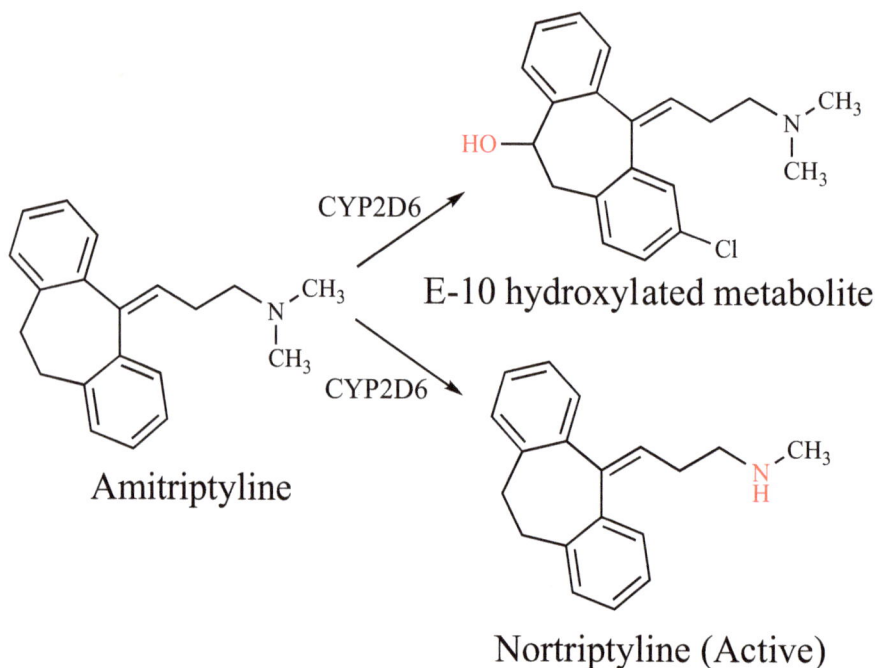

Fig. (7). Metabolism of amitriptyline.

Protriptyline (Vivactil™)

Protriptyline is a secondary amine TCA that has a greater affinity for NET over SERT. It has reduced sedative effects and a faster onset of action than other TCAs. Protriptyline undergoes slow absorption and reaches peak plasma concentrations in 6-12 h. It is highly tissue bound and is less affected by first-pass metabolism (10-25% or oral dose) than other TCA medications [25, 26].

Trimipramine (Surmontil™)

Trimipramine is a derivative of imipramine and possesses a dihydrodibenzazepine ring. Trimipramine has a branched side chain that reduces its affinity for both SERT and NET. Trimipramine is rapidly absorbed following oral administration from the gastrointestinal tract and reaches its peak plasma concentration in 2-4 h. Its elimination half-life is 24 h, which is comparatively shorter than for many other TCAs. The introduction of a methyl group creates an asymmetric center and trimipramine is marketed as a racemic mixture. The (+)- and the (−)-enantiomers of trimipramine are metabolized in a stereoselective manner, with the (+)-trimipramine undergoing an *N*-demethylation reaction *via* CYP2C19 and the (−)-trimipramine enantiomer metabolized selectively to 2-hydroxytriimipramine by CYP2D6 (Fig. **8**). Further, genetic polymorphisms in CYP2D6 and CYP2C19 result in variations in pharmacokinetics and plasma drug concentrations. Trimipramine, because of its tertiary amine, has the same anticholinergic and sedative side effects as other similar TCAs but is unique in that it lacks β-adrenergic activity [20, 27].

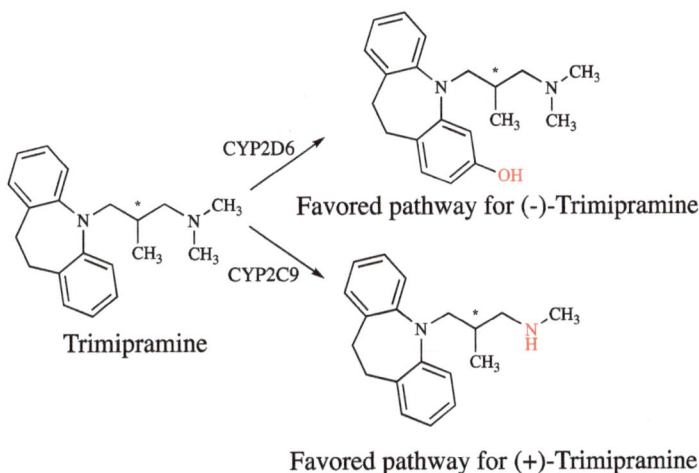

Favored pathway for (-)-Trimipramine

Trimipramine

Favored pathway for (+)-Trimipramine

Fig. (8). Metabolism of trimipramine.

Doxepin (Prudoxin™)

Doxepin is a tertiary amine dibenzoxazepine derivative with oxygen replacing one of the ethylene carbons in the bridge. The oxygen introduces asymmetry into the tricyclic ring system, resulting in the generation of *E*-(trans) and *Z*(cis)- geometric stereoisomers. Doxepin is a mixture of *E-Z* (85:15) isomers, where the (*E*)-isomer inhibits NET while the (*Z*)-isomer causes inhibition of SERT. Doxepin is metabolized primarily by CYP2D6 and CYP2C9 to its major active metabolite desmethyldoxepin (Fig. **9**) [18, 28].

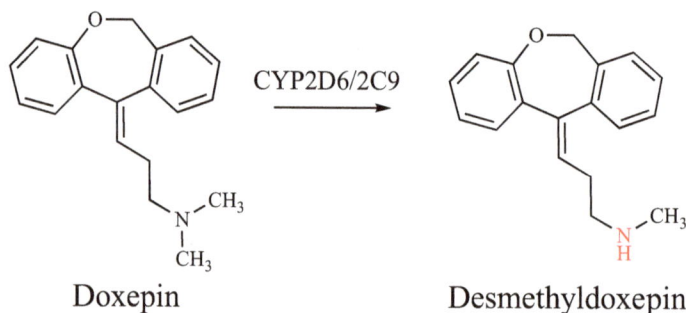

Doxepin   Desmethyldoxepin

Fig. (9). Metabolism of doxepin.

Maprotiline (Ludiomil™)

Maprotiline contains a tetracyclic ring with a central lipophilic carbocyclic bicyclooctadiene ring. Maprotiline is completely absorbed from the gastrointestinal tract upon oral administration and attains peak drug concentration in 8-24 h. Maprotiline is metabolized (Fig. **10**) by CYP2D6/ CYP2C19 to its major metabolite *N*-desmethylmaprotiline [29]. Maprotiline is also shown to undergo oxidative deamination, *N*-oxidation, aromatic and aliphatic hydroxylation and is excreted mostly as glucuronide conjugates. Maprotiline is highly selective for NET and does not exhibit anticholinergic side effects. Maprotiline is associated with cardiovascular side effects and has greater stimulatory effects that can lead to seizures in a dose-dependent manner [30].

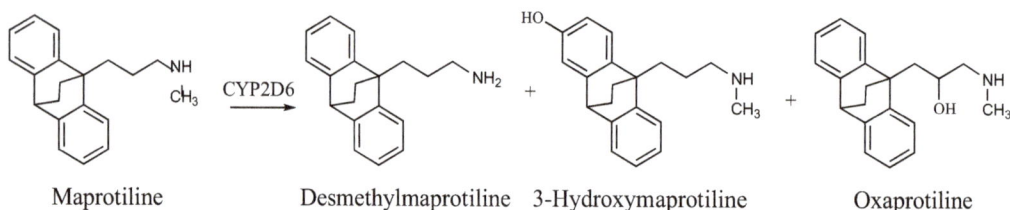

Maprotiline   Desmethylmaprotiline   3-Hydroxymaprotiline   Oxaprotiline

Fig. (10). Metabolism of maprotiline.

Amoxapine (Asendin™)

Amoxapine is an antidepressant that is also an *N*-desmethyl metabolite of the antipsychotic medication loxapine [31]. Amoxapine exhibits antipsychotic effects through its blockade of D_2 receptors. In amoxapine, the propylamine side chain is cyclized into a piperazine ring. Although amoxapine has similar effects as other secondary amine TCAs, its potency for inhibition of NET is comparatively weaker than other secondary amine TCAs. Amoxapine is rapidly absorbed from the gastrointestinal tract and reaches its peak plasma concentration within 3 h. Amoxapine has a half-life of 5-6 h and is metabolized by hydroxylation to its active 8- and 7-hydroxylated metabolites [32].

PHENYLALKYLAMINE SNRIS

Phenylalkylamine SNRI medications are commonly used in the modern-day treatment of depression and anxiety disorders. SNRI medications currently available on the market include venlafaxine, desvenlafaxine, duloxetine, and milnacipram. Among the nontricyclic phenylalkylamine SNRIs (Fig. **11**), *in vitro* and *in vivo* preclinical studies demonstrated that duloxetine is more potent than milnacipram, which is more potent than venlafaxine at inhibition of norepineprine and serotonin reuptake. SNRIs lack strong electron-withdrawing groups on the phenyl ring, unlike SSRI medications, that greatly decreases their affinity for SERT and allows norepipneprine reuptake inhibition, giving them their SNRI profile. However, similar to SSRIs, the opening of the tricyclic ring structure results in lower anticholinergic, antihistaminic, and antiadrenergic side effects compared to TCAs [18].

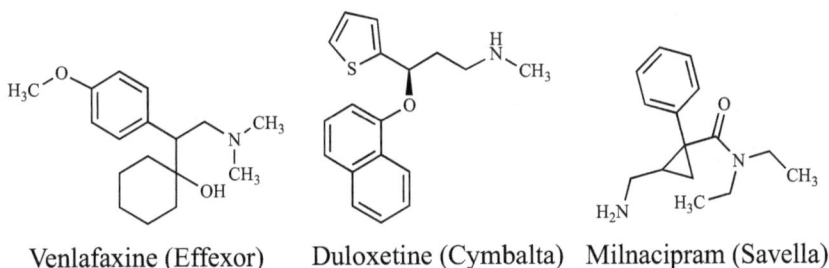

Venlafaxine (Effexor)   Duloxetine (Cymbalta)   Milnacipram (Savella)

Fig. (**11**). Phenylalkylamines antidepressants.

Venlafaxine (Effexor™)

Venlafaxine inhibits the reuptake of both serotonin and norepinephrine and was the first SNRI medication marketed in the U.S [5]. Venlafaxine has about 30 folds higher affinity at inhibiting SERT over NET [33]. Venlafaxine is well absorbed (90%) but has poor bioavailability of 15%. Venlafaxine has a short half-life of 4 h and it is associated with significant withdrawal symptoms that can occur within hours of discontinuation or a missed dose of the medication. Venlafaxine undergoes extensive first-pass hepatic metabolism, primarily by CYP2D6, to its major active *O*-desmethyl metabolite desvenlafaxine (Fig. **12**). Desvenlafaxine is also an SNRI medication available on the market. It has greater potency for SERT inhibition over NET. Other metabolic transformations involve a CYP3A4 mediated *N*-demthylation reaction. High variability in intrinsic oral clearance, four-folds less in poor metabolizers than in extensive metabolizers, of venlafaxine was observed due to CYP2D6 polymorphism. Venlafaxine is a weak inhibitor of CYP2D6 and, as a precaution, concurrent use of medications metabolized by CYP2D6 should be monitored for side effects and efficacy [34 - 36].

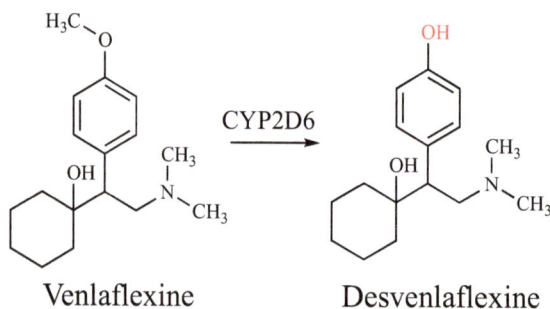

Fig. (12). Metabolism of venlafaxine.

Milnacipran (Savella™)

Milnacipran contains two asymmetric centers and is a racemic mixture of cis-isomers *d*-milnacipran (1*S*,2*R*) and *l*-milnacipran (1*R*,2*S*). Although the drug is used as a racemic mixture, the *d*-isomer is active and has a longer half-life than the 'inactive' *l*-isomer. Milnacipran acts by inhibiting the reuptake of both NE and 5-HT with equal potency [33]. Milnacipran has fewer known adverse effects than TCAs and SSRIs. It is rapidly absorbed and has high oral bioavailability (85%). Most of the administered drug is eliminated either unchanged in urine or as its *N*-glucuronide conjugate. Enzymes of the CYP class do not play a role in its metabolism, and the risk of interactions with drugs metabolized by CYP enzymes is minimal [37].

Duloxetine (Cymbalta™)

Duloxetine, marketed as a pure (*S*)-enantiomer, is a dual inhibitor of both SERT and NET with a 10-fold preference for the SERT [33]. Duloxetine is well absorbed and attains its peak plasma concentration in ~6 h of dosing. It has a large volume of distribution (1640 L) and an elimination half-life of 10-12 h. Duloxetine is *N*-demethylated by CYP2D6 to its active metabolite, *N*-desmethylduloxetine (Fig. **13**). Other metabolic transformations involve hydroxylation of the naphthyl ring at the 4-, 5-, or 6-positions by CYP1A2, which gets excreted in urine as phase II sulfate, glucuronide and *O*-methylated conjugates. Co-administration of a CYP1A2 inhibitor, such as fluvoxamine, is shown to cause clinically significant increases in duloxetine concentrations.

Duloxetine is a moderate inhibitor of CYP2D6 and co-administration of CYP2D6 metabolized drugs should be monitored [38].

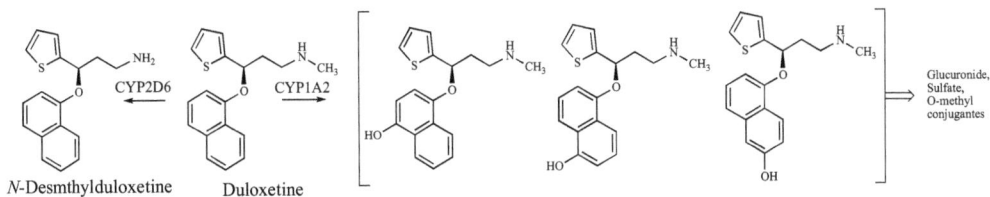

Fig. (13). Metabolism of duloxetine.

SELECTIVE NOREPINEPHRINE REUPTAKE INHIBITOR (NRIS)

Phenoxyphenylpropylamines (Fig. 14)

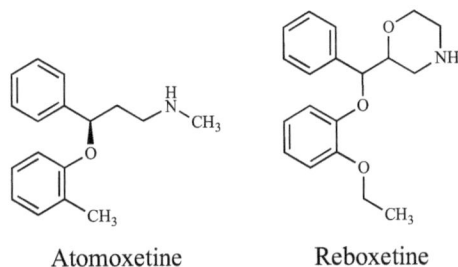

Atomoxetine   Reboxetine

Fig. (14). Phenoxyphenylpropylamine antidepressants.

This class of antidepressant drugs targets NE, as this neurotransmitter has long been thought to play a key role in the etiology of depression. In the clinical setting, selective NRIs may be advantageous in terms of short- and long-term efficacy and motivation in depressed patients but are also approved for the treatment of ADHD.

Mechanism of Action

NRI medications, such as atomoxetine, are highly selective NE reuptake inhibitors that increase intrasynaptic NE levels by blocking the norepinephrine transporter. This class of antidepressants can cause dose-dependent increases in extracellular levels of NE in the frontal cortex and hippocampus. In the LC, high concentrations of NRI agents such as reboxetine can inhibit the firing activity of brainstem NE neurons. This inhibition of NE neurons is thought to be mediated by somatodendritic alpha-2 adrenoceptors, as the inhibition of NE neurons caused by reboxetine can be reversed by alpha-2 antagonists.

Adverse Effects

Common side effects of NRIs such as atomoxetine include nausea/vomiting, insomnia, anxiety, agitation, increase in blood pressure, dizziness, dry mouth and drowsiness. If used for the treatment of depression, clinical studies have shown increased efficacy and remission of depression when used in combination with SSRI medications than if either agent is used alone.

Atomoxetine (Strattera™)

Atomoxetine is a selective norepinephrine reuptake inhibitor (NRI) having an electron-donating methyl group at the 2- (*ortho*) position, which provides selectivity for inhibition of norepinephrine reuptake over serotonin reuptake [18]. Atomoxetine, like fluoxetine, has a phenoxyphenylpropylamine pharmacophore, but the lack of a strong electron-withdrawing group on the phenoxy ring at the 4-position results in its reduced potency at SERT. Atomoxetine is used in the U.S. for the treatment of attention-deficit hyperactivity disorder (ADHD) and has an advantage over other medications used for this purpose such that it is not a habit-forming medication. The (*R*)-enantiomer is 9 times more potent than the (*S*)-enantiomer as an inhibitor of NET. Atomoxetine is rapidly and completely absorbed after oral administration and reaches peak plasma concentrations within 1-2 h of administration. Absolute oral bioavailability ranges from 63%-94% in poor and extensive metabolizers, respectively. Atomoxetine is highly bound to plasma albumin (99%) and has an elimination half-life of 3-7 h in extensive metabolizers, which could be prolonged to 21 h in poor metabolizers. Atomoxetine is metabolized (Fig. **15**) primarily by CYP2D6 to its major active metabolite 4-hydroxyatomoxetine, which undergoes *O*-glucuronide conjugation before elimination in urine [39].

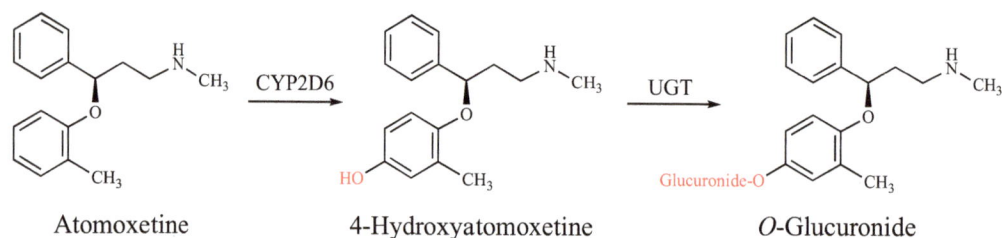

| Atomoxetine | 4-Hydroxyatomoxetine | *O*-Glucuronide |

Fig. (15). Metabolic transformation of atomoxetine.

Reboxetine (Edronax™)

Reboxetine is a selective norepinephrine reuptake inhibitor in which the propylamine side chain of atomoxetine is constrained into a morpholine ring. Like atomoxetine, reboxetine has an electron-donating, methoxy, substitution at the

2-(*ortho*)-position on the phenoxy ring and preferentially inhibits the reuptake of norepinephrine over serotonin [18]. Reboxetine is approved in Europe for the treatment of MDD. It is marketed as a racemic mixture of the *(R,R)-(−)-* and *(S,S)*-(+)-isomers of reboxetine. The *(S,S)*-(+)-enantiomer is two-fold more potent than its *(R,R)*-enantiomer. Reboxetine is well absorbed after oral administration with an absolute oral bioavailability of 94% and attains maximum plasma levels within 2-4 h. It is highly bound to plasma proteins (>97%), primarily to α1-acid glycoprotein, and has a volume of distribution of 32 L after oral administration. Reboxetine undergoes significant metabolic transformation and only 10% of the drug is detected unchanged in the urine. The metabolism of reboxetine is mediated primarily *via* CYP3A4 with *O*-desethylreboxetine being the major metabolite (Fig. **16**). The plasma half-life is ~12 h, which could be prolonged to 24 h in elderly patients and in patients with hepatic insufficiency [40].

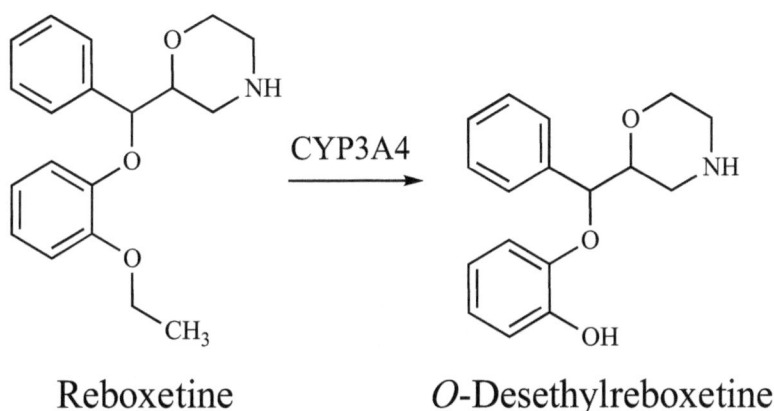

Reboxetine   *O*-Desethylreboxetine

Fig. (16). Metabolism of reboxetine.

SELECTIVE SEROTONIN REUPTAKE INHIBITORS (SSRIS)

SSRIs have become the most widely used medications for the treatment of depression. SSRIs are shown to be comparable or less effective than amitriptyline and TCAs. However, they are more popular than TCAs owing to their better tolerability and lower rates of treatment discontinuation due to undesirable side effects. SSRI medications are also approved for other treatment indications such as anxiety and OCD.

Mechanism of Action

SSRIs selectively block the neuronal reuptake of 5-HT and have less effect on the reuptake of NE. The efficacy of SSRIs supports the hypothesis that 5-HT dysfunction plays a significant role in the pathophysiology of depression.

Adverse Effects

SSRIs produce fewer sedative, autonomic and cardiovascular side effects compared to TCAs. Unlike TCAs, SSRIs are usually administered in the morning because they can increase alertness and if administered at bedtime, they may interfere with sleep. Common side effects include nervousness, dizziness and insomnia. In male patients, side effects also include sexual dysfunction in the forms of priapism and impotence, while in female patients, decreased libido is observed.

Phenoxyphenylalkylamines

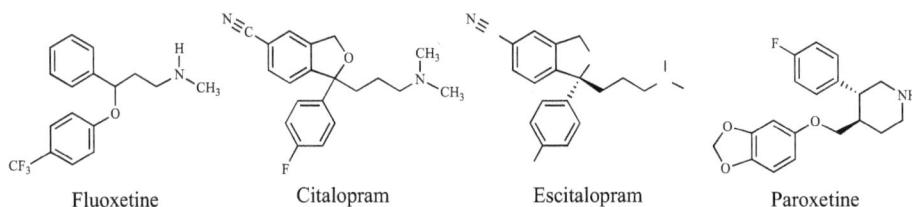

Fluoxetine   Citalopram   Escitalopram   Paroxetine

Fig. (17). Phenoxyphenylalkylamines antidepressants.

SAR of Phenoxyphenylalkylamines

• SSRIs (Fig. **17**) are derived from the opening of the TCA ring structure. Opening of the ring significantly reduces the steric bulkiness of the molecule, which appears to be a major basis for the relatively lower rate of anticholinergic, antihistaminic, and antiadrenergic activities of SSRIs compared to TCAs.
• The presence of strong electron-withdrawing substituents on the phenyl or the phenoxy ring is the basis for SERT inhibition selectivity. These substitutions are primarily at the 4-*para* position, although 3-*meta* substitutions are also tolerated.

Fluoxetine (Prozac™)

Fluoxetine is marketed as a racemic mixture of *(R)*- and *(S)*-fluoxetine. Fluoxetine selectivity for SERT inhibition depends on the position of the substituent on the phenoxy ring. Substitution of trifluoromethyl, an electron-withdrawring group, at the 4-*para* position confers fluoxetine affinity and selectivity for inhibition of serotonin reuptake [27]. Both enantiomers of fluoxetine have similar potency as inhibitors of serotonin reuptake both in *in vitro* and *in invo* uptake assays. Fluoxetine enantiomers are metabolized primarily by CYP2D6 *via* N-demethylation to their active desmethyl metabolite, *(R)*- and *(S)*-norfluoxetine (Fig. **18**). The *(S)*-norfluoxetine enantiomer is 1.5 fold more potent than the *(R)*-isomer in inhibiting serotonin reuptake [41]. Other minor metabolic transformations include *O*-delkylation reaction resulting in the inactive alcohol and keto metabolites. Both (*R*)- and (*S*)-norfluoxetine is less potent than the corresponding enantiomers of fluoxetine as inhibitors of NE uptake. Fluoxetine is well absorbed upon oral administration, is highly protein-bound (94%) and has a large volume of distribution (20-42 L/Kg). Although there can be a potential concern for drug-drug interactions, displacement of plasma bound drug is not shown to be clinically significant for fluoxetine. Maximum plasma half-life is reached within 4-8 h of oral administration. Fluoxetine has a long elimination half-life of 4-6 days, while norfluoxetine has an elimination half-life of 7-15 days. This long half-life confers an absence of withdrawal symptoms upon immediate discontinuation of the medication, a unique characteristic of fluoxetine among its SSRI counterparts. Concentrations of fluoxetine and norfluoxetine do not linearly follow their dose as they can inhibit their own metabolism. Fluoxetine and norfluoxetine are CYP2D6 inhibitors that can lead to an increase in their concentration. Therefore, when switching from fluoxetine to an MAOI medication, a washout period of at least 5 weeks should be given or a lower dose could be recommended [18]. Fluoxetine exhibits nonlinear pharmacokinetics and should be used with caution in patients with hepatic insufficiency [42, 23].

Disorder (OCD)

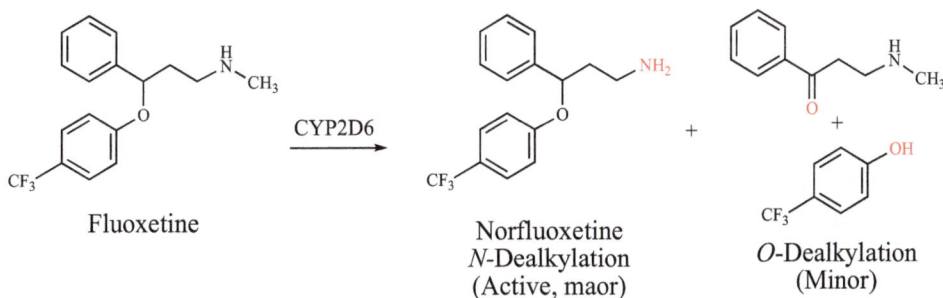

Fig. (18). Metabolic transformation of fluoxetine.

Paroxetine (Paxil™)

Paroxetine (Fig. **19**) has a phenylpropylamine side-chain constrained into a piperidine ring. Paroxetine is the most potent SSRI with no or minimal effects on dopamine and norepinephrine transporters. Paroxetine is 300 times more selective in blocking the reuptake of serotonin over that of norepinephrine [44]. Paroxetine has two chiral centers and is marketed as a single (3*S*,4*R*)-(−)-enantiomer. Paroxetine is almost completely absorbed from the gastrointestinal tract following oral administration, is widely distributed to tissues, and binds strongly to plasma proteins (93%-95%). High plasma protein binding is a cause of concern, but a change in its pharmacokinetics may not be clinically very significant. Compared to other SSRIs, paroxetine has a shorter plasma elimination half-life of 21 h, and as a result, a number of withdrawal symptoms upon discontinuation of the drug are observed. Paroxetine undergoes extensive first-pass metabolism with less than 50% of the dose reaching systemic circulation. Paroxetine is primarily metabolized by CYP2D6 (80%) *via* oxidative reaction to an inactive catechol intermediate, which is eliminated in urine as *O*-glucuronide conjugate Fig. (**19**). The catechol intermediate can also be converted to its ortho-quinoid metabolite that can react with nucleophilic centers of macromolecules causing hepatotoxicity. Paroxetine is a mechanism-based inhibitor of CYP2D6. Putative mechanism involves hydroxylation of the 1,3-dioxolane ring followed by abstraction of water from the hydroxymethylene metabolite to give a carbene intermediate that chelates with the iron (II) of the heme of CYP2D6. This is different from fluoxetine, whose inhibition of CYP2D6 is not mechanism-based. This increases the likelihood of a potential drug-drug interaction if paroxetine is coadministered with drugs metabolized by CYP2D6. For example, co-administration of paroxetine with imipramine or trimipramine is shown to cause reduced oral clearance and increased plasma concentrations of imipramine or trimipramine [44, 45].

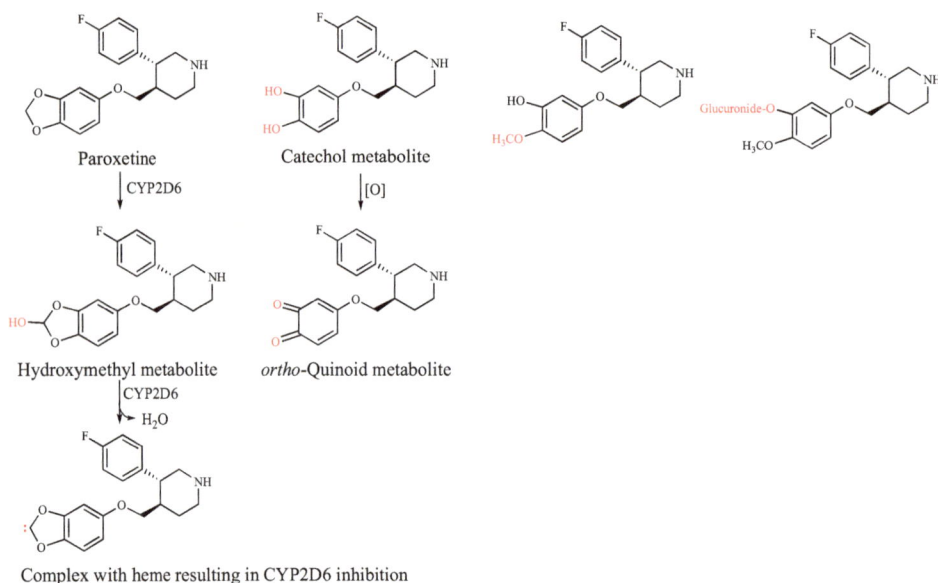

Complex with heme resulting in CYP2D6 inhibition

Fig. (19). Metabolism of paroxetine.

Citalopram (Celexa™)

Citalopram is a benzonitrile derivative (Fig. **20**). Among SSRIs, citalopram exhibits the greatest *in vitro* selectivity, about 2900 times, for inhibition of serotonin reuptake [41]. Citalopram consists of a chiral center and is marketed as a racemic mixture. In addition, its pure (*S*)-enantiomer, escitalopram, is also available. Therapeutic activity of racemic citalopram resides in the *S*-(+--enantiomer, which is 2-fold and 27 times more potent than the racemate and the (*R*)-enantiomer, respectively. Citalopram has an oral bioavailability of about 80%, likely due to its high lipophilicity and greater absorption. Escitalopram is rapidly absorbed after oral administration and attains a peak plasma concentration within 3-4 h of administration. Unlike other SSRIs, citalopram and escitalopram do not bind extensively to plasma proteins (56%) and are less likely to exhibit interactions due to the displacement of the drug from plasma protein. Escitalopram has an elimination half-life of 27-33 h, while citalopram has a half-life of about 37 h. Citalopram and escitalopram are metabolized to their significantly less active *N*-desmethyl metabolites (Fig. **20**) *via* enzymes CYP2C19, CYP2D6, and CYP3A4. Other metabolic transformations include MAO catalyzed oxidative deamination reactions yielding aldehyde metabolites that could be oxidized to their propionic acid derivatives [46 - 48].

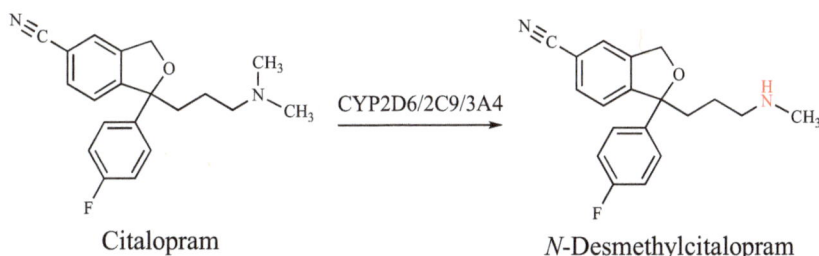

Citalopram → CYP2D6/2C9/3A4 → *N*-Desmethylcitalopram

Fig. (20). Metabolism of citalopram.

Phenylalkylamines

Sertraline (Zoloft™)

Sertraline has an alkylamine moiety constrained in a bicyclic phenylaminotetralin ring system. Sertraline is an SSRI that demonstrates 73 times greater selectivity for inhibition of serotonin reuptake than norepinephrine uptake [41]. Sertraline has two chloro substituents that increase SERT affinity. Sertraline contains two chiral centers and thus can exist in four possible stereoisomers; however, the *cis* (1*S*),(4*S*)-(+)-diastereomer is the one that is more potent and marketed. Sertraline is slowly absorbed upon oral administration and undergoes extensive first-pass metabolism by multiple CYP enzymes with contributions from CYP2B6, CYP2C9, CYP2C19, CYP2D6, and CYP3A4. A major metabolic transformation involves the formation of desmethylsertraline that is substantially less potent than the parent drug (Fig. **21**). Sertraline also undergoes MAO catalyzed oxidative deamination to its corresponding carbonyl derivative. Sertraline is extensively protein bound (98%) and co-administration of sertraline with highly plasma bound drugs can potentially result in proposed drug-drug interactions [49, 50]. However, for SSRIs, such interactions are rarely clinically significant.

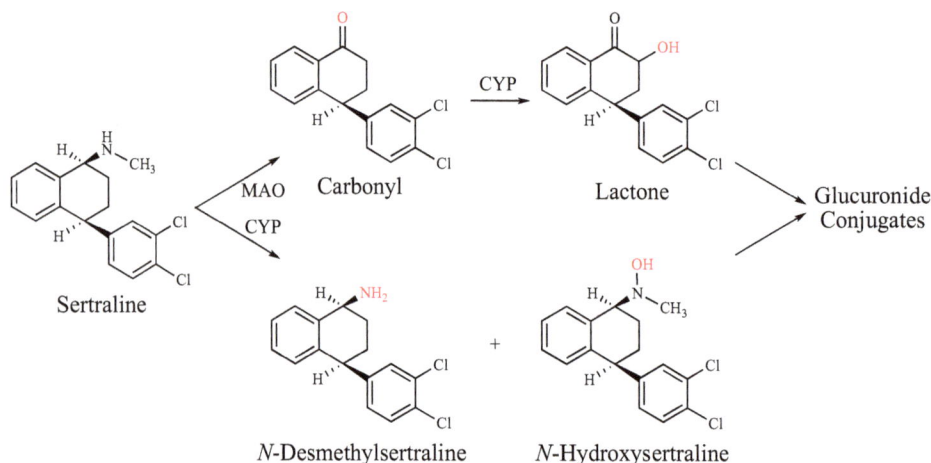

Fig. (21). Metabolism of sertraline.

Fluvoxamine (Luvox™)

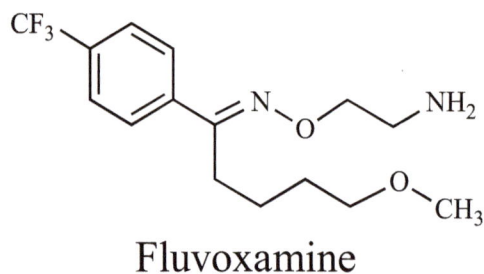

Fluvoxamine

Fig. (22). Structure of Fluvoxamine.

Fluvoxamine (Fig. **22**) is a non-tricyclic selective inhibitor of serotonin reuptake. The C=N double bond results in geometric isomerism in fluvoxamine. The 4-*para* substituted electron-withdrawing trifluoromethyl (CF$_3$) group imparts SERT affinity and selectivity. Fluvoxamine solutions should be protected from sunlight since UV-B light can lead to photoisomerization of the inactive (Z)-isomer [18]. Fluvoxamine is completely but slowly absorbed from the gastrointestinal tract and reaches peak plasma concentration in 2-8 h following oral administration.

Fluvoxamine does not extensively bind to plasma proteins (77%) and is unlikely to cause clinically relevant drug-drug interactions due to the displacement of protein-bound drugs. It is extensively metabolized and only 4% of the drug is excreted unchanged in urine. The plasma half-life of fluvoxamine is 15-20 h. Major metabolic transformation includes CYP2D6 catalyzed oxidative *O*-demethylation to the corresponding alcohol metabolite, which is subsequently oxidized to fluvoxamine acid. Fluvoxamine is a weak inhibitor of CYP2D6 and CYP3A4 [51, 52].

MONOAMINE OXIDASE INHIBITORS (MAOIS)

This class of agents has many potentially serious interactions with other drugs and food, and as a result, they are not considered drugs of choice in the treatment of depression. MAOIs are therefore often considered as an alternative form of therapy when patients have failed to respond to first-line therapies for depression and therefore have treatment-resistant depression.

Mechanism of Action

MAOIs bind irreversibly to the enzyme monoamine oxidase (MAO) which is responsible for the degradation of the biogenic amine neurotransmitters, NE, DA and 5-HT. The binding of MAOIs to MAO prevents the substrate from reaching the active site of the enzyme and increases the concentration of NE, DA and 5-HT in storage sites throughout the CNS. MAOIs are classified based on their selectivity for the two main types of MAOs; MAO-A mostly oxidizes 5-HT but can also metabolize NE and DA and MAO-B is responsible for the metabolism of DA. For this reason, the antidepressant effects of MAOI medications are believed to be due to the inhibition of MAO-A.

Adverse Effects

The major adverse effect reported with this class of antidepressant drugs is a hypertensive crisis. This crisis is characterized by some or sometimes all of the following symptoms: heart palpitations, headaches, neck stiffness, nausea/vomiting, sweating and photophobia. A hypertensive crisis can occur alone with MAOIs or following the administration of a sympathomimetic amine or food containing tyramine. These foods include many types of cheese, beer, some wines, some meats and fish. SSRIs, SNRIs, and TCAs should not be taken with MAOIs as both classes of drugs increase 5-HT levels in the brain and concurrent use can precipitate the serotonin syndrome. This syndrome is characterized by confusion, insomnia, seizures, hypertension, restlessness and agitation. MAOIs interact with SSRIs, TCAs and other antidepressant drugs and have the potential to cause severe toxicity when administered together.

Phenelzine and Tranylcypromine

Isoniazid is an antitubercular agent that results in the elevation of mood in patients with tuberculosis. Thus, in search of compounds with antidepressant properties, derivatives of isoniazid were synthesized. One of these derivatives was iproniazid, which possessed both antitubercular and antidepressant properties. Although iproniazid was not marketed due to hepatotoxicity, its antidepressant effect was associated with its ability to inhibit the MOA enzyme. MOA enzymes carry out the oxidative deamination reaction of amine-containing substrates, including the neutrotransmiters epinephrine, norepinephrine, dopamine, and serotonin. Further exploration of MAOIs led to the synthesis of hydrazine and non-hydrazine derivatives as antidepressant agents (Fig. **23**). Phenelzine and tranylcypromine are available for MDD. Both are irreversible inhibitors of MAO-A and MAO-B enzymes and cause an increase in free 5-HT and NE levels in the CNS, which is responsible for their antidepressant effect. Non-selective MAO-A and MAO-B agents are associated with several side effects and have the potential to cause hypertensive crises, following the ingestion of food rich in tyramine. Inhibition of MAO-A results in increases in the concentration of tyramine, an indirect sympathomimetic, which potentiates the release of catecholamines resulting in a rapid increase in blood pressure. For this reason, they rarely are a drug of first choice [53, 54].

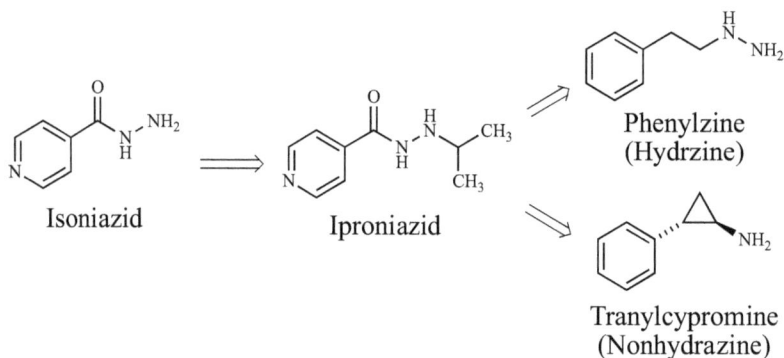

Fig. (23). Monoamine oxidase inhibitors.

MISCELLANEOUS AGENTS

Trazodone (Desyrel™)

Trazodone is a dual serotonin receptor (5-HT2) antagonist and serotonin reuptake inhibitor (SRI). Trazodone's efficacy is comparable to several SSRIs, including fluoxetine, paroxetine, and sertraline in relieving symptoms of MDD [55]. However, its use for depression is limited due to drowsiness being one of the most common side effects. Therefore, it is most commonly used as an off label-hypnotic for insomnia at low doses. Trazodone is rapidly absorbed after oral administration with an oral bioavailability of 65% and time to peak plasma concentration of about 1 h [56]. Trazodone has a mean elimination half-life of 3-6 h and is mostly metabolized by CYP3A4 catalyzed oxidative hydroxylation, *N*-dealkylation and *N*-oxidation reactions followed by conjugation reactions (Fig. **24**). m-chlorophenylpiperazine (mCPP) is the major active metabolite of trazodone that has stimulant and hallucinogenic properties [57, 58]. Use of trazodone is associated with hepatotoxicity, possibly due to its reactive epoxide and iminoquinone metabolites. Being a CYP3A4 substrate, co-administration of trazodone with a CYP3A4 inducer or inhibitor should be monitored.

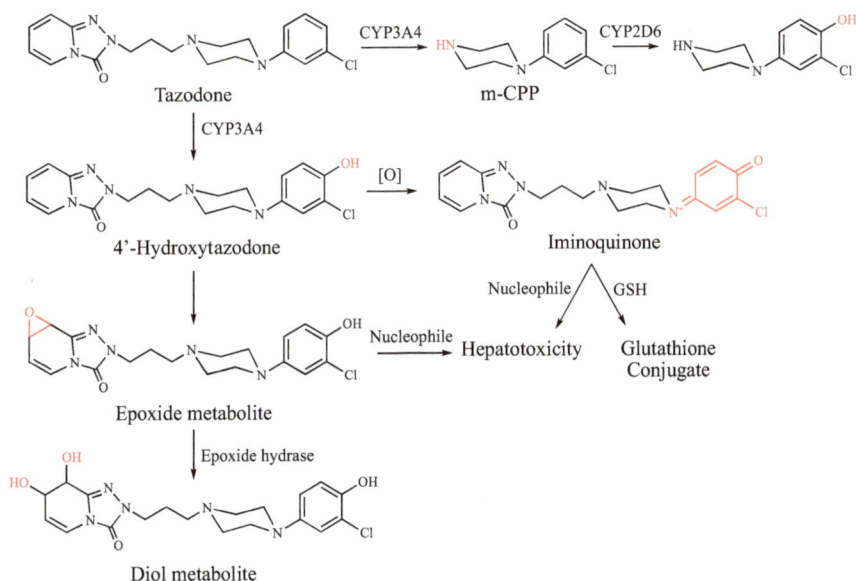

Fig. (24). Metabolism of trazodone.

Mirtazapine (Remeron™)

Mirtazapine is a noradrenergic and specific serotonergic antidepressant (NASSA) marketed as a racemic mixture [59]. Its efficacy is similar to TCAs and other antidepressants and SSRIs. It is rapidly well absorbed and attains peak plasma concentration within 2 h after oral administration. It has an elimination half-life of 20-40 h and is metabolized by CYP2D6/1A4 to 8-hydroxymirtazapine and by CYP3A4 to its *N*-desmethyl and *N*-oxide metabolites, followed by glucuronide conjugation (Fig. **25**). The (−)(*R*)-enantiomer attains greater peak plasma concentration as its elimination half-life is twice as long as the (+)(*S*)-enantiomer [60]. Common side effects of mirtazapine include an increase in appetite and somnolence. As a result, this medication is commonly used in older adults with depression, as the symptoms of depression in this population often include sleep disturbances and a decrease in appetite.

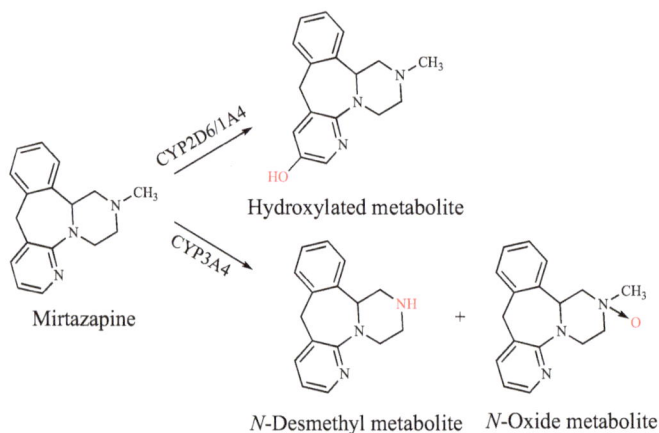

Fig. (25). Metabolism of mirtazapine.

Bupropion (Wellbutrin™)

Bupropion is marketed as a racemic mixture. The antidepressant effects of bupropion are mediated by inhibition of the reuptake of noradrenaline and dopamine (NDRI) [61]. Bupropion is also a nicotine antagonist and is marketed for smoking cessation, as well. Bupropion does not exhibit clinically significant sedative or anticholinergic side effects. It is well absorbed after oral administration and attains a peak plasma concentration within 2-3 h [62]. It also exhibits biphasic pharmacokinetics with a mean terminal phase half-life of 14 h and a mean distribution phase half-life of 3-4 h. Bupropion is a major substrate of CYP2B6. The (S)-isomer is selectively hydroxylated by CYP2B6 to an active and major metabolite hydroxybupropion, which undergoes cyclization to a morpholinol metabolite (Fig. 26). Therefore, concomitant use of bupropion with CYP2B6 inhibitors/inducers should be monitored. Bupropion is also a strong inhibitor of CYP2D6.

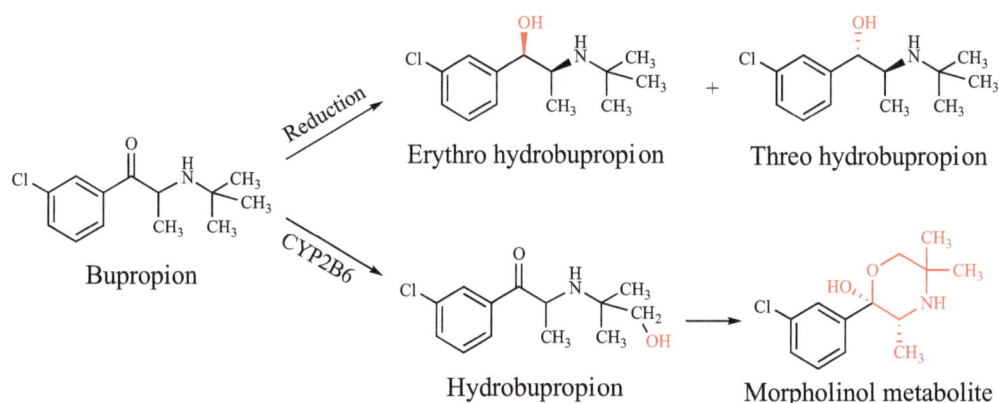

Fig. (26). Metabolism of bupropion.

CASE STUDIES

Case 1

OL is an 84-year-old female who presents to an outpatient primary care provider. She presents with her daughter who states that the reason for the visit is that the patient has symptoms of depression. These symptoms include loss of interest in usual activities such as attending events at the local senior center and excessive irritability. Additionally, OL has not been sleeping at night and refuses to eat most of the meals provided to her. OL has lost 8 pounds since her last visit and her current BMI is 18.5. OL's past medical history includes uncontrolled hypertension and a history of alcohol abuse. Her labs are noncontributory at this visit. Current medications include a multivitamin, hydrochlorothiazide 25mg PO daily and lisinopril 20mg PO daily. Her blood pressure remains elevated.

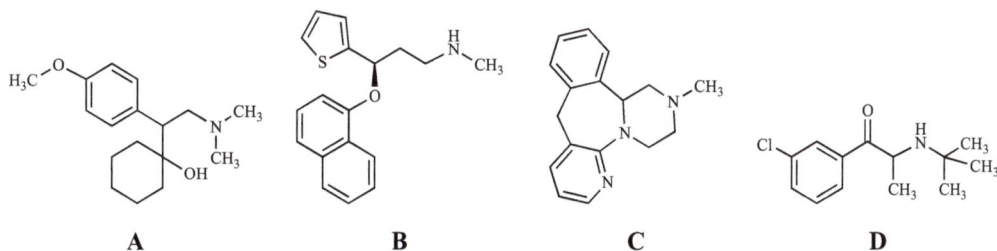

Q1. What antidepressant medication would aid the patient with increasing appetite and sleep?
Q2. What mechanism of the medication chosen for the above question increases appetite and sleep?

Q3. What role does the patient's uncontrolled hypertension play in which class of medication you would or would not choose?

Q4. Which of the following medications would be inappropriate for the patient based on the potential for appetite suppression?

Case 2

JW is a 44-year-old male with depression and is currently taking escitalopram for depression. He reports that he does not feel his current medication regimen is effective in controlling his symptoms of depression. In the past, he has also tried duloxetine and bupropion for appropriate lengths of time with no effect. His physician wants to start with him an MAOI medication today for treatment-resistant depression.

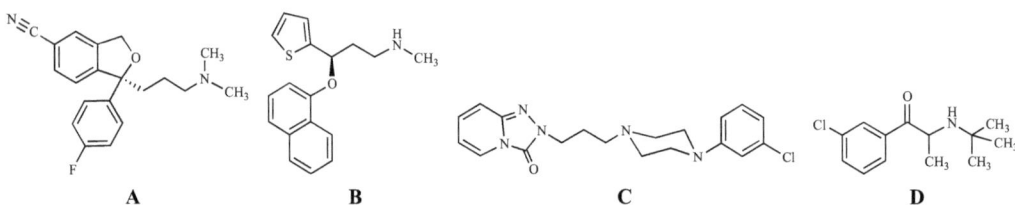

Q1. Which of the above structures represent medications that JW has tried and failed?

Q2. What is the risk of starting an MAOI medication immediately?

Q3. What types of symptoms could represent a serious medical condition if MAOI and SSRIs are taken together?

Q4. What other classes of medications has the patient not yet tried for treatment of his depression?

Case 3

ML is a 30-year-old female suffering from anxiety and depression currently on SSRI treatment for 4 months. She comes to the clinic today complaining of sexual side effects including decreased libido and anorgasmia. She wants to change to a medication that will have less chance of causing this side effect. Her past medical history includes hypertension, hyperthyroidism, and severe insomnia. Her blood pressure at this visit is 148/96. Her physician has set her blood pressure at less than 130/80.

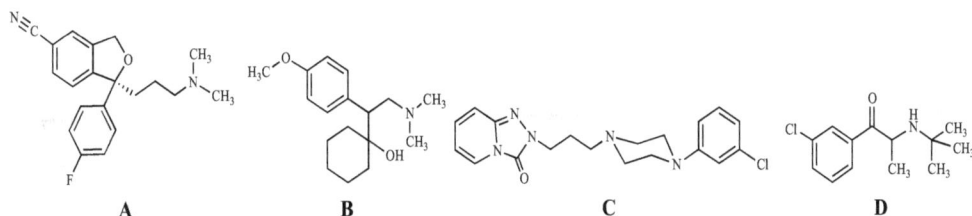

Q1. Which of the structures represents a medication that the patient is on now? What side effect of this medication is affecting this patient? What other serious side effects should be monitored when a patient is on this medication?

Q2. Which of the above structures represents a medication(s) that the patient should avoid due to known side effects that could exacerbate the patient's other medical conditions?

Q3. Which of the above medications would be an appropriate option for the patient at this time? Why?

DRUG DISCOVERY CASE STUDY

Discovery of SSRIs and Fluoxetine

It was realized during the 1960s that the TCAs acted by inhibiting the reuptake of norepinephrine and serotonin (5-HT). In 1969, psychiatrists Paul Kielholz, Izyaslav Lapin and Gregory Oxenkrug suggested that increased serotonergic activity in the brain accounted for the mood-elevation effect, while increased noradrenergic activity was responsible for the motor and energizing effects. This idea led to the search for SSRIs by different groups of scientists. Then, the effects of antihistamines on serotonin and norepinephrine uptake in tissues were examined by Arvid Carlsson, and he identified diphenhydramine affecting 5-HT uptake selectively. He then collaborated with Peder Berntsson and Hans Corrodi to develop a pheniramine analog as a potent SSRI in 1971, which was marketed in 1982 in Europe as zimelidine by Astra. It was withdrawn the following year due to reports of Guillaine–Barre´ syndrome that slowly disappeared after ceasing the medication. The second SSRI indalpine (an antihistamine analog), developed by Gerard Le Fur and his colleagues, was also withdrawn shortly after its introduction due to the occurrence of agranulocytopenia in a few patients. Fluvoxamine was the next SSRI that remained in the market for some time but there were concerns of potentially increasing suicidal behavior. Several diphenhydramine analogs were developed by Eli Lilly and found *N*-methy--phenoxyphenylpropylamine to be twice as potent at inhibiting the uptake of 5-HT as it was at inhibiting norepinephrine uptake. Later a series of its analogs were synthesized to finally discover the most frequently prescribed antidepressant drug fluoxetine (Prozac®) that was marketed in 1988 (Fig. **27**) [63]. Fluoxetine is still in the market due to its higher potency but with a black box warning stating that it may lead to suicidal thoughts in children and young adults.

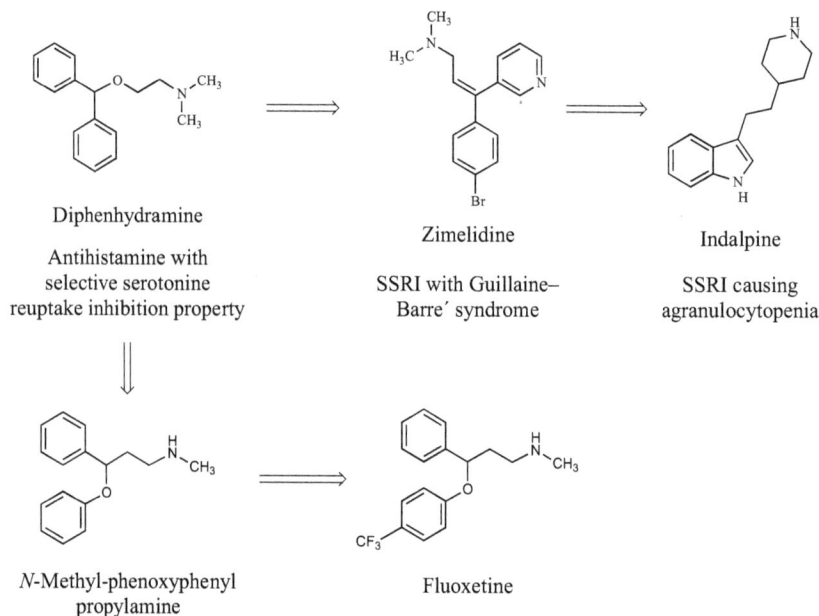

Diphenhydramine

Antihistamine with selective serotonine reuptake inhibition property

Zimelidine

SSRI with Guillaine–Barre´ syndrome

Indalpine

SSRI causing agranulocytopenia

N-Methyl-phenoxyphenyl propylamine

Fluoxetine

Fig. (27). Discovery of SSRIs and fluoxetine.

STUDENT SELF STUDY GUIDE

1. What are the consequences of ring geometry on activity with the isosteric replacement of S with -CH2CH2-?
2. What are the common structural features of TCAs?
3. What is the effect of ring substitution by an electron-withdrawing group on TCAs?
4. Activity towards NE vs 5HT transporter system of 1°, 2° and 3° amines on the side chain.
5. Classes of TCAs based on both ring system and side-chain amine with examples.
6. Structures and activity of miscellaneous antidepressants such as maprotiline, doxepin, amoxapine, mirtazapine.
7. What are SSRIs and NRIs? How can you generalize from structures?
8. How was SSRI developed from TCAs?
9. Is trazodone an SSRI? Why or why not?
10. What are the different classes of MAOIs?

11. SAR of hydrazine derivatives as antidepressants.
12. What are selective MAO-A and MAO-B inhibitors? What is their clinical significance?
13. Try solving all the clinically relevant case studies and discuss those in teams.
14. Learn the mechanism of action, structure-activity relationship and metabolism of all the drugs classes as well as individual drugs.

STUDENTS SELF-ASSESSMENT QUESTIONS

1. Sertraline is a_____

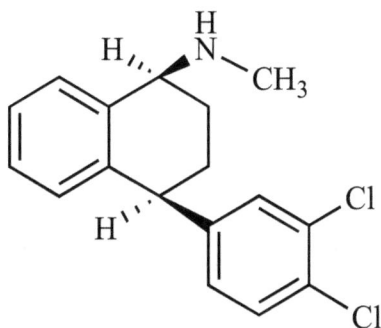

Sertraline

I) Norepinephrine reuptake inhibitor

II) Monoamine oxidase inhibitor

III) Selective serotonin reuptake inhibitor

A. I only

B. II only

C. III only

D. Both I and II

E. Both I and III

2. Chlorpromazine, shown below, contains _____

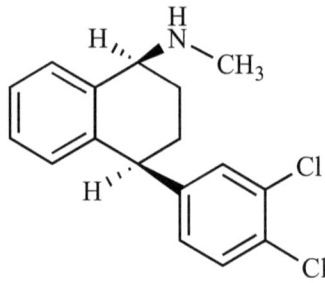

Sertraline

I) Piperidine ring

II) Piperazine ring

III) Phenothiazine ring

A. I only

B. II only

C. III only

D. Both I and III

E. Both II and III

3. Imipramine is a _____

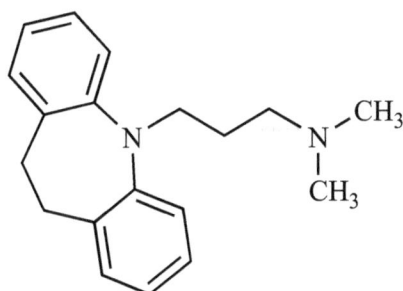

Imipramine

A. Tricyclic tertiary amine antidepressant

B. Tricyclic secondary amine antidepressant

C. Phenylalkylamines antidepressant

D. Phenoxyphenylpropylamines antidepressant

E. Phenothiazine antidepressant

4. Based on the SAR of antidepressants, identify selective norepinephrine reuptake inhibitor (NRI) from the structures shown below.

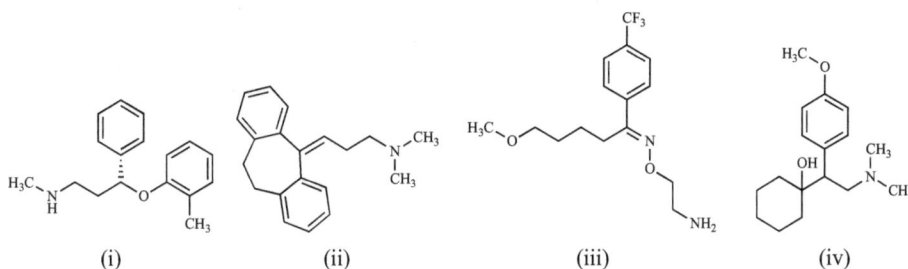

(i)	(ii)	(iii)	(iv)

.
.

A. Structures (i) and (iii)

B. Structures (i) and (iv)

C. Structures (ii) and (iii)

D. Structures (ii) and (iii)

E. Only Structure (i)

5. Which of the following metabolites (structures) could result from Fluoxetine metabolism?

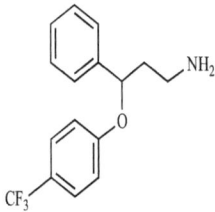 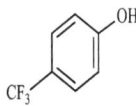 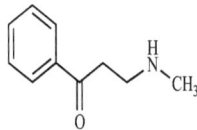 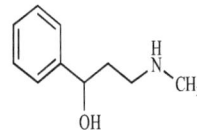

| (i) | (ii) | (iii) | (iv) |

A. Structure (i)

B. Structure (ii)

C. Structure (iii)

D. Structure (iv)

E. All of the above

6. Based on the SAR of tricyclic antidepressants, which of the following structures should have greater norepinephrine reuptake inhibition than inhibition of serotonin uptake?

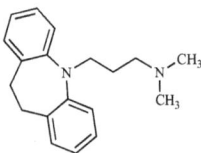 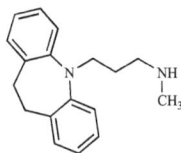 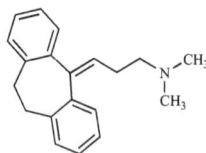 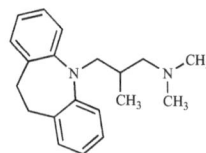

| (i) | (ii) | (iii) | (iv) |

A. Structure (i)

B. Structure (ii)

C. Structure (iii)

D. Structure (iv)

E. All of the above

7. Based on the SAR, rank the following antidepressant drug structures for their potential to exert anticholinergic and antihistaminic side effects. (Order is based on greatest to least side effect)?

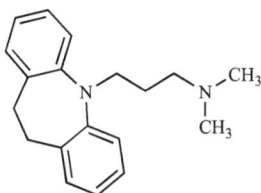
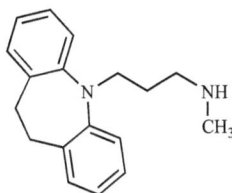
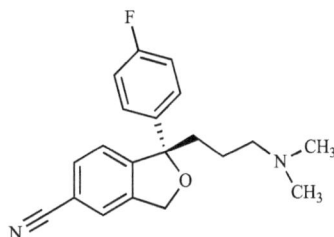

(i)   (ii)   (iii)

A. Structure (i) > Structure (iii) > Structure (ii)

B. Structure (i) > Structure (ii) > Structure (iii)

C. Structure (iii) > Structure (i) > Structure (ii)

D. None of the above drugs exhibit such side effects.

8. Identify the selective serotonin reuptake inhibitors from the structures below.

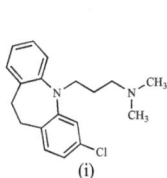
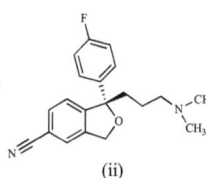
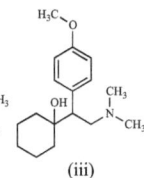
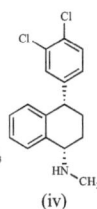
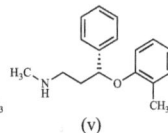

(i)   (ii)   (iii)   (iv)   (v)

A. Structures (i) and (iii)

B. Structures (ii) and (v)

C. Structures (iii) and (iv)

D. Structures (ii) and (iv)

E. Structures (i) and (ii)

9. Clomipramine cannot be metabolized by _____reaction

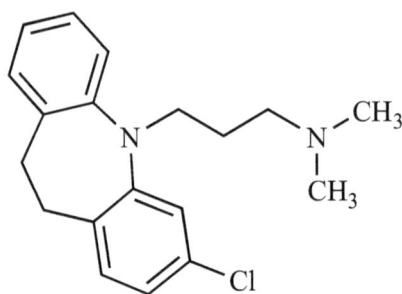

Clomipramine

A. *N*-oxidation

B. *N*-dealkylation

C. M Aromatic hydroxylation

D. *O*-dealkylation

E. Glucuronide conjugation

10. Co-administration of imipramine with fluoxetine can _____

A. Increase fluoxetine concentration

B. Decrease imipramine concentration

C. Increase imipramine concentration

D. Decrease fluoxetine concentration

E. Cannot cause change in the concentration of either drugs.

11. Which drug below has anticholinergic effects that owe to its adverse effects (*i.e.* blurred vision, constipation & dry mouth) often stated by patients taking them for the treatment of depression?

A. Fluoxetine

B. Sertraline

C. Fluvoxamine

D. Amitriptyline

12. Which of the following is true about buspirone?

A. Is effective in treating depression

B. Is cross-tolerant with benzodiazepines

C. Does not produce significant levels of sedation

D. Is a benzodiazepine

E. Has a rapid onset of action

13. Which of the following symptom(s) can be associated with changes in weight due to depression? (Select all that apply)

A. Increase in body aches

B. Increase in motivation

C. Increase in appetite

D. Increase in sleep

14. The older TCAs share all of the following adverse effects expect which one?

A. Orthostatic hypotension

B. Sedation

C. Seizures

D. Weight gain

E. Sexual dysfunction

15. What is the MOA of Strattera?

A. Highly selective NE reuptake inhibitor blocks the norepinephrine transporter (NET)

B. Moderately selective NE reuptake inhibitor blocks the norepinephrine transporter (NET)

C. Highly selective 5-HT reuptake inhibitor blocks the serotonin transporter (SERT)

D. Has a greater selectivity SERT then NET

CONSENT FOR PUBLICATION

Not applicable.

CONFLICT OF INTEREST

The authors confirm that the contents of this chapter have no conflict of interest.

ACKNOWLEDGEMENTS

Declare none.

REFERENCES

[1]   López-Muñoz F, Alamo C. Monoaminergic neurotransmission: the history of the discovery of antidepressants from 1950s until today. Curr Pharm Des 2009; 15(14): 1563-86.
        [http://dx.doi.org/10.2174/138161209788168001] [PMID: 19442174]

[2]   Kuhn R. The treatment of depressive states with G 22355 (imipramine hydrochloride). Am J Psychiatry 1958; 115(5): 459-64.
        [http://dx.doi.org/10.1176/ajp.115.5.459] [PMID: 13583250]

[3]   López-Muñoz F, Álamo C. History of the discovery of antidepressant drugs. In: López-Muñoz F, Srinivasan V, de Berardis D, Álamo C, Kato TA, Eds. Neuroprotective Agents and Antidepressant Therapy. New Delhi: Springer India 2016; pp. 365-83.

[4]   Schildkraut JJ. The catecholamine hypothesis of affective disorders: a review of supporting evidence. Am J Psychiatry 1965; 122(5): 509-22.
        [http://dx.doi.org/10.1176/ajp.122.5.509] [PMID: 5319766]

[5]   W Sneader, Ed. Drug Discovery. A History. West Sussex, England: John Wiley & Sons Ltd 2005.

[6]   Wong DT, Horng JS, Bymaster FP, Hauser KL, Molloy BB. A selective inhibitor of serotonin uptake: Lilly 110140, 3-(p-trifluoromethylphenoxy)-N-methyl-3-phenylpropylamine. Life Sci 1974; 15(3): 471-9.
        [http://dx.doi.org/10.1016/0024-3205(74)90345-2] [PMID: 4549929]

[7]   7. Hirschfeld RM: History and evolution of the monoamine hypothesis of depression. J Clin Psychiatry 2000; 61 (Suppl. 6): 4-6.

[8]   López-Muñoz F, Alamo C. Monoaminergic neurotransmission: the history of the discovery of

antidepressants from 1950s until today. Curr Pharm Des 2009; 15(14): 1563-86.
[http://dx.doi.org/10.2174/138161209788168001] [PMID: 19442174]

[9]　Moret C, Briley M. The importance of norepinephrine in depression. Neuropsychiatr Dis Treat 2011; 7 (Suppl. 1): 9-13.
[PMID: 21750623]

[10]　Kalia M. Neurobiological basis of depression: an update. Metabolism 2005; 54(5) (Suppl. 1): 24-7.
[http://dx.doi.org/10.1016/j.metabol.2005.01.009] [PMID: 15877309]

[11]　Maletic V, Robinson M, Oakes T, Iyengar S, Ball SG, Russell J. Neurobiology of depression: an integrated view of key findings. Int J Clin Pract 2007; 61(12): 2030-40.
[http://dx.doi.org/10.1111/j.1742-1241.2007.01602.x] [PMID: 17944926]

[12]　Manji HK, Drevets WC, Charney DS. The cellular neurobiology of depression. Nat Med 2001; 7(5): 541-7.
[http://dx.doi.org/10.1038/87865] [PMID: 11329053]

[13]　Hervás I, Artigas F. Effect of fluoxetine on extracellular 5-hydroxytryptamine in rat brain. Role of 5-HT autoreceptors. Eur J Pharmacol 1998; 358(1): 9-18.
[http://dx.doi.org/10.1016/S0014-2999(98)00579-2] [PMID: 9809863]

[14]　Commons KG, Linnros SE. Delayed antidepressant efficacy and the desensitization hypothesis. ACS Chem Neurosci 2019; 10(7): 3048-52.
[http://dx.doi.org/10.1021/acschemneuro.8b00698] [PMID: 30807103]

[15]　Nogrady T. Medicinal Chemistry: A Biochemical Approach. New York, USA: Oxford University Press 1985; p. 29.

[16]　Berken GH, Weinstein DO, Stern WC. Weight gain. A side-effect of tricyclic antidepressants. J Affect Disord 1984; 7(2): 133-8.
[http://dx.doi.org/10.1016/0165-0327(84)90031-4] [PMID: 6238068]

[17]　Daniels TC, Jorgensen EC, Eds. Wilson and Gisvold's Textbook of Organic Medicinal and Pharmaceutical Chemistry. Pennsylvania: Wolters Kluwer Health 1982; 383.

[18]　Lemke TL, Zito SW, Roche VF, Williams DA. Essentials of Foye's principles of medicinal chemistry. Philadelphia: Wolters Kluwer 2017; p. 641.

[19]　Gillman PK. Tricyclic antidepressant pharmacology and therapeutic drug interactions updated. Br J Pharmacol 2007; 151(6): 737-48.
[http://dx.doi.org/10.1038/sj.bjp.0707253] [PMID: 17471183]

[20]　Lapierre YD. A review of trimipramine. 30 years of clinical use. Drugs 1989.38(Suppl1):17-2, & 49-50.

[21]　Sallee FR, Pollock BG. Clinical pharmacokinetics of imipramine and desipramine. Clin Pharmacokinet 1990; 18(5): 346-64.
[http://dx.doi.org/10.2165/00003088-199018050-00002] [PMID: 2185906]

[22]　Balant-Gorgia AE, Gex-Fabry M, Balant LP. Clinical pharmacokinetics of clomipramine. Clin Pharmacokinet 1991; 20(6): 447-62.
[http://dx.doi.org/10.2165/00003088-199120060-00002] [PMID: 2044329]

[23]　Gupta SK, Shah JC, Hwang SS. Pharmacokinetic and pharmacodynamic characterization of OROS and immediate-release amitriptyline. Br J Clin Pharmacol 1999; 48(1): 71-8.
[http://dx.doi.org/10.1046/j.1365-2125.1999.00973.x] [PMID: 10383563]

[24]　Bowden CL, Koslow SH, Hanin I, Maas JW, Davis JM, Robins E. Effects of amitriptyline and imipramine on brain amine neurotransmitter metabolites in cerebrospinal fluid. Clin Pharmacol Ther 1985; 37(3): 316-24.
[http://dx.doi.org/10.1038/clpt.1985.46] [PMID: 2578912]

[25]　Ziegler VE, Biggs JT, Wylie LT, *et al.* Protriptyline kinetics. Clin Pharmacol Ther 1978; 23(5): 580-4.

[http://dx.doi.org/10.1002/cpt1978235580] [PMID: 639433]

[26]   Biggs JT, Holland WH, Sherman WR. Steady-state protriptyline levels in an outpatient population. Am J Psychiatry 1975; 132(9): 960-2.
[http://dx.doi.org/10.1176/ajp.132.9.960] [PMID: 1155634]

[27]   Kirchheiner J, Müller G, Meineke I, Wernecke KD, Roots I, Brockmöller J. Effects of polymorphisms in CYP2D6, CYP2C9, and CYP2C19 on trimipramine pharmacokinetics. J Clin Psychopharmacol 2003; 23(5): 459-66.
[http://dx.doi.org/10.1097/01.jcp.0000088909.24613.92] [PMID: 14520122]

[28]   Meyer-Barner M, Meineke I, Schreeb KH, Gleiter CH. Pharmacokinetics of doxepin and desmethyldoxepin: an evaluation with the population approach. Eur J Clin Pharmacol 2002; 58(4): 253-7.
[http://dx.doi.org/10.1007/s00228-002-0448-3] [PMID: 12136371]

[29]   Brachtendorf L, Jetter A, Beckurts KT, Hölscher AH, Fuhr U. Cytochrome P450 enzymes contributing to demethylation of maprotiline in man. Pharmacol Toxicol 2002; 90(3): 144-9.
[http://dx.doi.org/10.1034/j.1600-0773.2002.900306.x] [PMID: 12071336]

[30]   Alkalay D, Wagner WE Jr, Carlsen S, *et al.* Bioavailability and kinetics of maprotiline. Clin Pharmacol Ther 1980; 27(5): 697-703.
[http://dx.doi.org/10.1038/clpt.1980.99] [PMID: 7371367]

[31]   Lydiard RB, Gelenberg AJ. Amoxapine--an antidepressant with some neuroleptic properties? A review of its chemistry, animal pharmacology and toxicology, human pharmacology, and clinical efficacy. Pharmacotherapy 1981; 1(3): 163-78.
[http://dx.doi.org/10.1002/j.1875-9114.1981.tb02538.x] [PMID: 6152816]

[32]   Calvo B, García MJ, Pedraz JL, Mariño EL, Domínguez-Gil A. Pharmacokinetics of amoxapine and its active metabolites. Int J Clin Pharmacol Ther Toxicol 1985; 23(4): 180-5.
[PMID: 3997304]

[33]   Montgomery SA. Tolerability of serotonin norepinephrine reuptake inhibitor antidepressants. CNS Spectr 2008; 13(7) (Suppl. 11): 27-33.
[http://dx.doi.org/10.1017/S1092852900028297] [PMID: 18622372]

[34]   Amchin J, Zarycranski W, Taylor KP, Albano D, Klockowski PM. Effect of venlafaxine on the pharmacokinetics of risperidone. J Clin Pharmacol 1999; 39(3): 297-309.
[PMID: 10073330]

[35]   Amchin J, Zarycranski W, Taylor KP, Albano D, Klockowski PM. Effect of venlafaxine on CYP1A2-dependent pharmacokinetics and metabolism of caffeine. J Clin Pharmacol 1999; 39(3): 252-9.
[PMID: 10073324]

[36]   Fukuda T, Yamamoto I, Nishida Y, *et al.* Effect of the CYP2D6*10 genotype on venlafaxine pharmacokinetics in healthy adult volunteers. Br J Clin Pharmacol 1999; 47(4): 450-3.
[http://dx.doi.org/10.1046/j.1365-2125.1999.00913.x] [PMID: 10233212]

[37]   Puozzo C, Panconi E, Deprez D. Pharmacology and pharmacokinetics of milnacipran. Int Clin Psychopharmacol 2002; 17 (Suppl. 1): S25-35.
[http://dx.doi.org/10.1097/00004850-200206001-00004] [PMID: 12369608]

[38]   Knadler MP, Lobo E, Chappell J, Bergstrom R. Duloxetine: clinical pharmacokinetics and drug interactions. Clin Pharmacokinet 2011; 50(5): 281-94.
[http://dx.doi.org/10.2165/11539240-000000000-00000] [PMID: 21366359]

[39]   Sauer JM, Ring BJ, Witcher JW. Clinical pharmacokinetics of atomoxetine. Clin Pharmacokinet 2005; 44(6): 571-90.
[http://dx.doi.org/10.2165/00003088-200544060-00002] [PMID: 15910008]

[40]   Fleishaker JC. Clinical pharmacokinetics of reboxetine, a selective norepinephrine reuptake inhibitor for the treatment of patients with depression. Clin Pharmacokinet 2000; 39(6): 413-27.

[http://dx.doi.org/10.2165/00003088-200039060-00003] [PMID: 11192474]

[41]   Wong DT, Bymaster FP, Engleman EA. Prozac (fluoxetine, Lilly 110140), the first selective serotonin uptake inhibitor and an antidepressant drug: twenty years since its first publication. Life Sci 1995; 57(5): 411-41.
[http://dx.doi.org/10.1016/0024-3205(95)00209-O] [PMID: 7623609]

[42]   Altamura AC, Moro AR, Percudani M. Clinical pharmacokinetics of fluoxetine. Clin Pharmacokinet 1994; 26(3): 201-14.
[http://dx.doi.org/10.2165/00003088-199426030-00004] [PMID: 8194283]

[43]   Bergstrom RF, Lemberger L, Farid NA, Wolen RL. Clinical pharmacology and pharmacokinetics of fluoxetine: a review. Br J Psychiatry Suppl 1988; (3): 47-50.
[http://dx.doi.org/10.1192/S0007125000297286] [PMID: 3074865]

[44]   Foster RH, Goa KL. Paroxetine : a review of its pharmacology and therapeutic potential in the management of panic disorder. CNS Drugs 1997; 8(2): 163-88.
[http://dx.doi.org/10.2165/00023210-199708020-00010] [PMID: 23338224]

[45]   Jornil J, Jensen KG, Larsen F, Linnet K. Identification of cytochrome P450 isoforms involved in the metabolism of paroxetine and estimation of their importance for human paroxetine metabolism using a population-based simulator. Drug Metab Dispos 2010; 38(3): 376-85.
[http://dx.doi.org/10.1124/dmd.109.030551] [PMID: 20007670]

[46]   Rampono J, Kristensen JH, Hackett LP, Paech M, Kohan R, Ilett KF. Citalopram and demethylcitalopram in human milk; distribution, excretion and effects in breast fed infants. Br J Clin Pharmacol 2000; 50(3): 263-8.
[http://dx.doi.org/10.1046/j.1365-2125.2000.00253.x] [PMID: 10971311]

[47]   Sangkuhl K, Klein TE, Altman RB. PharmGKB summary: citalopram pharmacokinetics pathway. Pharmacogenet Genomics 2011; 21(11): 769-72.
[http://dx.doi.org/10.1097/FPC.0b013e328346063f] [PMID: 21546862]

[48]   Baumann P. Clinical pharmacokinetics of citalopram and other selective serotonergic reuptake inhibitors (SSRI). Int Clin Psychopharmacol 1992; 6 (Suppl. 5): 13-20.
[http://dx.doi.org/10.1097/00004850-199206005-00002] [PMID: 1431018]

[49]   DeVane CL, Liston HL, Markowitz JS. Clinical pharmacokinetics of sertraline. Clin Pharmacokinet 2002; 41(15): 1247-66.
[http://dx.doi.org/10.2165/00003088-200241150-00002] [PMID: 12452737]

[50]   Mandrioli R, Mercolini L, Raggi MA. Evaluation of the pharmacokinetics, safety and clinical efficacy of sertraline used to treat social anxiety. Expert Opin Drug Metab Toxicol 2013; 9(11): 1495-505.
[http://dx.doi.org/10.1517/17425255.2013.816675] [PMID: 23834458]

[51]   Perucca E, Gatti G, Spina E. Clinical pharmacokinetics of fluvoxamine. Clin Pharmacokinet 1994; 27(3): 175-90.
[http://dx.doi.org/10.2165/00003088-199427030-00002] [PMID: 7988100]

[52]   DeVane CL, Gill HS. Clinical pharmacokinetics of fluvoxamine: applications to dosage regimen design. J Clin Psychiatry 1997; 58(58) (Suppl. 5): 7-14.
[PMID: 9184622]

[53]   Fiedorowicz JG, Swartz KL. The role of monoamine oxidase inhibitors in current psychiatric practice. J Psychiatr Pract 2004; 10(4): 239-48.
[http://dx.doi.org/10.1097/00131746-200407000-00005] [PMID: 15552546]

[54]   Stahl SM, Felker A. Monoamine oxidase inhibitors: a modern guide to an unrequited class of antidepressants. CNS Spectr 2008; 13(10): 855-70.
[http://dx.doi.org/10.1017/S1092852900016965] [PMID: 18955941]

[55]   Haria M, Fitton A, McTavish D. Trazodone. A review of its pharmacology, therapeutic use in depression and therapeutic potential in other disorders. Drugs Aging 1994; 4(4): 331-55.

[http://dx.doi.org/10.2165/00002512-199404040-00006] [PMID: 8019056]

[56]   Kale P, Agrawal YK. Pharmacokinetics of single oral dose trazodone: a randomized, two-period, cross-over trial in healthy, adult, human volunteers under fed condition. Front Pharmacol 2015; 6: 224.
[http://dx.doi.org/10.3389/fphar.2015.00224] [PMID: 26483693]

[57]   Jauch R, Kopitar Z, Prox A, Zimmer A. [Pharmacokinetics and metabolism of trazodone in man (author's transl)]. Arzneimittelforschung 1976; 26(11): 2084-9.
[PMID: 1037253]

[58]   Rotzinger S, Fang J, Baker GB. Trazodone is metabolized to m-chlorophenylpiperazine by CYP3A4 from human sources. Drug Metab Dispos 1998; 26(6): 572-5.
[PMID: 9616194]

[59]   Anttila SA, Leinonen EV. A review of the pharmacological and clinical profile of mirtazapine. CNS Drug Rev 2001; 7(3): 249-64.
[http://dx.doi.org/10.1111/j.1527-3458.2001.tb00198.x] [PMID: 11607047]

[60]   Timmer CJ, Sitsen JM, Delbressine LP. Clinical pharmacokinetics of mirtazapine. Clin Pharmacokinet 2000; 38(6): 461-74.
[http://dx.doi.org/10.2165/00003088-200038060-00001] [PMID: 10885584]

[61]   Stahl SM, Pradko JF, Haight BR, Modell JG, Rockett CB, Learned-Coughlin S. A Review of the neuropharmacology of bupropion, a dual norepinephrine and dopamine reuptake inhibitor. Prim Care Companion J Clin Psychiatry 2004; 6(4): 159-66.
[http://dx.doi.org/10.4088/PCC.v06n0403] [PMID: 15361919]

[62]   Findlay JW, Van Wyck Fleet J, Smith PG, *et al.* Pharmacokinetics of bupropion, a novel antidepressant agent, following oral administration to healthy subjects. Eur J Clin Pharmacol 1981; 21(2): 127-35.
[http://dx.doi.org/10.1007/BF00637513] [PMID: 6804243]

[63]   Sneader W. Drugs originating from the screening of organic chemicals.Drug Discovery A History. West Sussex, England: John Wiley & Sons Ltd 2005.
[http://dx.doi.org/10.1002/0470015535]

CHAPTER 5

Sedatives, Hypnotics and Anxiolytics

Donald Sikazwe[*]

Department of Pharmaceutical Sciences, Feik School of Pharmacy, University of the Incarnate Word, San Antonio, TX, USA

Abstract: The major objective of this chapter is to concisely explain and equip pharmacy students with the chemical and pharmacological knowledge of traditional/conventional and newer sedative-hypnotics and anxiolytics, that is, barbiturates, benzodiazepines and non-benzodiazepine agents. Upon studying this book chapter, students will be able to:

• Categorize Chemically/Pharmacologically sedative-hypnotics and anxiolytics.

• Explain the mechanisms by which barbiturates, benzodiazepines, and non-benzodiazepine sedative-hypnotics and anxiolytics exert their pharmacological effects.

• Summarize the benzodiazepine and barbiturate structure-activity relationships (SAR).

• Describe the key pharmacokinetic (ADMET) characteristics of individual drug molecules.

Keywords: Anxiolytics, Barbiturates, Benzodiazepines, GABA receptor, GABA$_A$ receptor agonists, Hypnotics, Inverse agonists and antagonists, Orexins, Partial agonists, Ramelteon, Sedatives, Structure-activity relationships, Z-drugs.

HISTORICAL BACKGROUND

Sedative, hypnotics and anxiolytics are part of the CNS depressant group of drugs with clinical utility in anxiety, insomnia, muscle relaxation, seizures, alcohol detoxification, and even anesthesia. Earlier xenobiotic agents possessing such pharmacological properties included *ethanol, bromide salts, chloral hydrate,* and *paraldehyde* [1 - 3]. The barbiturate era, for the above medical indications and epilepsy, started in the early 1900s with the discovery of *barbital* (in 1903) and *phenobarbital* (in 1912) and has to date witnessed the chemical synthesis of more than 2,500 barbiturates [2]. Drawbacks to barbiturate pharmacotherapy include

[*] **Corresponding author Donald Sikazwe:** Department of Pharmaceutical Sciences, Feik School of Pharmacy, University of the Incarnate Word, San Antonio, TX 78209, USA; Tel: 210-883-1174; Fax: 210-822-1516; E-mail: sikazwe@uiwtx.edu

M. O. Faruk Khan & Ashok E. Philip (Eds.)

narrow therapeutic indices (a toxicity risk), higher potential for abuse, dependence, and significant overdose/ drug-related suicides. After a prolonged barbiturate market dominance, drug research led to the discovery of the anti-anxiety drug *meprobamate*. This drug was launched in 1955 and sold under *Miltown* and *Equanil* brand names [3]. Although less toxic at therapeutic doses, excessive use of meprobamate agent can also lead to dependence. The search for even much safer sedative-hypnotics, with lower abuse and toxicity liabilities, led to the discovery of benzodiazepine (BZD) compounds. *Chlordiazepoxide*, the 1st BZD, was introduced in 1960, became the model chemical template for the BZD drug class, and quickly inspired the discovery/development of more than fifty known analogs, the first of which was *diazepam* [3, 4]. Diazepam reigned from the 1960s through 1970s and in that time-period achieved the most prescribed benzodiazepine drug status in the US [3]. To date, benzodiazepines remain widely prescribed, although they are gradually being replaced by the newer non-benzodiazepine sedative-hypnotics and anxiolytics entering the market. A brief comparison of benzodiazepine and barbiturate pharmacological effects reveals that they both possess similar sedative-hypnotic properties with the major difference being that benzodiazepines have demonstrated a substantially safer or improved therapeutic index. Benzodiazepines have therefore supplanted barbiturates in the treatment of anxiety and sleep disorders.

State of the art: In order to optimize drug activity and minimize adverse effect liabilities of the classical sedative-hypnotics and anxiolytic agents, we have now entered the era of structurally diverse and even mechanistically different newer agents. Newer agents like the non-benzodiazepine z-drugs (*zolpidem, zaleplon, eszopiclone*), *buspirone* and *ramelteon* have slowly been trickling into the US market since the late 1980s [5, 6]. The above agents implicate additional diverse receptor targets or sub-targets and call for the discovery/development of novel and receptor-selective small molecules. In fact, 2014 brought to the market new and mechanistically different molecules (*suvorexant, lemborexant*, and others in development) targeting hypocretin or orexin (OX_1/OX_2) receptors [7a]. That aside, (Fig. **1**) illustrates sedative-hypnotics and anxiolytics consistently found in the top 100 National Association of Chain Drug Stores (NACDS) 2018-19 factbook and 200 pharmacy times drug lists [7b & 7c].

INTRODUCTORY CONCEPTS

To equip pharmacy students with the chemical and pharmacological knowledge of *classical/traditional/conventional* and *newer* sedative-hypnotics and anxiolytics, this chapter will highlight clinically relevant aspects of drug structure, drug mechanisms of action, the chemical basis of drug action and pharmacokinetics or ADMET (Absorption, Distribution, Metabolism, Elimination and Toxicity). This has been done purposely to confine the subject matter to medicinal chemistry and facilitate easier comprehension. Related or cross-over topics (anesthesia, antidepressants, analgesia, antihistamines, *etc.*) have also been avoided, especially because such topics are addressed elsewhere in the book. Broadly speaking, sedative-hypnotic and anxiolytic agents were developed to manage insomnia and stress-related anxieties. Below are some general descriptors of sedative-hypnotics and anxiolytics plus the respective treatment agents.

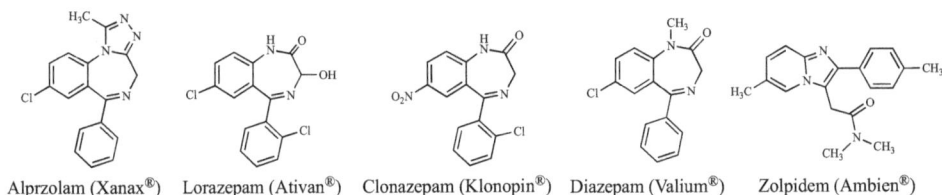

Alprzolam (Xanax®)   Lorazepam (Ativan®)   Clonazepam (Klonopin®)   Diazepam (Valium®)   Zolpidem (Ambien®)

Fig. (1). Effectual 100 or 200 top listed sedative-hypnotics and anxiolytics in the market [7b, c].

Sedative-hypnotics

Barbiturates, benzodiazepines, z-drugs, and ramelteon typify the pharmaco-therapeutic agents [1, 5, 8, 9]. Recently, *suvorexant* and *lemborexant* (both for insomnia) were added to the list [7a]. Sedatives calm or minimize excitement or nervousness. Agents that do not impair motor/mental function are desired. Hypnotic agents are sleep inducers with utility in insomnia. Ideal sedative-hypnotics should rapidly initiate and re-establish physiological sleep (*e.g.*, durations of non-rapid eye movement or NREM and rapid eye movement or REM), and lack: abuse liabilities, daytime sedation, drug discontinuation associated rebound insomnia, etc [5, 8]. Sedative-hypnotics are known to cause sedation at lower doses while hypnosis predominates at higher doses, so dosing is a key consideration (note that extreme doses of sedative-hypnotics may produce general anesthesia) [10].

Anxiolytics

Due to disease comorbidity and symptom overlap between depression and anxiety, selective serotonin reuptake inhibitors or SSRIs (*Fluoxetine, Paroxetine, Sertraline, Fluvoxamine, Citalopram, and Escitalopram*) and *serotonin-norepinephrine reuptake inhibitors or SNRIs (Venlafaxine and Duloxetine)* are now considered as 1st line treatment agents [11 - 14]. Since SSRIs and SNRIs are slow- acting and may take weeks to alleviate anxiety, *benzodiapines* (now second line-treatments) provide the fast-acting alternative. Other anxiolytic agents include *meprobamate,* and *buspirone* [2, 6]. The types of disorders treated /managed with anxiolytic agents are [14, 15]:

- Generalized Anxiety Disorder (GAD, most common anxiety disorder)
- Panic Disorder (PS)
- Social Anxiety Disorder (SAD)
- Posttraumatic Stress Disorder (PTSD)
- Obsessive–Compulsive Disorder (OCD)

Chemical-clinical considerations related to sedative-hypnotics and anxiolytics should include: *drug chemical classifications (e.g.*, barbiturates, benzodiazepines) plus their general mechanisms of action; *molecular weights or MWs* (these agents are characteristically lipophilic brain penetrant small molecules with less than 450 MWs); *pKa values* which determine drug abilities to form water-soluble salts and bonds with receptor active site functionalities (*i.e.*, amino acids); *lipophilicity* (expressed as log *P* values, influences drug duration of action and potency); *metabolism* (impacts drug dosing, duration of action, and toxicity due to elevations of plasma parent drug or metabolite concentrations). Most sedative-hypnotics and anxiolytics are metabolized by *cytochrome P450* (CYP) and *uridine diphosphate glucuronosyltransferases* (UGT) or glucuronidating enzymes, therefore, co-administration with enzyme inhibitors/inducers must be minimized or avoided.

Mechanisms of Action

The mechanisms of action attributed to the sedative-hypnotics and anxiolytics discussed herein can be divided into three major groupings:

- γ-amino butyric acid (GABA) receptor modulation
- Melatonin MT1/MT2 receptor activation
- 5-HT1$_A$ receptor activation

γ-Amino Butyric Acid (GABA) Receptor Modulation

GABA is a major central nervous system (CNS) inhibitory neurotransmitter. It precipitates neuronal inhibition *via* its actions at several GABA receptor types (GABA$_A$, GABA$_B$, GABA$_C$) [16]. The sedative-hypnotic and anxiolytic pharmacological effects of select older drugs are mainly mediated through GABA$_A$. Like GABA$_C$ and un-like GABA$_B$ (a G-protein coupled receptor or GPCR), GABA$_A$ is a ligand-gated ion channel (LGIC) or ionotropic receptor with the capacity to accommodate endogenous GABA and a wide collection of xenobiotics (drug molecules plus environmental chemicals) [16]. Sample xenobiotic known to interact with the GABA receptor include barbiturates, benzodiazepines, meprobamate, z-drugs, neurosteroids, ethanol, and general anesthetics (like isoflurane and propofol). These molecules exert their pharmacological effects by binding *allosterically* to particular GABA$_A$ receptor subunits and potentiating GABA's activity at the receptor (Fig. **2**) [17]. *Allosteric binding* refers to molecules binding or occupying topographically independent sites from the endogenous ligand's (in this case, GABA) binding site, also called the *orthosteric* site [17].

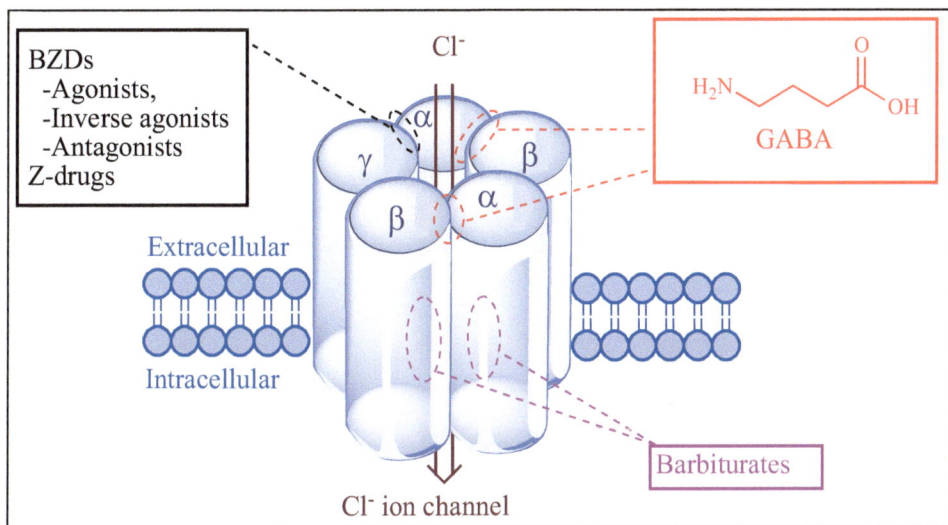

Fig. (2). GABA$_A$ receptor model depicting different molecular subunits (α, β, γ) plus the BZD, Z-drugs and GABA binding sites. BZDs and Z-drugs non-selectively bind to the α$_{1-3}$ subunits of GABA$_A$.

GABA$_A$ modulation involves alteration of receptor activity by inducing and stabilizing conformational changes which either enhance or decrease the receptor's affinity for GABA [18]. *Positive Allosteric Modulators* (*PAMs:* barbiturates, benzodiazepines, z-drugs, *etc.*) bind to their respective sites on the GABA$_A$ and enhance GABA's binding efficiency and response [17]. Ultimately, these molecules promote the influx of negatively charged chloride Cl$^-$ ions through the receptor ion channel, leading to inhibition of neuronal excitability or hyperpolarization. As indicated in the receptor model (Fig. **2**), molecules acting specifically at BZD receptor sites can also be designated as *agonists*, *inverse agonists* and *antagonists* [18]. While these pharmacological modes of action explain how these molecules interact with the *BZD binding sites*, students are advised that other GABA$_A$ receptor agonists, partial agonists, inverse agonists and antagonists exist, and are used for other disease state treatments or as investigational tools [19, 20]. For our purposes, BZD site agonists of interest include benzodiazepines and z-drugs. *Negative Allosteric Modulators (NAMs)* decrease Cl$^-$ ion conductance by inducing unfavorable receptor conformations for

GABA binding [17]. *NAM* examples include BZD receptor site carboline *inverse agonists* (ethyl-β-carboline-3-carboxylate or β-CCE and N-methyl-β-carboli-e-3-carboxamide) [21]. These compounds can inhibit the effects of benzo-diazepines and induce anxiety and seizures. Furthermore, BZD binding site antagonists, like flumazenil, are referred to as *Neutral Allosteric (NAs) modulators* [22]. Essentially, *NAs* have no net effect on GABA induced Cl⁻ ion conductance. To summarize, sedative-hypnotics and anxiolytics bind to $GABA_A$ and potentiate the neuronal inhibitory activity of synaptically available GABA. While GABA's binding to $GABA_A$ receptor is responsible for channel opening and chloride ion influx, higher dose barbiturates do not need GABA, instead, they can directly activate the receptor to open and prolong the duration of Cl⁻ ion influx [23]. On the other hand, benzodiazepines promote GABA activity and increase the frequency of ion channel opening by generating fast transient inhibitory postsynaptic currents (IPSCs) [24]. Since barbiturates, benzodiazepines and other sedative-hypnotics (*e.g.*, ethanol) act *via* a similar mechanism, they can promote or potentiate each other's pharmacological effects. To a certain extent, this helps explain why developing tolerance to one often implies developing cross-tolerance to another [25].

$GABA_A$ receptors are a complex family of trans-membrane hetero-pentameric proteins present throughout the central nervous system and in peripheral tissue. Literature is replete with molecular biology studies of $GABA_A$ receptor, however, our literature searches indicated that 19 $GABA_A$ subunit isoforms (α1-6, β1-3, γ1-3, δ, ε, θ, π) have already been characterized [22, 26]. The major configuration of this receptor consists of α, β and γ subunits in a ratio of 2:2:1. Abundances for the subunit combinations reportedly range from a high of 60% for the $\alpha_1\beta_2\gamma_2$ to 15-20% for the $\alpha_2\beta_3\gamma_2$, and 10-15% for the $\alpha_3\beta_3\gamma_2$ [22]. $GABA_A$-α1 subtypes are found in the brain cortex (plus most brain areas) and are involved in *sedation, anticonvulsant, and memory*. The $GABA_A$-α2 subfamily is involved in the sleep/wake cycle and exists in the hippocampus, amygdala, and basal ganglia. $GABA_A$-α3 subtypes, which exist in the cerebral cortex and reticular thalamic nucleus, are important in sleep, anxiolytic and antidepressant effects. The take home message is that the location of receptor subtypes suggests their function and their selective activation (*e.g.*, Z-drugs with high α1 affinity) or inhibition can result in different pharmacological effects.

Melatonin MT1/MT2 Receptor Activation

Melatonin (MLT) or N-acetyl-5-methoxytryptamine is the endogenous agonist for the MT1/MT2 GPCR superfamily [27, 28]. MLT is secreted by the pineal gland (mostly at night), is a hormone, and exerts many pharmacological effects by interacting with its receptors in the brain (the hypothalamus, thalamus, basal ganglia, cerebellum, hippocampus, and parts of the cerebral cortex), eyes, and periphery tissue (Fig. **3**) [27, 28]. The higher presence of M1/MT2 receptors in the hypothalamic suprachiasmatic nucleus (SCN, the circadian clock) indicates that melatonin influences the body's sleep-wake clock *via* these receptors, although its main function remains to regulate seasonal rhythms [27, 29]. MT1/MT2 gene deletion and antagonist studies suggest that both receptors play a role in circadian rhythm phase shifts and MT1 receptor activation results in a concentration-dependent inhibition of SCN neuronal firing [27, 29]. Overall, MLT plays a role in phase shifting the rhythms of the sleep-wake cycle. Normally, more MLT is synthesized at night than during the day and its levels decrease with age. Since ramelteon (a sedative-hypnotic drug) is a structural analog of MLT, it also acts by activating MT1/MT2 receptors. Melatonin is biosynthesized from serotonin or 5-hydroxytryptamine (5HT) under the influence of both polymorphic N-acetytransferase (NAT) activity and the circadian homeostasis/cycle/rhythm/clock which emanates from the brain's SCN [27, 30]. Since MT1 and MT2 receptor activations are involved in sleep induction and maintenance, they have become pharmaceutical targets for developing therapeutic agents against insomnia.

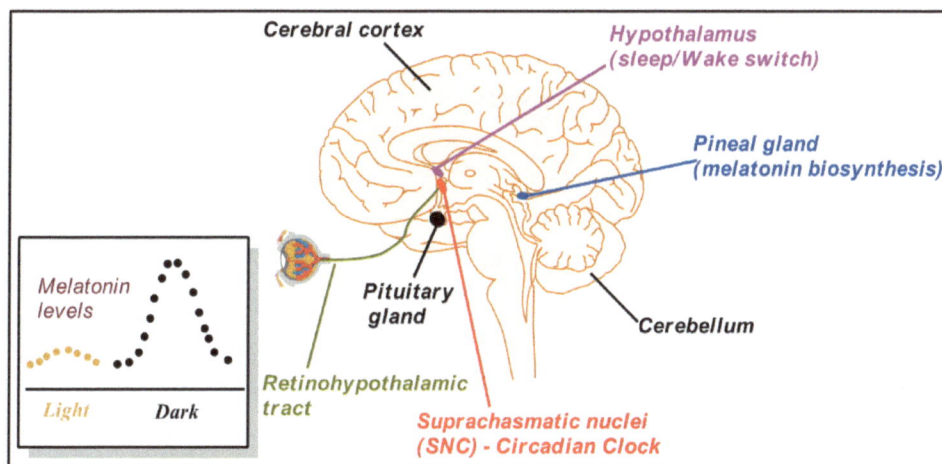

Fig. (3). A model of melatonin biosynthetic and impacted regions of the brain, and its day and night levels.

Pineal gland MLT synthesis is modulated by light and detailed mechanisms of which are elaborated elsewhere, suffice it to say that MLT is biosynthesized from 5HT in a two-step process – NAT enzyme-catalyzed acetylation of amino (-NH$_2$) group; and hydroxyindole-*O*-methyltransferases (HIOMT) catalyzed *O*-methylation (Fig. **4**) [30].

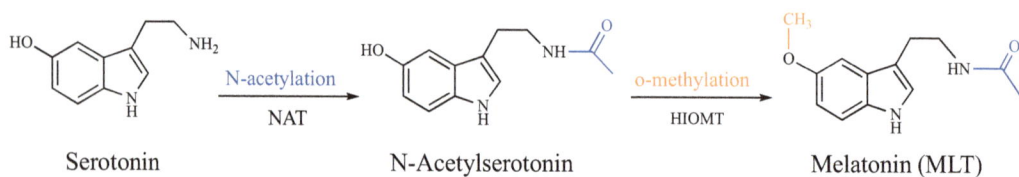

Fig. (4). MLT biosynthesis *via* N-acetylserotonin.

5-HT1$_A$ Receptor Activation

Partial agonist action at serotonin 1$_A$ or 5-hydroxytryptamine1$_A$ (abbreviated as 5-HT1$_A$) receptors, explains the anxiolytic activity of buspirone [31]. In other words, buspirone exhibits both agonist and antagonist activities and therefore does not fully activate 5-HT1$_A$ receptors. Animals lacking 5-HT1$_A$ gene exhibit increased fear. Unlike GABA$_A$ receptor modulation, 5-HT1$_A$ partial agonism produces little sedation and the propensity for dependence or abuse is highly diminished [31]. 5-HT activity is mediated through activation of members of a large family of 5-HT receptor proteins that have been divided into seven subfamilies (5-HT$_{1-7}$, with different functions) on the basis of amino acid sequence homologies and signaling mechanisms [32]. Due to the myriad pharmacological effects involving serotonin receptors, the serotonergic system continues to be a rich target for designing/developing many CNS active agents including the widely prescribed atypical antipsychotics, anti-migraine pharmacotherapeutics, antidepressants, and now the anxiolytics.

BARBITURATES

Barbiturates are chemical derivatives of barbituric acid or 2,4,6-trioxohexahydropyrimidine (Fig. **5**) and they exert their sedative-hypnotic effects by promoting the inhibitory actions of GABA [1, 12, 33]. They possess sedative-hypnotic, anxiolytic, anesthetic, anticonvulsant effects, and act *via* allosteric modulation of GABA$_A$. Today, however, they are infrequently used as sedative-hypnotics due to their toxicity (narrow therapeutic index), greater CNS depression, and abuse liabilities. Nonetheless, barbiturates continue to find clinical utility in other disorders (*e.g.*, phenobarbital's use in hyperbilirubinemia and the relief of intracranial pressure in traumatic brain injury) [1].

Barbituric acid itself has no CNS depressant effects but alkyl and aromatic R$_5$/R$_5$, substituents impart sedative hypnotic as well as anti-epileptic activities in the derivatives [2, 33, 34]. C2 carbonyl (C=O) barbiturates are called *oxy*barbiturates while those bearing a sulfur atom (C=S) at C2 are referred to as *thio*barbiturates [33, 34]. Overall, *thio*-babiturates are more lipophilic than their *oxy*-counterparts. The sulfur group also confers the rapid onset of action and reduces drug terminal half-life (*e.g.* from >30 to <15 hours) [33, 35]. *Unsubstituted* and electron-withdrawing group (EWG) C5 *di-substituted* barbiturates are weak acids (pka 4 - 8), exhibit lower H_2O solubility, and are absorbed slowly orally [36]. These barbiturates form sodium (Na) salts in high (pH >12 pH) solutions (*e.g.*, sodium hydroxide or NaOH solutions). Lowering the pH of these alkaline drug solutions can lead to incompatibility issues and the formation of insoluble barbiturate precipitates (cloudy aqueous solutions). Also, alkalizing urinary pH with sodium bicarbonate (Na_2CO_3) often promotes barbiturate excretion in urine.

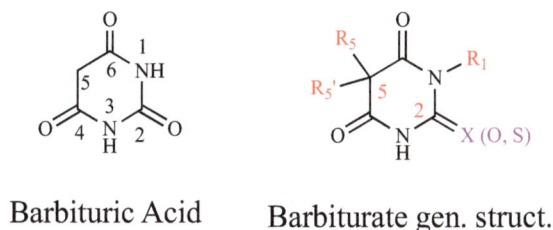

Barbituric Acid   Barbiturate gen. struct.

Fig. (5). Barbituric Acid and barbiturate drugs general structure.

Lower dose barbiturates positively and allosterically modulate $GABA_A$ receptors and are indicated for anxiety. Higher doses of barbiturates are hypnotic, and can directly activate $GABA_A$ in the absence of GABA (the mechanism of which is still unclear), cause cardiovascular and respiratory depression and may be fatal. Very high barbiturate doses or concentrations block the Cl^- ion conductance thereby limiting the extent of drug response [37]. In addition to barbiturate abuse/overdose/addiction/withdrawal syndrome liabilities, this class of molecules is known for its ability to induce CYP450 enzymes as well as some phase II enzymes [38]. As a matter of fact, their enzyme induction ability is a cause for concern in polypharmacy that contributes to many drug-drug interactions (DDIs) associated with barbiturate pharmacotherapy. Enzyme induction entails increased enzyme protein biosynthesis/activity and often leads to sub-optimal pharmacotherapy. This can imply dose adjustments in order to achieve drug therapeutic concentrations in plasma or a change in drug therapy.

Barbiturates are also grouped according to their duration of action (DOA) [12, 36]. Long-acting agents (*e.g.*, phenobarbital) exhibit DOAs of greater than 6 hours, intermediate-acting agents like amobarbital and butabarbital, last between 3 to 6 hours while short-acting barbiturates (pentobarbital, secobarbital, *etc.*) have DOAs of less than 3 hours. Again, their ability to elicit physiological addictions and toxicities in adults and neonates has significantly deterred the clinical use of barbiturates. Table **1** illustrates a few of the barbiturates for short-term clinical use today [1, 2].

Table 1. Clinically Used Sedative-Hypnotic Barbiturates.

Barbiturates	MW	DOA (h)	Key Enzymes[a]
Phenobarbital (Luminal®)	232.24	>6*	CYP450; UGT; SULT[*a]
Amobarbital (Amytal®)	226.28	3-6*	CYP450; UGT[*a]
Butabarbital (Butisol®)	212.12	3-6*	CYP450; UGT[*a]
Pentobarbital (Nembutal®)	226.28	<3*	CYP450[*a]
Secobarbital (Seconal®)	238.29	<3*	CYP450[*a]

* Data from Liu [36];
[*a] Data from Liu and Dailymed [36, 39].

Individual Barbiturate Drugs (Mechanism, Metabolism, Drug Interactions)

Clinical barbiturates are mostly sodium (Na) salts whose solution forms exist in *keto-enol* tautomeric equilibria (Fig. **6**). C5 substituents (*i.e.*, R_5' and R_5) introduce differences in potency and distribution pharmacokinetics and therefore the duration of action. Because barbiturates are weak acids, their excretion rates can be altered by urine pH (higher or alkaline pH favors ionization and enhanced renal excretion while lower or acidic pH decreases excretion and enhances tubular reabsorption). Barbiturates are generally classified according to their duration of action (DOA) and C5 substitutions groups determine lipophilicity. Lipophilicity and route of administration impact both DOA and drug onset of action, in fact, sedating barbiturates require log *P* values of 2 for optimal activity [40]. Highly lipophilic (higher log *P* values, longer chain C5 alkyl substituents) barbiturates exhibit *rapid onset* and short DOAs due to equilibration facilitated tissue redistribution from the brain to other fatty tissue. Lipophilic barbiturates also cross the placenta during pregnancy and distribute into breast milk. Barbiturates, especially long-lived ones, induce hepatic 1A2, 2C9, 2C19, 3A4 and UGT enzymes [38, 41]. The net result of enzyme induction is the accelerated metabolism of both xenobiotics and endobiotics (steroid hormones, cholesterol, bile salts, and vitamins). Enzyme induction also contributes to barbiturate *tolerance* due to increased barbiturate metabolism [25, 38]. Additionally, prolonged use of barbiturates can desensitize and down-regulate $GABA_A$ leading to *tolerance* [42]. Overall, drug-metabolizing enzyme (DME) induction and inhibition are sources of pharmacokinetic or metabolism-based DDIs for barbiturates.

Long Acting Barbiturates (DOA> 6 h)

Phenobarbital (Luminal) [1, 10, 36]

- Substitution: *N*-methyl plus C-5 substituents (one ethyl- and one phenyl).
- Is a positive allosteric modulator of $GABA_A$ receptor.

- A sedative-hypnotic although it is mainly clinically used as an anti-epileptic agent.
- Like other barbiturates, this agent induces CYP and glucuronidating enzymes. Enzyme induction is a cause of most pharmacokinetic DDIs associated with phenobarbital.
- Exhibits relatively lower lipophilicity (log P 1.46) and plasma binding versus other barbiturates.
- Is inactivated by CYP450 catalyzed *para*-aromatic hydroxylations or *p*-ArOH and subsequent phase II metabolism *via* glucuronidation and sulfation reactions (Fig. **7**).

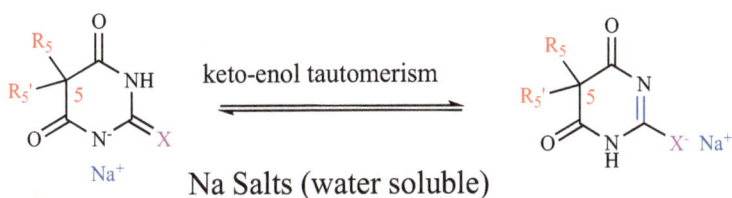

Fig. (6). Tautomeric salt forms of barbiturates.

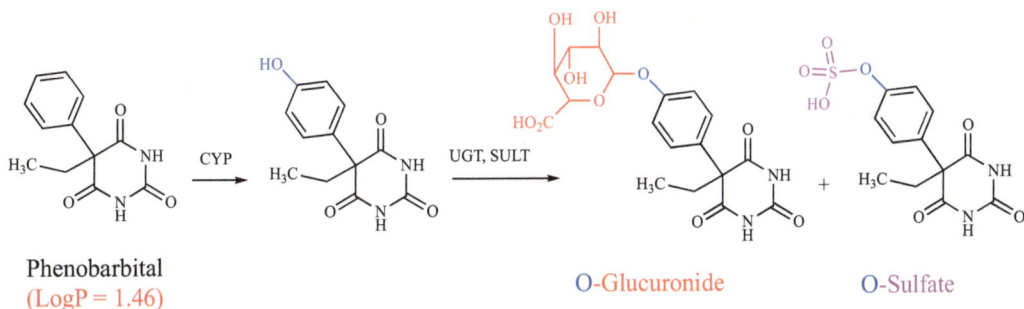

Fig. (7). Phenobarbital and its metabolites.

Intermediate Acting Barbiturates (DOA 3-6h)

Amobarbital (Amytal) and Butabarbital (Butisol) [1,10,36]

- Primarily used as sedative hypnotics.
- Substitutions: Butyl and Ethyl alky chains C5 substitutions are present.
- Exhibit log *P* values of 1.6 - 2, and therefore are more lipophilic than phenobarbital.
- Are metabolized *via* hydroxylation (red arrows) and subsequent conjugation into glucuronides and sulfates (Fig. **8**). Amobarbital can undergo ω-1 or ω (or terminal carbon) oxidations, while Butabarbital is metabolized on its butyl chain. Terminal alcohol intermediates can be oxidized to aldehydes and

carboxylic acids before elimination.

- Metabolism to glucuronide and sulfate conjugates makes these molecules hydrophilic, less lipid-soluble, thereby inactivates them and facilitates renal excretion.

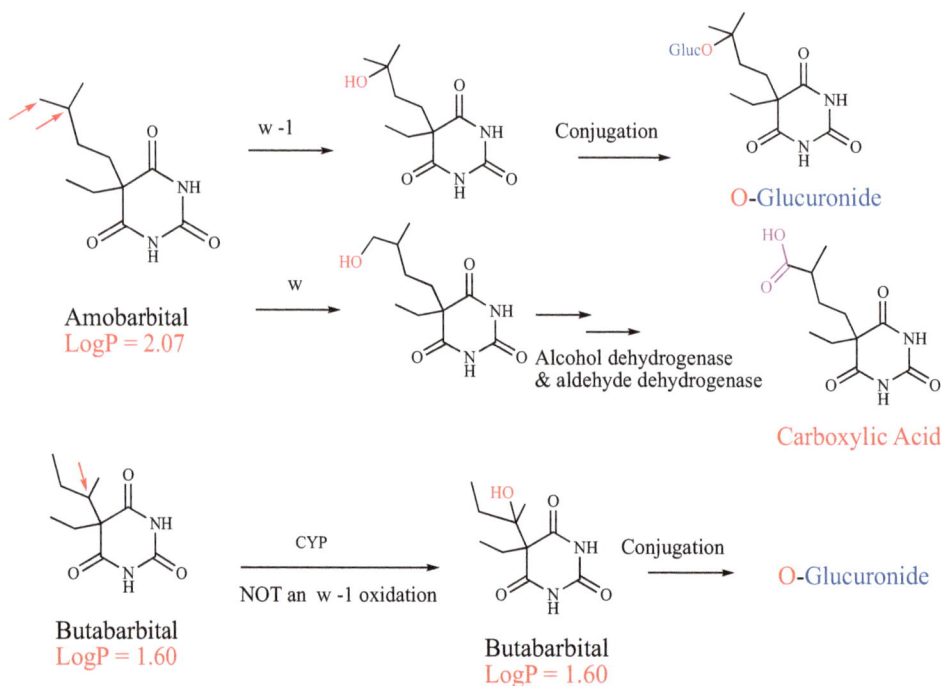

Fig. (8). Amobarbital and Butabarbital metabolic biotransformations.

Short Acting Barbiturates (DOA< 3 h)

Pentobarbital (Nembutal) and Secobarbital (Seconal) [1, 10, 36]

- Are sedative hypnotics used to induce anesthesia (quick onset and very short DOA).
- Substitutions: C5 groups (*ethyl* and *allyl* or five carbon *alkyls*) are present.
- Exhibit log *P* values of greater than 2 and are the most lipophilic barbiturates.
- Their metabolic fates or profiles are similar to those of the intermediate acting agents, and are therefore inactivated in a similar fashion. Rapid metabolism and tissue redistribution account for their short DOA.
- Pentobarbital itself undergoes ω-1 oxidation (red arrow). Secobarbital (Seconal), on the other hand, can undergo either ω-1 oxidation on its butyl chain (blue arrow) or olefinic oxidation to a vicinal diol (OH groups on adjacent carbons) (Fig. **9**).

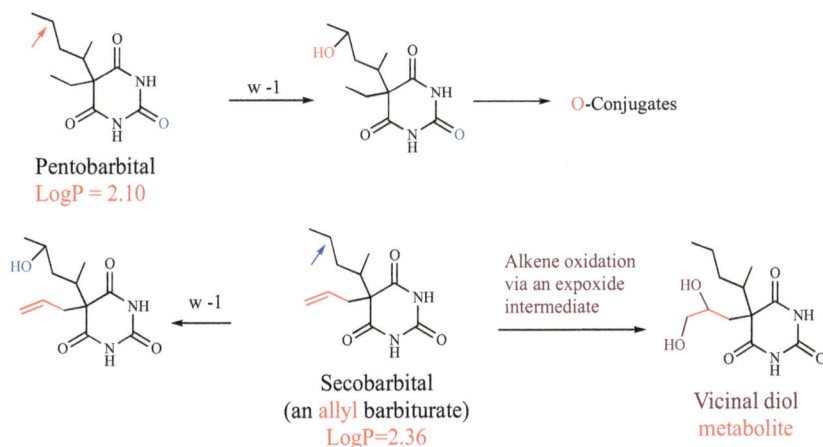

Fig. (9). Pentobarbital and Secobarbital metabolism.

Barbiturate SAR

The structure-activity relationships (SAR) for barbiturates may be summed up as follows (Fig. **10**) [10, 36]:

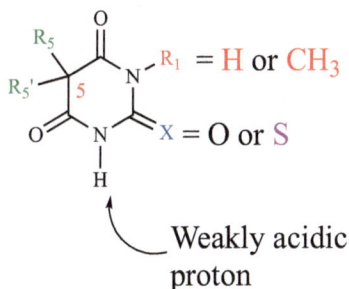

Fig. (10). Barbiturate SAR.

- The unsubstituted barbituric acid lacks sedative-hypnotic activity.
- Alkyl R_1 groups, when present, enhance lipophilicity.
- R_5/R_5' or 5,5-di-substituents impart *lipophilicity*, *activity* and *DOA*. R_5/R_5' groups may be alkyl or aryl. To be active, alkyl chain lengths need to be < 6 carbons.
- Electron donating groups (EDGs) increase barbiturate pKa (pKa >7) and *vice versa* for electron-withdrawing groups (EWGs). Changes in pKa values influence water solubility.
- Replacement of "O" with "S" enhances lipophilicity and affords barbiturates with a quick onset of action.

BENZODIAZEPINES

The benzodiazepine drug family came into existence in 1957 with the discovery of Chlordiazepoxide (marketed as Librium in 1960) which was soon followed by an even more popular Diazepam (Valium) in 1963 [4, 43]. Since then, various BZD containing structures have been synthesized and presented in the literature, however, the molecules described in this chapter can be described as belonging to two extreme chemical classifications: the *2-keto (C=O)* and the *di- or tri-azole* derivatives (Fig. **11**). 2-Keto derivatives typify *"class A"* BZDs while the *diazole* (also called imidazole) and *tri-azole* containing derivatives are members of the *"class B"* or "fused ring" or "annelated" series [44]. For the most part, annelation enhances BZD receptor site binding affinities expressed as K_i values in nanomolar (nm) ranges (*e.g.*, Midazolam K_i = 3.3 nm, and Triazolam K_i = 2.8 nm) versus un-annelated agents (*e.g.*, Diazepam Ki= 5 nm) [44].

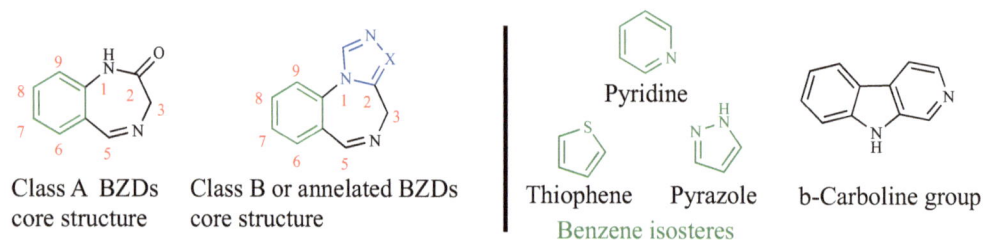

Class A BZDs core structure   Class B or annelated BZDs core structure

Pyridine

Thiophene   Pyrazole   b-Carboline group

Benzene isosteres

Fig. (11). Benzodiazepine general or core structures, benzene moiety isosteres and the carboline group.

Residing somewhere between the above BZD class extremes are other diverse structures that incorporate, for instance, benzene *isosteres* (*e.g.*, pyridine, thiophene, pyrazole), *3-hydroxy (OH)* and *β-carboline* functionalities. The chemistry (*i.e.*, diverse chemical structures, synthetic approaches, pharmacophoric elements, stereochemistry, and SAR or structure-activity relationships) of BZDs has been reviewed extensively by others [45, 46]. More importantly, it is now widely acknowledged that *heterogeneity* in the benzodiazepine binding sites, on $GABA_A$, accounts for the ability of these sites to accommodate structurally distinct drug molecules.

Classical BZDs share similar distribution profiles although their metabolic and elimination pharmacokinetics may differ. Liver CYP450 enzymes facilitate most phase I biotransformations of BZDs resulting in oxygenated species that can further rearrange or decompose to yield active and inactive metabolites. Follow up phase II biotransformations *via* uridine diphosphate glucuronosyltransferases (UGTs), as well as sulfotransferases (STs), afford hydrophilic glucuronides and sulfates, respectively, which can be eliminated in urine. The long-acting characteristic of some BZDs (*e.g.*, diazepam) can be explained by the formation of *N1*-dealkylated active metabolites which, unlike the parent drug, further undergo slower metabolism and therefore accumulate in tissues. Shorter acting BZDs are capable of undergoing aliphatic hydroxylations and subsequent rapid glucuronidations to inactive hydrophilic conjugates. Depending on patient needs, there may be advantages or disadvantages to using longer and shorter acting BZDs. Table **2** illustrates some of the benzodiazepines in clinical use today.

Table 2. Clinically Encountered BZDs.

Benzodiazepines	MW	DOA (h)	Key Enzymes
Diazepam (Valium®)	*271.72*	*4 - 6[b]*	*CYP3A4; CYP2C19[c]*
Oxazepam (Serax®)	*286.72*	*-*	*UGT[d]*
*Estazolam (ProSom®)	*294.74*	*6 - 10[a]*	*CYP2D6; CYP3A4[a]*
*Temazepam (Restoril®)	*300.74*	*6 - 10[a]*	*CYP3A4; UGT[a]*
*Flurazepam (Dalmane®)	*386.90*	*10 - 20[a]*	*CYP2D6; CYP3A4[a]*
*Quazepam (Doral®)	*385.80*	*10 - 20[a]*	*CYP2D6; YP3A4[a]*
Clorazepate (Tranxene®)	*408.92*	*-*	*CYP3A4; UGT[d]*
Lorazepam ((Ativan®)	*321.16*	*4 - 6[b]*	*UGT[c]*
Alprazolam (Xanax®)	*308.77*	*3 - 5[b]*	*CYP3A4; UGT[d]*
Midazolam (Versed®)	*325.77*	*0.5 - 1[b]*	*CYP3A4; UGT[c]*
*Triazolam (Halcion®)	*343.21*	*2 - 5[a]*	*CYP3A4 [a]*
Flumazenil (BZD antagonist)	*303.29*	*1[d]*	*Esterases; UGT[d]*

* FDA approved BZDs for insomnia [5];
[a] Pharmacokinetics data by Bain [5];
[b] Pharmacokinetic data by Bisaga [47];
[c] Data by Saari *et al* [24];
[d] Dailymed and PubChem data [39]; ˙ Missing data.

Mechanistically, BZDs *positively* and *allosterically* potentiate GABA$_A$ receptors. This mechanism of action underlies their sedative-hypnotic and even anti-anxiety properties. Other clinically useful pharmacological effects attributed to BZDs include seizure suppression and muscle relaxation. Unlike other sedative-hypnotics, the anxiolytic effects of BZDs selectively occur at lower doses resulting in minimal sedation and motor incapacity.

Individual Benzodiazepine Drugs (Mechanisms, Metabolism, and Drug Interactions)

Classical benzodiazepines and *annelated BZDs* (Fig. **11**) bind allosterically to GABA$_A$ and modulate the affinity of the receptor for its natural ligand GABA [10,

24, 36, 48, 49]. Anxiolytic drug concentrations are lower than those needed for their sedative-hypnotic effects. These agents are therefore particularly suitable for treating anxiety-related insomnia [50]. Most oral BZDs are lipophilic, they undergo extensive and rapid absorption with high bioavailabilities (80-100%). BZDs are also grouped according to their duration of action. In general, long-acting BZDS exhibit 24 hours or longer half-lives. Half-lives of intermediate-acting agents range from 5 to 24 hours, whereas that of the ultra-short active ones are less than 5 hours [48]. BZDs are for the most part well tolerated, however, excessive/residual sedation plus other dosing related side effects are mainly due to the accumulation of parent drug and active metabolites. BZDs are involved in numerous drug-drug interactions (DDIs) with oral contraceptives, certain antibiotics, antidepressants and azo-antifungal inhibitors of CYP450 enzymes in the liver. CYP450 inhibitors reduce the rate of elimination of the CYP450 dependent benzodiazepines and can lead to excessive systemic drug accumulation and elevated side effects. CYP450 inducers (*e.g.*, rifampicin carbamazepine and phenytoin), on the other hand, can accelerate the elimination of BZDs and decrease their effectiveness [51]. Increased sedation, impaired motor coor-dination, and suppressed breathing occur when BZDs are concurrently consumed with alcohol, opioids, and other CNS depressants, because these agents potentiate their action. Representative BZDs and their pharmacokinetic profiles are described below.

Long-acting BZDS ($t_{1/2}$ >24 hours)

Diazepam (Valium) [10, 24, 52]

- Is a classical "Class A" BZD and a C2 keto-derivative of Chlordiazepoxide. This molecule is a $GABA_A$ positive allosteric modulator with clinical application in various anxiety states.
- Is lipophilic (log P = 2.8) and readily crosses the blood-brain barrier (BBB) into the brain. Diazepam is rapidly absorbed and possesses long half-life (approx. 46 h) which increases with age.
- Undergoes oxidative biotransformations (Fig. **12**) to several pharmacologically active metabolites including Nordiazepam, Temazepam and Oxazepam. These metabolites contribute to the overall long duration of action of diazepam and excessive sedation.

Flurazepam (Dalmane) [5, 10, 52]

- Belongs to "Class A" BZD sedative-hypnotics with an overall long elimination $t_{1/2}$ of about 75 h.
- The parent drug itself is lipophilic (log P = 4.4) and exhibits short elimination ($t_{1/2}$ ~ 2h), however, its 3A4 catalyzed N-dealkylation and hydroxylation lead to

longer-lived active metabolites (Fig. **13**). These metabolites, therefore, account for flurazepam's overall long DOA, sedating effects (days after drug discontinuation), and slow drug elimination.

- The *N*-dealkylated metabolite has an approximate elimination $t_{1/2}$ of 47-100 h (longer in the elderly) *vs* 2-4 h for the hydroxylated metabolite due to rapid glucuronidation.

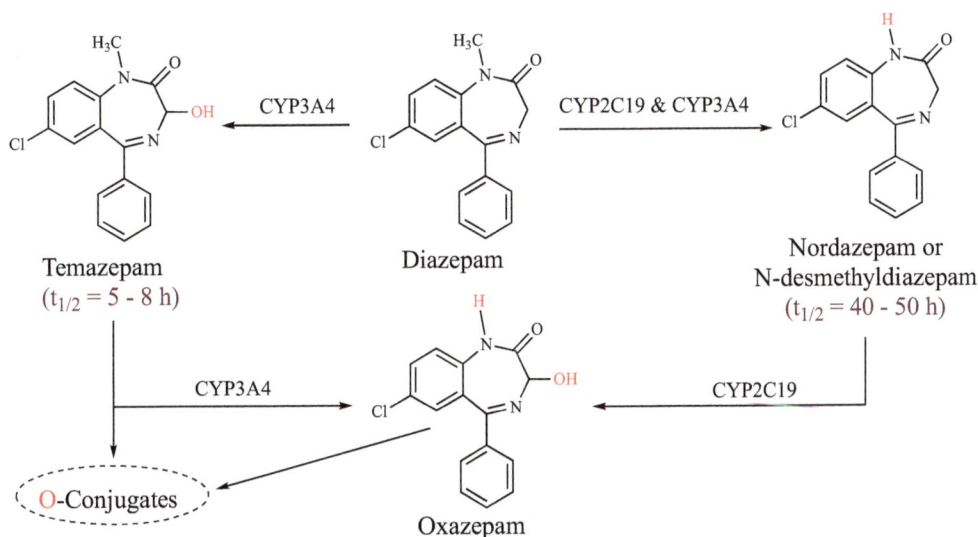

Temazepam
($t_{1/2}$ = 5 - 8 h)

Diazepam

Nordazepam or
N-desmethyldiazepam
($t_{1/2}$ = 40 - 50 h)

O-Conjugates

Oxazepam

Fig. (12). Diazepam's metabolic pathway.

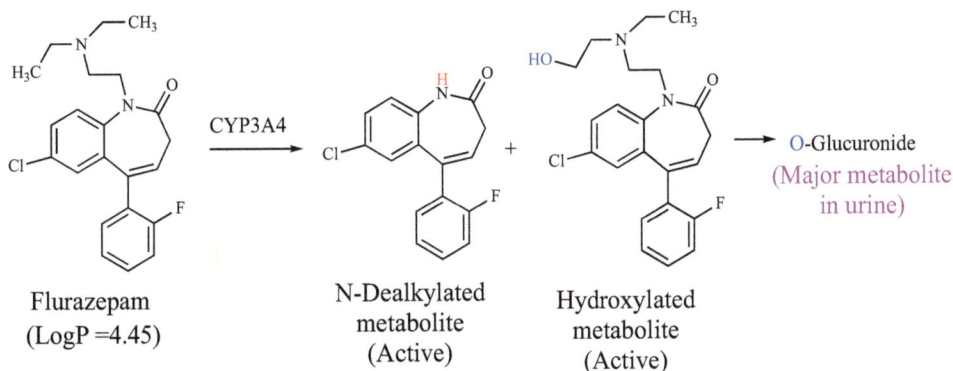

Flurazepam
(LogP =4.45)

N-Dealkylated
metabolite
(Active)

Hydroxylated
metabolite
(Active)

O-Glucuronide
(Major metabolite
in urine)

Fig. (13). Flurazepam biotransformation pathway.

Quazepam (Doral) [10, 39, 53]

- Is a lipohillic *thio*benzodiazepine with a long DOA. Quazepam Is a "Class A" trifluoroethyl BZD for insomnia.
- The drug's long DOA is due to the formation of *oxo* or *carbonyl* long-acting

metabolites *via oxidative desulfuration* and *N*-dealkylation reactions. Phase II metabolism ultimately inactivates these metabolites.

- *Oxidative desulfuration* of quazepam affords *N*-dealkylated 2-oxoquazepam metabolite ($t_{1/2\sim}$ 40 h) and its follow up metabolite *N*-dealkylated 2-oxoquazepam ($t_{1/2}\sim$73 h). These active metabolites contribute to the excessive sedation associated with this drug. Both these active metabolites undergo inactivation through OH group insertions at the circled carbon 3 (also called C3 metabolic hydroxylations), and then excreted as glucuronide conjugates in urine (Fig. **14**).
- Notably, 3A4 and UGT inhibitors can lead to higher plasma levels of quazepam.

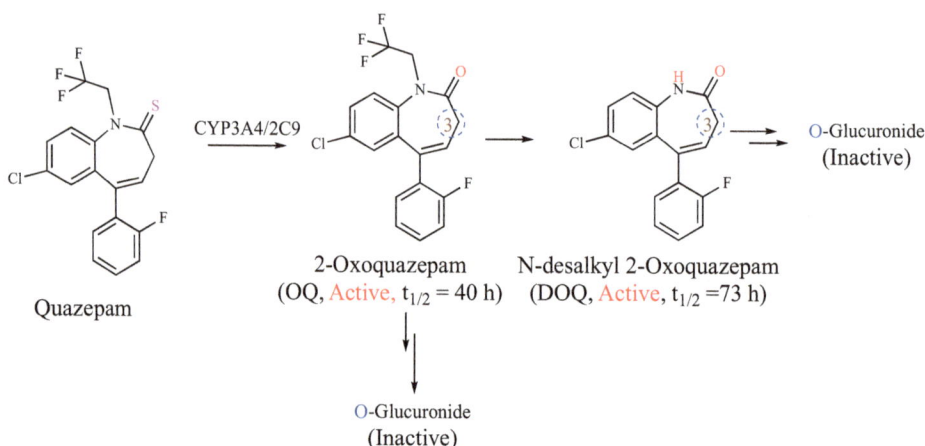

Quazepam

2-Oxoquazepam
(OQ, Active, $t_{1/2}$ = 40 h)

N-desalkyl 2-Oxoquazepam
(DOQ, Active, $t_{1/2}$ =73 h)

O-Glucuronide
(Inactive)

O-Glucuronide
(Inactive)

Fig. (14). Quazepam phase I and phase II bioconversions.

Clorazepate Dipotassium (Tranxene) [39, 54]

- Is yet another "Class A" BZD - the only hydrophilic or polar BZD. This drug is also used for treating various anxiety states.
- Is a *dipotassium* salt *prodrug* designed to be water-soluble and undergoes rapid acid-catalyzed decarboxylation in the stomach to generate two active metabolites.
- The first active metabolite is Nordiazepam (N-desmethyl-diazepam, $t_{1/2}$ > 40 hours). Nordazepam undergoes slow hydroxylation to clorazepate's second active metabolite called Oxazepam (Fig. **15**).

Intermediate Acting BZDs ($t_{1/2}$ 5-24 Hours)

Lorazepam (Ativan) [24, 39]

- Is a highly lipophilic (log *P* = 4.0) "Class A" BZD or 1,4-benzodiazepine, and a synthetic derivative of Oxazepam.
- Is well absorbed (90% oral bioavailability, highly distributed (0.8 -1.3 l/kg), and

readily inactivated *via* glucuronidation (Fig. **16**).

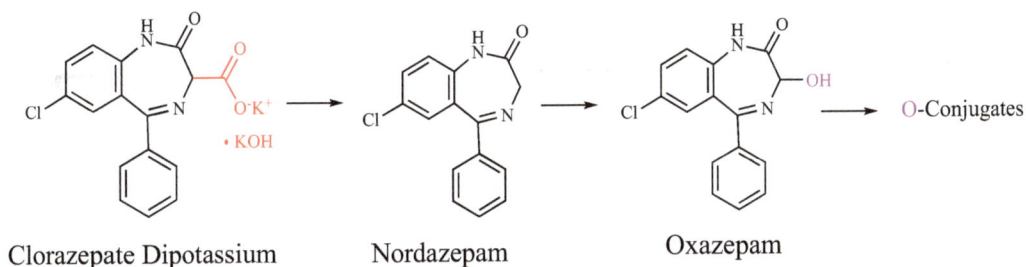

Clorazepate Dipotassium   Nordazepam   Oxazepam

Fig. (15). Clorazepate's bioconversion to active phase I and inactive phase II conjugates.

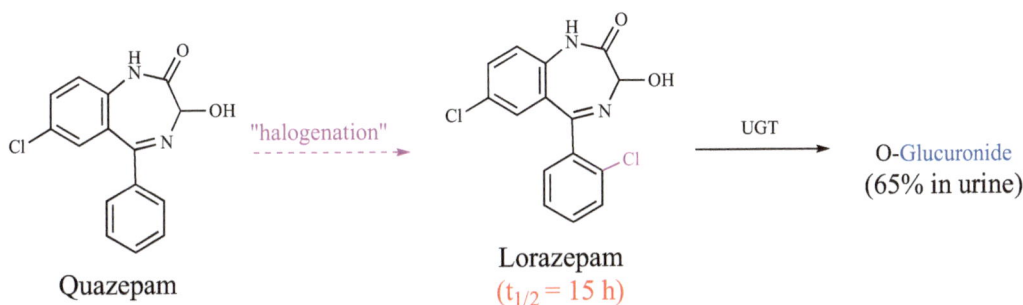

Quazepam   Lorazepam
($t_{1/2}$ = 15 h)

Fig. (16). Lorazepam inactivation plus its relationship to quazepam.

Estazolam (Prosom) [10, 39]

- Is a "Class B" or *1,2-Annelated* BZD or 1,4-triazolobenzodiazepine with a $t_{1/2}$ of 10-24 h. This molecule has a log P = 3.8.
- Undergoes extensive biotransformations which include oxidation to a hydrophilic, weakly active or low GABA$_A$ affinity *4'-hydroxyestazolam* (main metabolite) and inactivations by UGTs to O-glucuronides (Fig. **17**). The minor, *1-oxoestazolam*, metabolite is inactive and also forms glucuronides.
- The short DOA by estazolam is due to metabolic inactivation. The *triazolo* ring prevents C3 oxidations to the long-lived metabolites observed with "class A" BZD structures.
- Since estazolam relies on 3A4 for its metabolism, ketoconazole and itraconazole and other 3A4 inhibitors must be avoided.

Alprazolam (Xanax) [52, 55, 56]

- Is a very lipophilic (log P = 3.2) 1,4-triazolobenzodiazepine with a $t_{1/2}$ = 12 h.
- Incorporates a *triazole* group, which is an acidic moiety and a carboxylic acid *isostere* (alprazolam's pka is 2.4). Triazole ring *methyl* group hydroxylation determines the drug's duration of action since it seems to be the limiting step in

the deactivation of alprazolam.
• Exhibits a shorter elimination half-life due to rapid O-glucuronidation (Fig. **18**).
  Drug metabolite accumulations have not been observed.

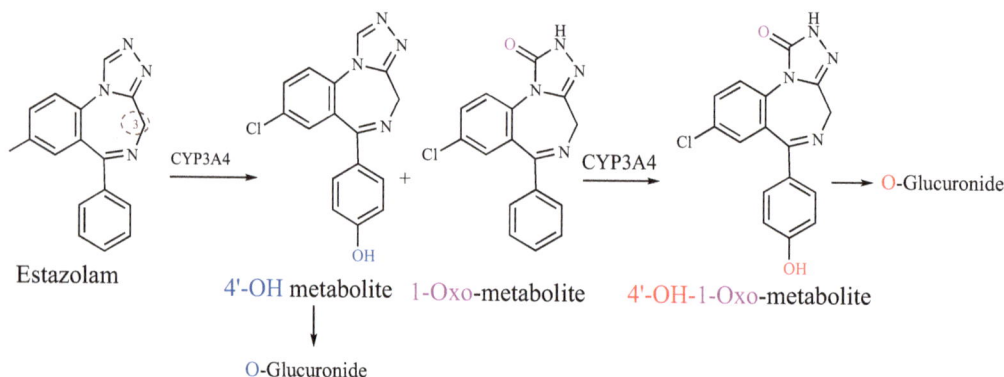

Fig. (17). Estazolam's metabolic pathway.

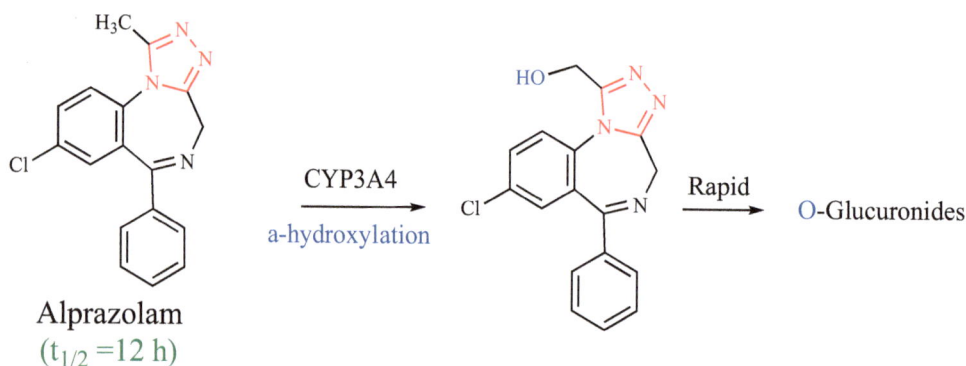

Fig. (18). Alprazolam's deactivation pathway.

Short-acting BZDS (t_{1/2} < 5 Hours)

Oxazepam (Romazicon) [39]

• Is a "Class A" *3-hydroxybenzodiazepinone* for short-term treatment of anxiety.
  Oxazepam's log *P*-value is 2.2.
• Is a common active metabolite of several BZDs (*e.g.*, chlordiazepoxide,
  diazepam, temazepam, chlorazepate) and exhibits an elimination half-life of 4-8
  h.
• Exhibits a short duration of action and less cumulative effects due to rapid
  glucuronidation. Oxazepam's pharmacokinetics are less impacted by age.
• Does not require CYP mediated hydroxylation since it already contains a C3-OH
  moiety, however, oxazepam depends on UGTs for inactivation (Fig. **19**).

Temazepam (Restoril) [10, 39, 52, 56]

- Is a very short acting ($t_{1/2}$ 0.4-0.6 h) lipophilic (log P = 2.2) sedative hypnotic belonging to the "Class A" *3-hydroxybenzodiazepinones*.
- Is not dependent on 3A4 phase metabolism because it already has C3-OH functionality. The C3-OH group facilitates drug inactivation through rapid glucuronidation (Fig. **20**). In fact, 90% of urinary temazepam is detected in the form of glucuronides.
- Has no appreciable active metabolites and therefore no cumulative effects.

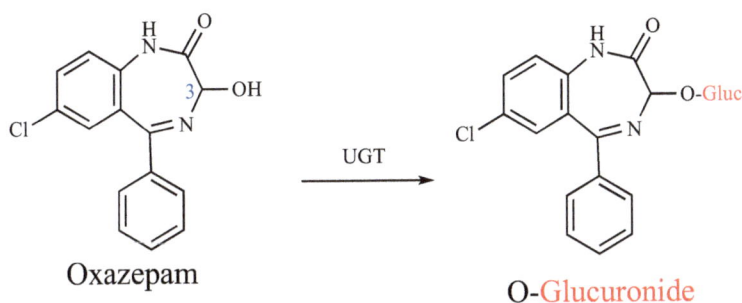

Oxazepam   O-Glucuronide

Fig. (19). Oxazepam's rapid UGT facilitated metabolism.

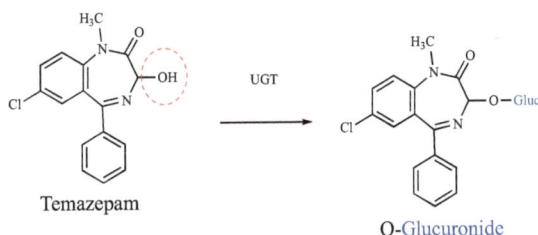

Temazepam   O-Glucuronide

Fig. (20). Temazepam phase II metabolism.

Midazolam (Versed) [24, 44]

- A lipophilic (log P = 3.8) molecule which belongs to the *1,2-annelated* or "Class B" BZD drugs.
- Its structure embeds an imidazole ring, as such the molecule is an *imidazobenzodiazepine*. This ring is weakly acidic (pKa~6) and undergoes a reversible azepine ring opening to form water-soluble acidic salts at pH<4. As such, midazolam solutions are buffered to acidic pH of 3.5. At pH > 4 (*e.g.* physiological pH 7.4) the ring closes, the drug retains its lipophilic properties, and can traverse lipid membranes (Fig. **21**).
- Undergoes imidazole *methyl* hydroxylation and glucuronidation before excretion

(Fig. **22**), as such, the imidazole ring *methyl* group hydroxylation imparts the short DOA into this molecule.

- Is an ultra-short acting ($t_{1/2} \sim 2$ - 5 h) BZD due to rapid glucuronidation.
- Only 50% orally bioavailable due to 1st pass effect.

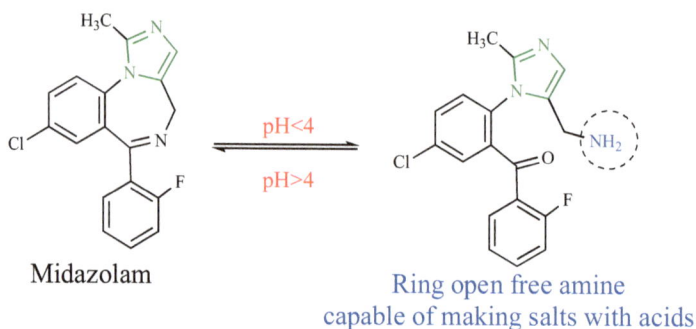

Midazolam   Ring open free amine
capable of making salts with acids

Fig. (21). pH Mediated Midazolam ring-opening and closure.

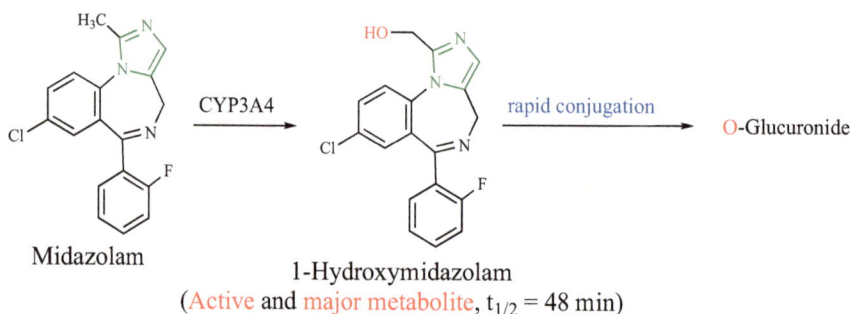

Midazolam   1-Hydroxymidazolam
(Active and major metabolite, $t_{1/2} = 48$ min)

Fig. (22). Midazolam metabolic reactions.

Triazolam (Halcion) [10, 39]

- Is also a lipophilic (log $P = 2.4$) "Annelated" short-acting ($t_{1/2} \sim 4$ h) BZD with a metabolic profile similar to midazolam.
- Undergoes extensive metabolism, resulting in *α-hydroxytriazolam* and *4-hydroxytriazolam* are the key active and inactive metabolites, respectively. The two metabolites experience further biotransformations and account for multiple inactive glucuronides which are excreted in the urine (Fig. **23**).
- The *triazole* ring accounts for triazolam's short DOA because its hydroxylation ultimately leads to drug inactivation *via* glucuronidation .

Flumazenil (Romazicon®) [24, 39]

- Flumazenil is <u>NOT an antianxiety BZD</u>. However, it is a GABA$_A$ BZD receptor site antagonist with utility in reversing BZD and even *z-drug* toxicity or overdose.
- Is a lipophilic (log P = 2.1) ester BZD. Chemically, it is an imidazoben-zodiazepine and belongs to "class B" BZDs. This molecule exhibits poor oral bioavailability because of 1st pass metabolism.
- Is ultra-short acting ($t_{1/2}$ ~ 40 - 80 minutes) due to rapid ester moiety hydrolysis to carboxylic acids and *acyl-* (or carboxylic acid) glucuronides (Fig. **24**). Owing to its short-acting nature, Flumazenil is infused to avoid rebound BZD toxicity.
- Mechanistically, Flumazenil binds to the BZD binding site on the GABA$_A$ receptor and competitively inhibits BZD and Z-drugs from binding.

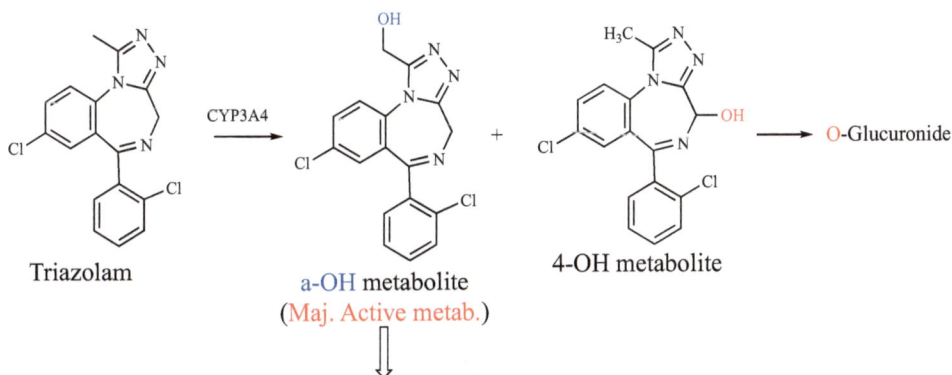

Fig. (23). Triazolam's metabolic scheme.

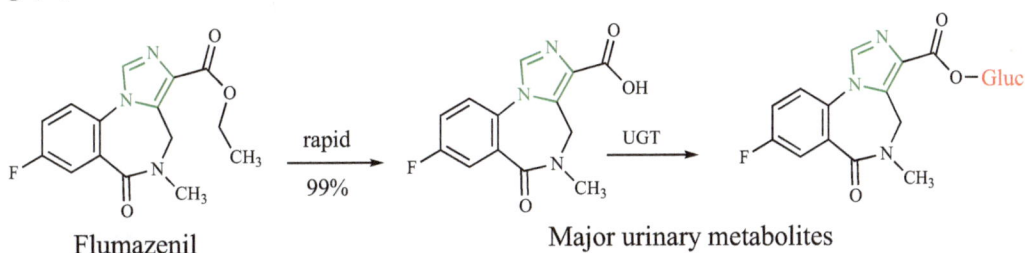

Fig. (24). Hydrolytic and conjugation deactivating reactions of flumazenil.

Benzodiazepine SAR

The following structural features influence the activity of BZD drugs (Fig. **25**) [10, 44]:

- Phenyl or benzene or heteroaromatic isosteres are required for π-π stacking binding interactions within the BZD site.
- C6, C8 & C9 substitutions diminish activity.
- Electron withdrawing groups or EWGs (*e.g.*, F, Cl, NO_2) are required at C7.
- C2 keto-functional group (C=O) is optimal for BZD activity.
- C3 alkyl groups lower BDZ activity but structures with C3-OH retain activity.
- OH groups at C3 impart polarity, and BZD structures possessing this group retain activity. The OH group also facilitates phase II conjugations (*e.g.*, glucuronidations). Note that *non-polar* BZDs are highly protein-bound.
- Ring C *is NOT required for binding*, BUT when present can influence BZD activity. EWGs at C2' or C6' enhance activity, while C4' substitutions diminish it.

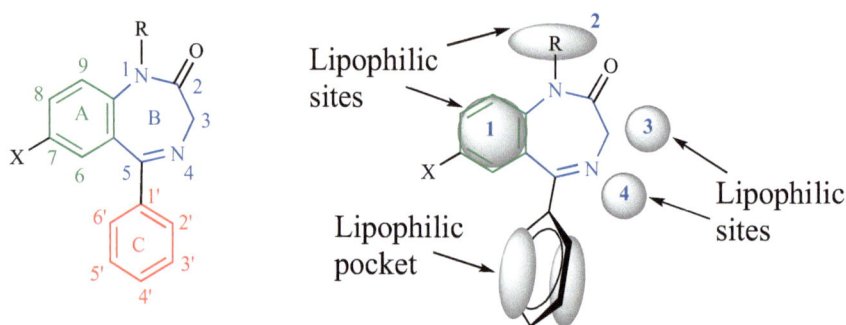

Fig. (25). BZD general structure featuring ring C (left). The structure on the right illustrates binding sites.

NON-BENZODIAZEPINES

This class of sedative-hypnotics comprises several older plus newer structurally and mechanistically dissimilar agents. Representative and clinically available agents from this class of molecules are listed in Table **3**.

Table 3. Clinically Available Non-BZD Sedative-Hypnotics and Anxiolytics.

Non-Benzodiazepines	MW	DOA (h)	Key Enzymes
Zolpidem (Ambien®)	307.40	3 - 8[a]	3A4 [a]
Zaleplon (Sonata®)	305.34	2 - 4[a]	3A4; Aldehyde oxidase [a]
Eszoplicone (Lunesta®)	388.81	5 - 8 [a]	3A4; 2E1; 1A2 [a]
Meprobamate (Miltown®)	218.25	4 - 6[c]	CYP450; UGT[b]
Ramelteon (Rozerem®)	259.35	6 - 8[a]	3A4; 1A2[a]
Buspirone (BuSpar®)	385.51	2 - 3[b]	3A4[c]
Suvorexant (Belsomra®)	450.93	-	3A4;UGT[d]
Lemborexant (Dayvivo®)	410.42	-	3A4[e]

[a]Pharmacokinetic values from Bain [5];

[b]Data by Douglas *et* al [57];
[c]Data from Bisaga [47];
[d]Dailymed data [70];
[e]Access data [71]; ‌Missing data.

Z-drugs, Zolpidem and Zaleplon act *via* α1-containing $GABA_A$ whereas Eszopiclone (the *S-isomer* or *enantiomer* of Zopiclone) targets α1, α2 and α3 - endowed $GABA_A$ receptors [58]. These agents are well-tolerated and have proven to be more efficacious over the long term in diverse patient cohorts. Meprobamate, a polymorphic CYP2C19 dependent major metabolite of Carisoprodol (a muscle relaxant used for acute musculoskeletal pain), was introduced in the 1950s and is indicated for anxiety management [59]. Meprobamate allosterically potentiates $GABA_A$ receptors and at higher doses promotes Cl^- ion conductance in the absence of GABA [60]. Ramelteon, on the other hand, possesses agonist activity for the sleep/wake MT_1/MT_2 melatonin receptors in the SCN [29]. This agent selectively binds to MT_1 with higher affinity than the endogenous ligand melatonin, itself. Originally approved for GAD in 1986, Buspirone is an azpirone class anxiolytic with a lower propensity for sedation, motor impairment, and dependence [31]. Unlike benzodiazepines, buspirone exerts its pharmacological action *via* inhibition and downregulation of $5\text{-}HT1_A$ receptors. Two recent additions, Suvorexant (2014) and Lemborexant (2019), act *via* a promising new mechanism as *orexin* (OX_1/OX_2) G protein-coupled receptor antagonists [69]. The orexin pipeline already comprises structurally dissimilar molecules in various clinical trial stages for narcolepsy and other CNS disorders. Aside from the side effect or off-target issues associated with using older sedative-hypnotics and anxiolytics, the need for mechanistically different molecules is also being driven by the 2019 FDA required boxed warnings for injury risks from sleep walking related to the z-drugs [69].

Individual Non-benzodiazepine Drugs (Mechanisms, Metabolism, Drug Interactions)

This heterogeneous group of agents includes z-drugs (zolpidem, zaleplon and eszopiclone) and meprobamate, which are all positive allosteric modulators (PAMs) of $GABA_A$ receptor [2]. With the exception of meprobamate, the remaining agents exhibit some selectivity in their interactions with $GABA_A$ subunits and are primarily used as sleep aids. In other words, these agents possess minimal anxiolytic or anticonvulsant effects. Ramelteon, the melatonin receptor agonist, exhibits predominant hypnotic effects while buspirone (the $5HT_{1A}$ partial agonist) has predominant anxiolytic effects [51]. Suvorexant and Lemborexant are dual orexin (OX_1/OX_2) receptor antagonists (DORAs). These agents competitively block orexin neuropeptides "A" and "B", whose levels are higher during wakefulness and drop significantly when asleep [70, 71]. Blocking orexin agonist activity at OX_1/OX_2 diminishes receptor activation and results in sleep induction.

Zolpidem Tartrate (Ambien®) [5, 8, 10, 51, 61]

- Is an *Imidazopyridine* sleep-inducing molecule, the 1st subtype-selective agent with high affinity (K_i = 20nM) for α_1 containing (*i.e.*, $\alpha_1\beta_2\gamma_2$ & $\alpha_1\beta_3\gamma_2$) BZD/GABA$_A$ receptor sites.
- Is orally bioavailable (70%) with lipophilicity (log$P$ = 2.6) as a contributory factor. Zolpidem is rapidly absorbed and readily eliminated ($t_{1/2}$ = 2.5 h).
- Undergoes extensive 3A4 biotransformations, with the carboxylic acid major (80%) urinary metabolite (Fig. **26**). The drug exhibits **no** repeated-dose drug accumulations.
- Contains *methyl* groups (CH_3) that are equally vulnerable to 3A4 catalyzed hydroxylations.
- CYP3A4 inhibitors (ketoconazole, erythromycin, cimetidine, *etc*.) impair zolpidem's clearance while the inducers (rifampin, phenytoin, carbamazepine, *etc*.) reduce the drug's hypnotic effects due to sub-therapeutic plasma levels. Also, caffeine potentiates the effects of zolpidem *via* a paradoxical mechanism.

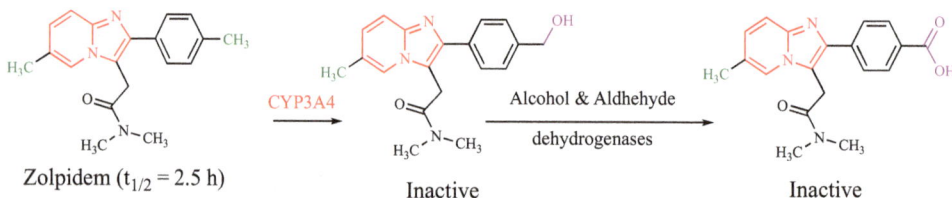

Fig. (26). Zolpidem's structure, metabolic pathway and the enzymes involved.

Zaleplon (Sonata®) [5, 8, 10, 51, 62]

- Is chemically a *Pyrazolopyrimidine* used to induce sleep. This agent selectively targets α_1 containing BZD/GABA$_A$ receptor sites.
- Undergoesquick absorption with a rapid onset. It also rapidly excreted (elimination $t_{1/2}$ = 1 h) despite the dose. The above pharmacokinetic behavior helps explain this drug's short duration of action.
- First pass effect on zaleplon accounts for the drug's low (30%) PO bioavailability. Aldehyde oxidase (AO) plays a significant role in the drug's metabolic deactivation while 3A4 has minor involvement. Animal studies indicate that 3A4 can compensate for low AO activity and significantly metabolize the drug, too. Therefore, it can be rationalized that drugs capable of simultaneously inhibiting AO and 3A4 may effect zaleplon's duration of action.
- Note that AO's extensive metabolism of zaleplon affords 5-oxozaleplon as the major inactive metabolite (Fig. **27**).

- Cimetidine and Raloxifene are inhibitors of aldehyde oxidase, their co-administration would lead to higher plasma or systemic levels of zaleplon.

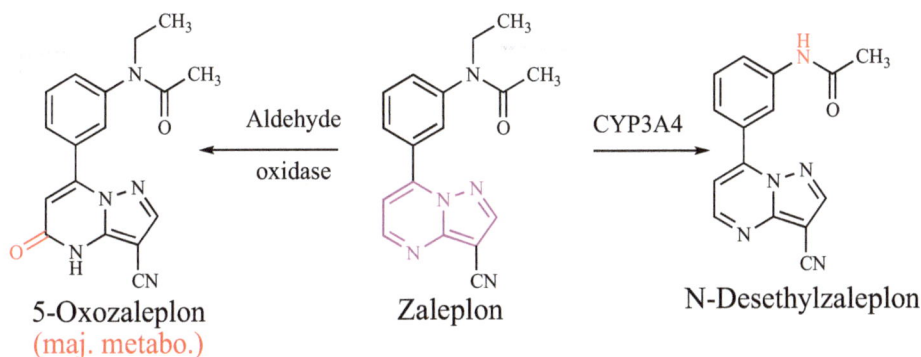

Fig. (27). Zaleplon's partial metabolic scheme indicating two of the several inactive metabolites.

Eszopiclone (Lunesta®) [5, 8, 10, 51]

- Chemically belongs to *Cyclopyrrolone* hypnotic agents for insomnia.
- Is described as a *"superagonist"* at BZD α1β2γ2 and α1β2γ3 binding sites on GABA$_A$.
- Eszopiclone or *S*-Zopiclone is a hypnotic *eutomer* with a 6h half-life and may be chemically obtained from racemic Zopiclone (**R/S**) using chiral separation techniques.
- Exhibits **no** drug accumulation on repeated dosing and is devoid of next-day sedation. The drug is extensively metabolized by 3A4 and 1A2 to an *active* N-oxide and *inactive N-des*methyl metabolites (Fig. **28**).
- Inhibitors of CYP3A4 (*e.g.*, itraconazole, clarithromycin, nefazodone, ritonavir, nelfinavir) can increase plasma levels of eszopiclone and rifampicin, a potent inducer of CYP3A4 does the opposite. Co-administration with ethanol leads to additive impairment of psychomotor performance.

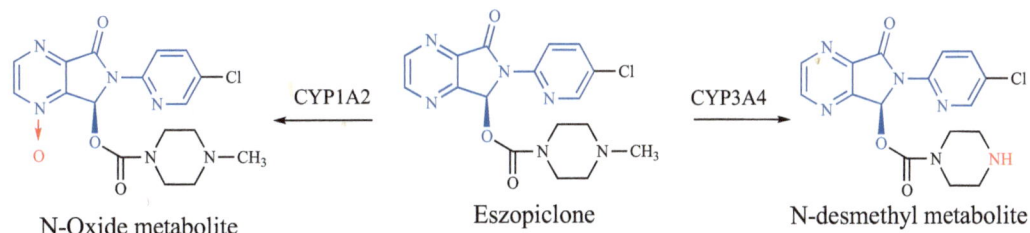

Fig. (28). Oxidative metabolic reactions of Eszopiclone.

Meprobamate (Equanil) [2, 57, 59]

- Is a $GABA_A$ receptor modulator primarily prescribed for *anxiety* but widely used as a *sedative-hypnotic*. Like barbiturates, meprobamate can open the $GABA_A$ Cl⁻ ion channel directly without GABA. It is a *1,3-propane diol* derivative, chemically classified as a *bis-carbamate* (two carbamate groups in the drug structure).

- Is an *active* and *major* metabolite of Carisoprodol (a muscle relaxant for acute musculoskeletal pain) with a long $t_{1/2}$ of 6 - 17 hours. This metabolic reaction relies on *polymorphic* 2C19. Rapid metabolizer 2C19 phenotypes would experience high systemic levels of meprobamate if administered with carisoprodol. The reverse would be true for poor metabolizer phenotypes.

- Undergoes rapid absorption, crosses the placenta and distributes into breast milk. Meprobamate is extensively metabolized by the liver into *inactive* hydroxymeprobamate and glucuronides (only 10 - 20% of the drug is eliminated unchanged in urine, (Fig. **29**).

- Exhibits *additive* CNS depression when co-administered with other CNS depressants (*e.g.*, alcohol, narcotics, and barbiturates).

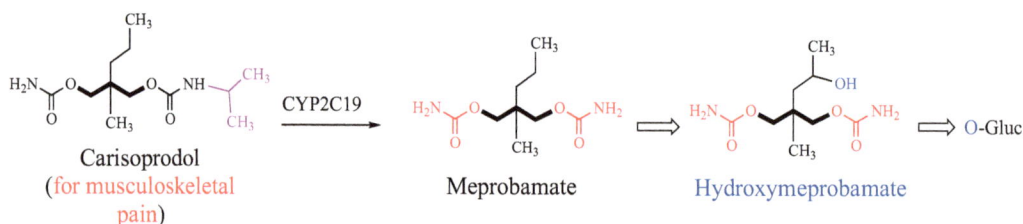

Fig. (**29**). Meprobamate metabolic scheme featuring carisoprodol's bioconversion.

Ramelteon (Rozerem®) [10, 51, 63 - 65]

- Is a *dihydrobenzofuran* melatonin (MT1/MT2) receptor agonist indicated for insomnia and has no abuse liability. It is lipophilic and a rapidly absorbed *"conformationally constrained analog"* of melatonin. The constraint is essential because it orients ramelteon's oxygen *electron* lone pair critical for receptor binding (Fig. **30**).

- The *S*-isomer is the *eutomer* (more active isomer), therefore stereochemistry influences ramelteon's receptor binding affinity.

- Extensive 1st pass metabolism explains this drug's poor (2%) oral bioavailability.

- Its metabolic pathways involve CYP1A2 (major), CYP3A4 & CYP2C19, plus lactone hydrolysis. Only the OH-metabolite is active (Fig. **31**).

- Fluvoxamine (CYP1A2 inhibitor), other CYP enzyme inhibitors (*e.g.*, Fluconazole, Ketoconazole, Fluoxetine), and theophylline (a CYP1A2 substrate that competes with Ramelteon) can increase systemic levels of Ramelteon. Rafampin, a CYP inducer, can reduce drug levels.

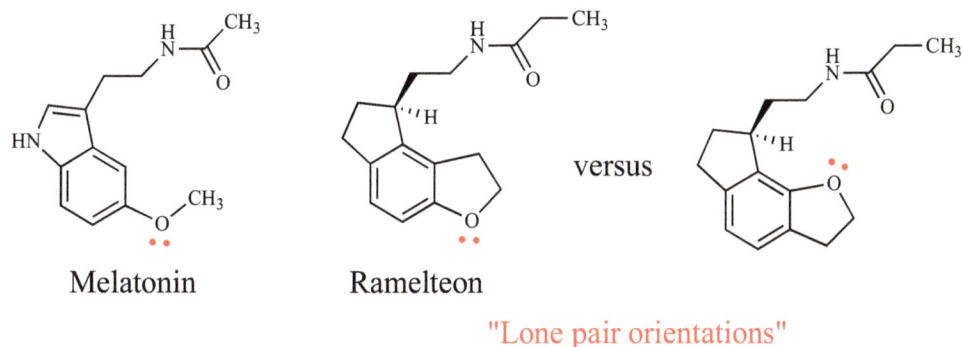

versus

"Lone pair orientations"

Fig. (30). Structures of melatonin and ramelteon illustrating oxygen electron lone-pair orientations.

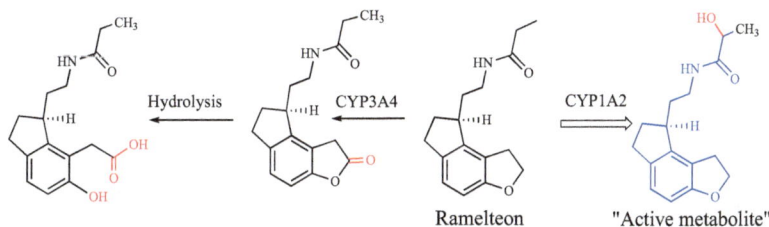

Fig. (31). Ramelteon metabolism *via* CYP1A2 and CYP3A4.

Buspirone (Buspar®) [6, 31, 51]

- Is an *Azapirone* miscellaneous anxiolytic agent used in generalized anxiety disorder (GAD).
- Is the only anxiolytic on the US market whose mechanism of action involves partial agonism at *septohippocampal* 5-HT$_{1A}$ receptors in the brain. 5-HT$_{1A}$ anxiolytics lack muscle relaxant, sedative, and anticonvulsant activities and do not impair psychomotor functioning.
- Exhibits a slower onset of effect (takes 1 to 3 weeks, due to receptor down-regulation) compared to BZDs and poor (5%) oral bioavailability due to extensive 1st pass metabolism. Renal disease and hepatic cirrhosis slow down buspirone excretion and metabolism, respectively.
  - ○ Relies on CYP3A4 (and to a less extent CYP2D6) for its extensive metabolism. Key active metabolites (Fig. **32**): *1-(2-pyrimidinyl)-piperazine* or **1-PP,***N*-oxide, and *6'-hydroxybuspirone.***1-PP** is an α$_2$-adrenergic antagonist and 5-HT1$_A$ partial agonist. This metabolite may contribute to buspirone's overall activity and DOA. CYPs 2D6/3A4 also bio-convert buspirone to *6'-hydroxybuspirone* whose clinical utility is unknown.

Curiously, *6'-hydroxybuspirone* blood levels rise to 40 times higher than the parent drug.

○ Strong CYP3A4 inhibitors (*e.g.*, Erythromycin and Itraconazole) and grape fruit juice can enhance the levels of buspirone in systemic circulation.

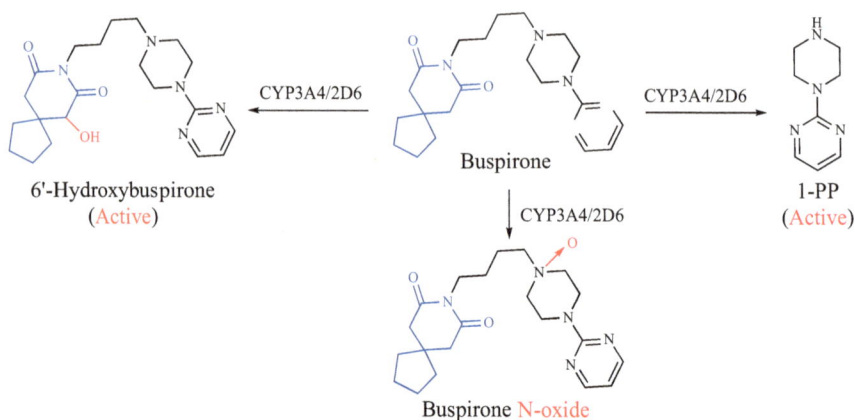

Fig. (32). Buspirone biotransformations indicating key active metabolites.

Suvorexant (Belsomra®) [70]

- Is a sleep-inducing *Diazepane Amide* with utility in insomnia (maintains both latency and sleep). Potential abuse liability, hence Suvorexant is a schedule IV controlled drug.
- Is a high affinity and competitive dual orexin (OX_1/OX_2) receptor antagonist (DORA). It inhibits orexin "A" and "B" type neuropeptides, which promote wakefulness, from binding to their receptors.
- Exhibits 80% PO bioavailability, is well absorbed and crosses the BBB (log P = 3.6) with $t_{1/2}$ of 12 h.
- Suvorexant is extensively metabolized by 3A4 (key CYP450 enzyme) and UGTs (minor role) to several inactive –OHs, -COOH & -Glucuronides (Fig. 33). Drug interactions may occur when taken together with strong 3A4 inducers or inhibitors. Also, the drug/metabolites may transfer into mammary milk in nursing mothers.

Lemborexant (Dayvigo®) [71]

- Is a recently introduced *Pyrimidine* **DORA** and sleep-inducing molecule for insomnia. It also competitively antagonizes OX_1 and OX_2 receptors.
- Leborexant has exhibited low PO bioavailability in animal studies - suggesting first-pass effect. The molecule is lipophilic (cLog P = 3), possesses a $t_{1/2}$ = 17-19

h, and its *1R*, *2S*-enantiomer is more active.

- Is primarily metabolized by 3A4, and one major metabolite (M10, with comparable affinity to parent drug at OX_1/OX_2) has been identified. Drug interactions may be expected if co-administered with strong 3A4 inducers and inhibitors.
- Note: at the time of our literature search for this molecule, the drug was very new, some human pharmacokinetics data and the active metabolite (M10) structure were not available in open access journals or databases (Fig. **34**).

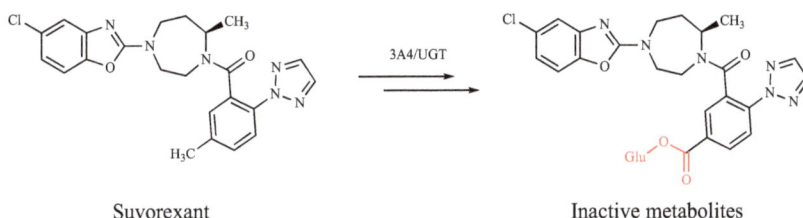

Fig. (33). Suvorexant key metabolizing phases I and II enzymes leading to inactive metabolites.

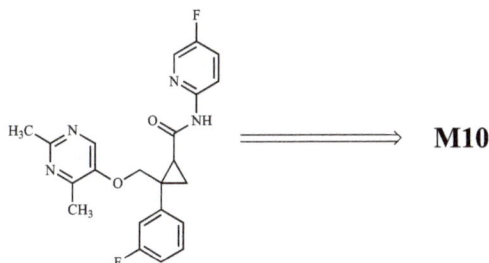

Fig. (34). Lemborexant biotransformation route to its key active metabolite M10 (structure unavailable).

CASE STUDIES

Case 1

Geena is a 55 YO male who recently immigrated to the US with a two weeks supply of phenobarbital and the antibiotic doxycycline. He notices that despite being compliant in taking the two prescriptions, his infection is not improving. He stops by your pharmacy and enquires from you the reason the infection is not responding to treatment.

Explanation:

....

....

....

....
....

Case 2

Patient Z is a 27 YO woman who goes to an outpatient clinic with complaints of insomnia. She suffers from an obsessive-compulsive disorder and has been seen frequently by a psychiatrist. She is currently taking Eszopiclone and is seeking a dosage adjustment and advice on whether to switch medications. Explain Eszopiclone's mechanism of action and the effects of taking this medication with alcohol.

....
....
....
....
....
....
....
....

....
....
....
....
....

Case 3

Dr. Treeo is head of pharmacy at *Calm Waters Hospital* and *your PharmD preceptor*. Among his duties at the hospital is the maintenance of drug inventories. Dr. Treeo recently received two boxes of some back-ordered sedative-hypnotics and would like to train his PharmD interns in all manners of identifying drugs.

Intern's assignment: Using your drug structure expertise, chemically categorize the following core drug structures found in the present and past sedative-hypnotics and anxiolytics.

DRUG DISCOVERY CASE STUDIES

Case 1: Meprobamate Discovery [3]

In 1945, British Drug Houses Ltd (BDH) chemists were searching for *gram-*

negative anti-microbial agents using *phenoxetol* or *phenoxyethanol* as the lead molecule (Fig. **35**).

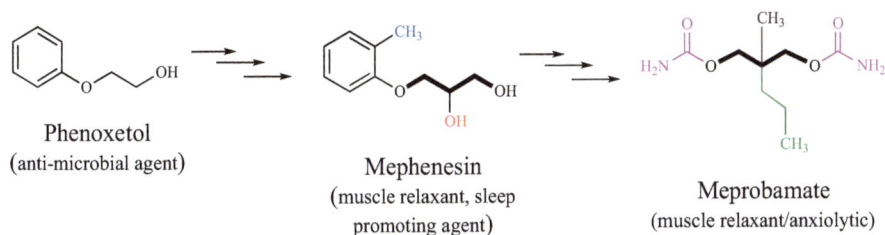

Fig. (35). Illustration of some of the design and synthetic leaps taken to arrive at meprobamate.

When Frank Berger observed that administration of small quantities of *phenoxetol analogs* to mice/rats/guinea pigs induced muscle relaxation and sleep, he focused his attention one particular analog, an old drug called *Mephenesin* or 3-(--methoxyphenyl)-1,2-propanediol), which exhibited the best safety margin and produced the most muscle relaxant effects. In 1948, E. R. Squibb introduced Mephenesin on the clinical market as *Tolserol*, to be used for muscle relaxation under light anesthesia. However, Mephenesin's undesirable shorter duration of action due to rapid metabolic deactivation plus pronounced effects on the spinal cord led Frank to seek alternative compounds. Structure deconstruction/re-construction of Mephenesin gave rise to Meprobamate or 2-methyl-2-n-prop--1,3-propanediol dicarbamate. This compound demonstrated eight times longer duration of action versus Mephenesin. Synthetic work for this molecule was conducted by B. J. Ludwig (in 1950, at Wallace Laboratories, US), and in 1955 the drug entered the US market as a muscle relaxant and anxiolytic agent under two trade names: *Miltown* (by Wallace Laboratories) and *Equanil* (by Wyeth Laboratories, US). This molecule reigned during the 1950s until Diazepam came on the market. Actually, Meprobamate partly inspired the discovery of benzodiazepines.

Case 2: Chlordiazepoxide/Diazepam Discovery [3, 4, 66]

In search of novel tranquilizers in the 1950's, Leo Sternbach (a chemist at Hoffman-La Roche, USA) reached back into his earlier 1930's postdoctoral unfruitful work on *benz-heptoxdiazine dye* chemistry. Structural manipulation of benz-heptoxdiazine, in 1955, led to the synthesis of a variety of derivatives, amongst which were *quinazoline N-oxides* possessing disappointing pharmacological properties (Fig. **36**).

This line of research seemed to be yielding no good results, Leo and co-workers even shifted their efforts to synthesizing antibiotics. According to Leo *"this intensive work, of little practical value, finally led, in April 1957, to a hopeless situation."* *Serendipity* (Circa 1957): In their attempt to clean-up the glassware they had piled up, containing various mother liquors, Leo's co-worker (Earl Reeder), alerted him to a few nice crystals of a compound labeled **Ro 5-0690** that had formed in flasks from the shelved 1955 stabilization experiments involving quinazoline-N-oxides and methylamine (CH_3NH_2). To their surprise, pharmacological testing of these crystals yielded positive sedating, muscle relaxation, and anxiolytic results. Structural analysis of the crystals led to them to conclude that an un-expected *benzodiazepine-N-oxide* compound had formed. Within 2.5 years (in 1960) Chlordiazepoxide was introduced on the market under the trade name Librium. This encouraging news inspired further structural investigations on chlordiazepoxide and spurred the generation of many BZDs in use today. For instance, the desire to formulate a non-bitter tasting syrup/elixir for pediatric and geriatric patients led to the removal of the *oxide* feature, and the introduction of the *C2 keto* (C=O) and *N1-methyl* groups. The end result of the aforementioned structural changes was a novel and an even more potent molecule called *Diazepam* (Valium) which was introduced in 1963 and soon became the blockbuster drug of the day.

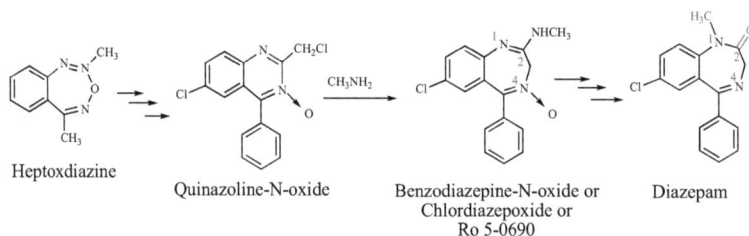

Fig. (36). Abbreviated synthetic scheme leading to chlordiazepoxide and diazepam.

Case 3: Ramelteon Discovery [65, 67, 68]

Aaron Leaner *et al* discovered melatonin, in 1958, and set out to investigate its potential utility in their skin diseases related research. They soon found out that melatonin administration did not reverse either *vitiligo* or melanocyte-stimulating hormone-induced *hyperpigmentation*. The intervening years witnessed other investigators establish the pineal gland's involvement in the biosynthesis of melatonin. Further understanding of melatonin's pharmacological effects was aided by the cloning and characterization of its receptors, which were classified in 1998 as MT_1, MT_2, and MT_3. Investigations linking melatonin's secretion to the circadian rhythm in the brain's hypothalamic suprachiasmatic nucleus (SCN), plus its ability to initiate sleep onset upon exogenous administration to healthy humans, provided further proof for the role of this agent in modulating sleep. However, due to melatonin's poor oral bioavailability, its non-selective effects, and short half-life, research efforts aimed at discovering molecules with improved pharmacological profiles were initiated. These efforts led to the discovery of melatonin's synthetic analog called Ramelteon (Rozerem) or (S)-N-[2-(1,6,-,8-tetrahydro-2Hindeno[5,4-b]furan-8-yl)ethyl]propionamide by Takeda Pharmaceutical Company (Fig. 37). In 2005, Ramelteon received FDA approval and entered the US clinical market for insomnia treatment. Among the advantages of Ramelteon are: rapid action and the lack of dependence or abuse liabilities.

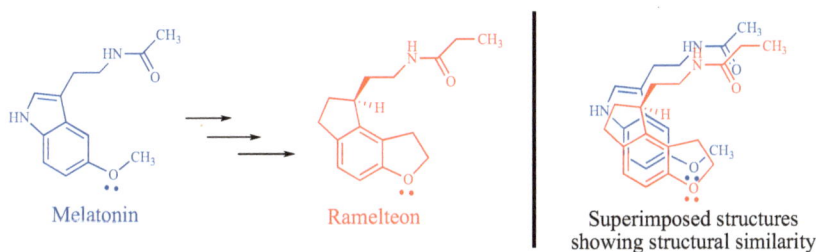

Melatonin   Ramelteon   Superimposed structures
                                                  showing structural similarity

Fig. (37). Structural modification of melatonin to form ramelteon plus structural similarities.

STUDENT SELF-STUDY GUIDE

- Define the terms *sedative*, *hypnotic* and *anxiolytic*.
- Chemically categorize sedative-hypnotic and anxiolytic drugs.
- Classify the barbiturates by duration of action (DOA) and rationalize what ADME parameters influence DOA
- Classify the benzodiazepines by duration of action (DOA) and rationalize what ADME parameters influence DOA
- Describe the mechanisms of action of the different sedative-hypnotic and anxiolytic drugs.
- What is allosteric modulation?
- Describe PAMs, NAMs and NAs.
- Describe the SAR elements of BZDs and Barbiturates.
- What is the influence of lipophilicity (log *P*) on sedative-hypnotic and anxiolytic drug activity?
- Characterize drug-metabolizing enzyme induction and inhibition, also called pharmacokinetic DDIs and their impact on pharmacotherapeutic outcomes.

STUDENT SELF-ASSESSMENT QUESTIONS

1. The acronym GABA stands for:

…………..

2. All of the following descriptors apply to GABA, *except*:

A. A GABA receptor ligand

B. A xenobiotic agent

C. An amino acid molecule

D. A neurotransmitter

3. Diazepam can be appropriately mechanistically categorized under:

E. PAMs

F. NAMs

G. NAs

H. Inverse agonists

4. Give two examples of annelated BZDs.

a)…………………………………………………………...

b)…………………………………………………………..

5. <u>**SELECT ALL THAT APPLY:**</u> **BDZs and Z-Drugs fall into a heterogeneous group of drugs that produce pharmacological effects via**
…………………………………………..

I. Inhibition of $GABA_A$

J. Activation of $GABA_A$

K. Inhibition of GABA

L. Potentiation of GABA

M. Enhancement of Cl- entry

6. According to the SAR of BZDs, is Ring C required for activity?

YES……. **NO**……..

7. TRUE or FALSE: Nordazepam metabolism affords Oxazepam.

8. TRUE or FALSE: Barbiturates are weak bases

9. TRUE or FALSE: Zolpidem (*log* P = 3.8) has good oral bioavailability

10. Name two contributory factors to the short duration of action of some barbiturates

a)………………………………………………………..

b)………………………………………………………..

11. What is the main idea behind *conformationally* constraining the oxygen atom in Ramelteon's structure?

Answer: …………………………………………………………………………..

………………………………………………………………………………………..

………………………………………………………………………………………………

………………

………………………………………………………………………………………………

………………

………………………………………………………………………………………………

………………

12. Discuss buspirone's metabolism and its potential impact on the parent drug's duration of action.

Answer:

……………………………………………………………………………………………

……………………………………………………………………………………………

• Trevor AJ. Sedative-Hypnotic Drugs. In: Katzung BG, eds. *Basic & Clinical-Pharmacology, 14e Ed.* New York, NY: McGraw-Hill; 2018.

• Moniri NH. Sedative-Hypnotics. In: Lemke TL, Williams DA, eds. *Foye's Principles of Medicinal Chemistry, 8th ed.* Philadelphia, PA: Lippincott Williams & Wilkins; 2019.

• Liu S. Central Nervous System Depressants. In: Beale Jr JM, Block JH, eds. *Wilson and Gisvold's textbook of Organic Medicinal and Pharmaceutical Chemistry, 12ᵗʰ ed.* Philadelphia, PA: Lippincott Williams & Wilkins; 2011.

- Lopez-Munoz FL, Ucha-Udabe R, Alamo C. The history of barbiturates a century after their clinical introduction. *Neuropsychiatr Dis Treat.* 2005: 1(4), 329-343.

- Proctor A, Bianchi MT. Clinical Pharmacology in Sleep Medicine. *ISRN Pharmacol.* 2012; 2012:914168 (doi:10.5402/2012/914168)

- Chadwick B, Waller DG, Edwards JG. Potentially hazardous drug interactions with psychotropics. *Adv Psychiatr Treat.* 2005; 11: 440-449.

CONSENT FOR PUBLICATION

Not applicable.

CONFLICT OF INTEREST

The authors confirm that the contents of this chapter have no conflict of interest.

ACKNOWLEDGEMENTS

Declare none.

REFERENCES

[1] López-Muñoz F, Ucha-Udabe R, Alamo C. The history of barbiturates a century after their clinical introduction. Neuropsychiatr Dis Treat 2005; 1(4): 329-43. [PMID: 18568113]

[2] Sedative-Hypnotics. http://www.goldfrankstoxicology.com/chapters/GTE9_Chap74.pdf

[3] Ban TA. The role of serendipity in drug discovery. Dialogues Clin Neurosci 2006; 8(3): 335-44. [PMID: 17117615]

[4] López-Muñoz F, Alamo C, García-García P. The discovery of chlordiazepoxide and the clinical introduction of benzodiazepines: half a century of anxiolytic drugs. J Anxiety Disord 2011; 25(4): 554-62. [http://dx.doi.org/10.1016/j.janxdis.2011.01.002] [PMID: 21315551]

[5] Bain KT. Management of chronic insomnia in elderly persons. Am J Geriatr Pharmacother 2006; 4(2): 168-92. [http://dx.doi.org/10.1016/j.amjopharm.2006.06.006] [PMID: 16860264]

[6] Zhu M, Zhao W, Jimenez H, et al. Cytochrome P450 3A-mediated metabolism of buspirone in human liver microsomes. Drug Metab Dispos 2005; 33(4): 500-7. [http://dx.doi.org/10.1124/dmd.104.000836] [PMID: 15640381]

[7] aChoi Y, Raymer BK. Sleep modulating agents. Bioorg Med Chem Lett 2019; 29(16): 2025-33. [http://dx.doi.org/10.1016/j.bmcl.2019.06.043] [PMID: 31307886] bhttps://www.nacds.org/membership/resources/2020.chttps://www.pharmacytimes.com/contributor/sean-kane-pharmd/ 2018/02/ the-top-200-drugs-of-2018-which-drugs-are-making-an-impact2020.

[8] Ebert B, Wafford KA, Deacon S. Treating insomnia: Current and investigational pharmacological approaches. Pharmacol Ther 2006; 112(3): 612-29. [http://dx.doi.org/10.1016/j.pharmthera.2005.04.014] [PMID: 16876255]

[9]   Foral P, Dewan N, Malesker M. Insomnia: a therapeutic review for pharmacists. Consult Pharm 2011;
        26(5): 332-41.
        [http://dx.doi.org/10.4140/TCP.n.2011.332] [PMID: 21733814]

[10]   Moniri NH. Sedative-Hypnotics.Foye's Principles of Medicinal Chemistry. 7th ed., Philadelphia, PA:
        Lippincott Williams & Wilkins 2013.

[11]   Farach FJ, Pruitt LD, Jun JJ, Jerud AB, Zoellner LA, Roy-Byrne PP. Pharmacological treatment of
        anxiety disorders: current treatments and future directions. J Anxiety Disord 2012; 26(8): 833-43.
        [http://dx.doi.org/10.1016/j.janxdis.2012.07.009] [PMID: 23023162]

[12]   Dwivedi SK, Shrivastava D, Pandey G. Diagnosis of drugs on anxiety disorder: an overview. Int J of
        Pharm & Research Sci 2012; 1(1): 73-107.

[13]   Dunlop BW, Davis PG. Combination treatment with benzodiazepines and SSRIs for comorbid anxiety
        and depression: a review. Prim Care Companion J Clin Psychiatry 2008; 10(3): 222-8.
        [http://dx.doi.org/10.4088/PCC.v10n0307] [PMID: 18615162]

[14]   Stein M, Steckler T, Lightfoot JD, Hay E, Goddard AW. Pharmacologic treatment of panic disorder.
        Curr Top Behav Neurosci 2010; 2: 469-85.
        [http://dx.doi.org/10.1007/7854_2009_35] [PMID: 21309122]

[15]   Dell'osso B, Lader M. Do benzodiazepines still deserve a major role in the treatment of psychiatric
        disorders? A critical reappraisal. Eur Psychiatry 2013; 28(1): 7-20.
        [http://dx.doi.org/10.1016/j.eurpsy.2011.11.003] [PMID: 22521806]

[16]   Chebib M, Johnston GAR. GABA-Activated ligand gated ion channels: medicinal chemistry and
        molecular biology. J Med Chem 2000; 43(8): 1427-47.
        [http://dx.doi.org/10.1021/jm9904349] [PMID: 10780899]

[17]   Conn PJ, Christopoulos A, Lindsley CW. Allosteric modulators of GPCRs: a novel approach for the
        treatment of CNS disorders. Nat Rev Drug Discov 2009; 8(1): 41-54.
        [http://dx.doi.org/10.1038/nrd2760] [PMID: 19116626]

[18]   Nutt DJ, Malizia AL. New insights into the role of the GABA(A)-benzodiazepine receptor in
        psychiatric disorder. Br J Psychiatry 2001; 179: 390-6.
        [http://dx.doi.org/10.1192/bjp.179.5.390] [PMID: 11689393]

[19]   Krogsgaard-Larsen B. Frolund, U. Kristiansen, K. Frydenvang, B. Ebert. $GABA_A$ and $GABA_B$
        receptor agonists, partial agonists, antagonists and modulators:design and therapeutic prospects. Eur J
        Pharm Sci 1997; 5: 355-84.
        [http://dx.doi.org/10.1016/S0928-0987(97)10009-4]

[20]   Krogsgaard-Larsen P, Frølund B, Liljefors T, Ebert B. $GABA_{(A)}$ agonists and partial agonists: THIP
        (Gaboxadol) as a non-opioid analgesic and a novel type of hypnotic. Biochem Pharmacol 2004; 68(8):
        1573-80.
        [http://dx.doi.org/10.1016/j.bcp.2004.06.040] [PMID: 15451401]

[21]   Polc P. Electrophysiology of benzodiazepine receptor ligands: multiple mechanisms and sites of
        action. Prog Neurobiol 1988; 31(5): 349-423.
        [http://dx.doi.org/10.1016/0301-0082(88)90014-7] [PMID: 2851856]

[22]   Rudolph U, Knoflach F. Beyond classical benzodiazepines: novel therapeutic potential of $GABA_A$
        receptor subtypes. Nat Rev Drug Discov 2011; 10(9): 685-97.
        [http://dx.doi.org/10.1038/nrd3502] [PMID: 21799515]

[23]   Greenfield LJ. Molecular mechanisms of antiseizure drug activity at $GABA_A$ receptors: Seizure.. Eur J
        Epilepsy 2013.
        [http://dx.doi.org/10.1016/j.seizure.2013.04.015]

[24]   Saari TI, Uusi-Oukari M, Ahonen J, Olkkola KT. Enhancement of GABAergic activity:
        neuropharmacological effects of benzodiazepines and therapeutic use in anesthesiology. Pharmacol

Rev 2011; 63(1): 243-67.
[http://dx.doi.org/10.1124/pr.110.002717] [PMID: 21245208]

[25]   Khanna JM, Kalant H, Chau A, Shah G. Rapid tolerance and crosstolerance to motor impairment effects of benzodiazepines, barbiturates, and ethanol. Pharmacol Biochem Behav 1998; 59(2): 511-9.
[http://dx.doi.org/10.1016/S0091-3057(97)00477-2] [PMID: 9477002]

[26]   Sieghart W. Structure, pharmacology, and function of GABA$_A$ receptor subtypes. Adv Pharmacol 2006; 54: 231-63.
[http://dx.doi.org/10.1016/S1054-3589(06)54010-4] [PMID: 17175817]

[27]   Vanecek J. Cellular mechanisms of melatonin action. Physiol Rev 1998; 78(3): 687-721.
[http://dx.doi.org/10.1152/physrev.1998.78.3.687] [PMID: 9674691]

[28]   Dubocovich ML, Delagrange P, Krause DN, Sugden D, Cardinali DP, Olcese J. International Union of Basic and Clinical Pharmacology. LXXV. Nomenclature, classification, and pharmacology of G protein-coupled melatonin receptors. Pharmacol Rev 2010; 62(3): 343-80.
[http://dx.doi.org/10.1124/pr.110.002832] [PMID: 20605968]

[29]   Cardinali DP, Srinivasan V, Brzezinski A, Brown GM. Melatonin and its analogs in insomnia and depression. J Pineal Res 2012; 52(4): 365-75.
[http://dx.doi.org/10.1111/j.1600-079X.2011.00962.x] [PMID: 21951153]

[30]   Zawilska JB, Skene DJ, Arendt J. Physiology and pharmacology of melatonin in relation to biological rhythms. Pharmacol Rep 2009; 61(3): 383-410.
[http://dx.doi.org/10.1016/S1734-1140(09)70081-7] [PMID: 19605939]

[31]   Loane C, Politis M. Buspirone: what is it all about? Brain Res 2012; 1461: 111-8.
[http://dx.doi.org/10.1016/j.brainres.2012.04.032] [PMID: 22608068]

[32]   Pytliak M, Vargová V, Mechírová V, Felšöci M. Serotonin receptors - from molecular biology to clinical applications. Physiol Res 2011; 60(1): 15-25.
[http://dx.doi.org/10.33549/physiolres.931903] [PMID: 20945968]

[33]   Pandit JJ. Intravenous anaesthetic agents. Anaesth Intensive Care Med 2007; 9(4): 154-9.
[http://dx.doi.org/10.1016/j.mpaic.2007.08.007]

[34]   Roper-Hall HT. The Barbiturates: Their Chemistry, Action, and Toxicology: (Section of Odontology). Proc R Soc Med 1936; 29(3): 275-81.
[http://dx.doi.org/10.1177/003591573602900338] [PMID: 19990586]

[35]   Cordato DJ, Herkes GK, Mather LE, Morgan MK. Barbiturates for acute neurological and neurosurgical emergencies--do they still have a role? J Clin Neurosci 2003; 10(3): 283-8.
[http://dx.doi.org/10.1016/S0967-5868(03)00034-1] [PMID: 12763328]

[36]   Liu S. Central Nervous System Depressants.Wilson and Gisvold's textbook of Organic Medicinal and Pharmaceutical Chemistry. 12th ed., Philadelphia, PA: Lippincott Williams & Wilkins 2011.

[37]   Rho JM, Donevan SD, Rogawski MA. Direct activation of GABA$_A$ receptors by barbiturates in cultured rat hippocampal neurons. J Physiol 1996; 497(Pt 2): 509-22.
[http://dx.doi.org/10.1113/jphysiol.1996.sp021784] [PMID: 8961191]

[38]   Ioannides C, Parke DV. Mechanism of induction of hepatic microsomal drug metabolizing enzymes by a series of barbiturates. J Pharm Pharmacol 1975; 27(10): 739-46.
[http://dx.doi.org/10.1111/j.2042-7158.1975.tb09393.x] [PMID: 241786]

[39]   ahttp://dailymed.nlm.nih.gov/dailymed/2020.bhttps://pubchem.ncbi.nlm.nih.gov/2020.

[40]   Hansch C, Steward AR, Anderson SM, Bentley D. The parabolic dependence of drug action upon lipophilic character as revealed by a study of hypnotics. J Med Chem 1968; 11(1): 1-11.
[http://dx.doi.org/10.1021/jm00307a001] [PMID: 5637185]

[41]   Musshoff F, Stamer UM, Madea B. Pharmacogenetics and forensic toxicology. Forensic Sci Int 2010; 203(1-3): 53-62.

[http://dx.doi.org/10.1016/j.forsciint.2010.07.011] [PMID: 20828952]

[42]   Ito T, Suzuki T, Wellman SE, Ho IK. Pharmacology of barbiturate tolerance/dependence: GABAA receptors and molecular aspects. Life Sci 1996; 59(3): 169-95.
[http://dx.doi.org/10.1016/0024-3205(96)00199-3] [PMID: 8699929]

[43]   Skolnick P. Anxioselective anxiolytics: on a quest for the Holy Grail. Trends Pharmacol Sci 2012; 33(11): 611-20.
[http://dx.doi.org/10.1016/j.tips.2012.08.003] [PMID: 22981367]

[44]   Gerecke M. Chemical structure and properties of midazolam compared with other benzodiazepines. Br J Clin Pharmacol 1983; 16 (Suppl. 1): 11S-6S.
[http://dx.doi.org/10.1111/j.1365-2125.1983.tb02266.x] [PMID: 6138062]

[45]   Archer GA, Sternbach LH. The Chemistry of Benzodiazepines. Chem Rev 1968; 68(6): 747-84.
[http://dx.doi.org/10.1021/cr60256a004]

[46]   Zhang W, Koehler KF, Zhang P, Cook JM. Development of a comprehensive pharmacophore model for the benzodiazepine receptor. Drug Des Discov 1995; 12(3): 193-248.
[PMID: 7662830]

[47]   Bisaga A. benzodiazepines and other sedatives and hypnotics In: Galanter M, Kleber HD, Eds. The American Psychiatric Publishing Textbook of Substance Abuse Treatment. Arlington, VA: The American Psychiatric Publishing, Inc 2008.

[48]   Greenblatt DJ, Shader RI, Divoll M, Harmatz JS. Benzodiazepines: a summary of pharmacokinetic properties. Br J Clin Pharmacol 1981; 11 (Suppl. 1): 11S-6S.
[http://dx.doi.org/10.1111/j.1365-2125.1981.tb01833.x] [PMID: 6133528]

[49]   Breimer DD. Pharmacokinetics and metabolism of various benzodiazepines used as hypnotics. Br J Clin Pharmacol 1979; 8(1): 7S-13S.
[http://dx.doi.org/10.1111/j.1365-2125.1979.tb00449.x] [PMID: 41545]

[50]   Amrein R, Eckert M, Haefeli H, Leishman B. Pharmacokinetic and clinical considerations in the choice of a hypnotic. Br J Clin Pharmacol 1983; 16 (Suppl. 1): 5S-10S.
[http://dx.doi.org/10.1111/j.1365-2125.1983.tb02265.x] [PMID: 6138081]

[51]   Mandrioli R, Mercolini L, Raggi MA. Metabolism of benzodiazepine and non-benzodiazepine anxiolytic-hypnotic drugs: an analytical point of view. Curr Drug Metab 2010; 11(9): 815-29.
[http://dx.doi.org/10.2174/138920010794328887] [PMID: 21189133]

[52]   Navia MA, Chaturvedi PR. Design principles for orally bioavailable drugs. Drug Discov Today 1996; 1(5): 179-89.
[http://dx.doi.org/10.1016/1359-6446(96)10020-9]

[53]   Miura M, Ohkubo T. *In vitro* metabolism of quazepam in human liver and intestine and assessment of drug interactions. Xenobiotica 2004; 34(11-12): 1001-11.
[http://dx.doi.org/10.1080/02772240400015214] [PMID: 15801544]

[54]   Frey HH, Scherkl R. Clorazepate, correlation between metabolism and anticonvulsant activity. Eur J Pharmacol 1988; 158(3): 213-6.
[http://dx.doi.org/10.1016/0014-2999(88)90069-6] [PMID: 2908106]

[55]   Griffin CE III, Kaye AM, Bueno FR, Kaye AD. Benzodiazepine pharmacology and central nervous system-mediated effects. Ochsner J 2013; 13(2): 214-23.
[PMID: 23789008]

[56]   Garzone PD, Kroboth PD. Pharmacokinetics of the newer benzodiazepines. Clin Pharmacokinet 1989; 16(6): 337-64.
[http://dx.doi.org/10.2165/00003088-198916060-00002] [PMID: 2567646]

[57]   Douglas JF, Ludwig BJ, Smith N. Studies on the metabolism of meprobamate. Exp Biol Med 1963; 112: 436-8.

[http://dx.doi.org/10.3181/00379727-112-28069]

[58]   Nutt DJ, Stahl SM. Searching for perfect sleep: the continuing evolution of GABA$_A$ receptor modulators as hypnotics. J Psychopharmacol (Oxford) 2010; 24(11): 1601-12.
[http://dx.doi.org/10.1177/0269881109106927] [PMID: 19942638]

[59]   Tse SA, Atayee RS, Best BM, Pesce AJ. Evaluating the relationship between carisoprodol concentrations and meprobamate formation and inter-subject and intra-subject variability in urinary excretion data of pain patients. J Anal Toxicol 2012; 36(4): 221-31.
[http://dx.doi.org/10.1093/jat/bks018] [PMID: 22511696]

[60]   Rho JM, Donevan SD, Rogawski MA. Barbiturate-like actions of the propanediol dicarbamates felbamate and meprobamate. J Pharmacol Exp Ther 1997; 280(3): 1383-91.
[PMID: 9067327]

[61]   Crestani F, Martin JR, Möhler H, Rudolph U. Mechanism of action of the hypnotic zolpidem *in vivo*. Br J Pharmacol 2000; 131(7): 1251-4.
[http://dx.doi.org/10.1038/sj.bjp.0703717] [PMID: 11090095]

[62]   Weitzel KW, Wickman JM, Augustin SG, Strom JG. Zaleplon: a pyrazolopyrimidine sedative-hypnotic agent for the treatment of insomnia. Clin Ther 2000; 22(11): 1254-67.
[http://dx.doi.org/10.1016/S0149-2918(00)83024-6] [PMID: 11117652]

[63]   Johnson MW, Suess PE, Griffiths RR. Ramelteon: a novel hypnotic lacking abuse liability and sedative adverse effects. Arch Gen Psychiatry 2006; 63(10): 1149-57.
[http://dx.doi.org/10.1001/archpsyc.63.10.1149] [PMID: 17015817]

[64]   Srinivasan V, Brzezinski A, Pandi-Perumal SR, Spence DW, Cardinali DP, Brown GM. Melatonin agonists in primary insomnia and depression-associated insomnia: are they superior to sedative-hypnotics? Prog Neuropsychopharmacol Biol Psychiatry 2011; 35(4): 913-23.
[http://dx.doi.org/10.1016/j.pnpbp.2011.03.013] [PMID: 21453740]

[65]   Miyamoto M. Pharmacology of ramelteon, a selective MT1/MT2 receptor agonist: a novel therapeutic drug for sleep disorders. CNS Neurosci Ther 2009; 15(1): 32-51.
[http://dx.doi.org/10.1111/j.1755-5949.2008.00066.x] [PMID: 19228178]

[66]   Sternbach LH. The benzodiazepine story. J Med Chem 1979; 22(1): 1-7.
[http://dx.doi.org/10.1021/jm00187a001] [PMID: 34039]

[67]   Wurtman RJ. Melatonin as a hormone in humans: a history. Yale J Biol Med 1985; 58(6): 547-52.
[PMID: 3914144]

[68]   Buysse D, Bate G, Kirkpatrick P. Fresh from the pipeline: Ramelteon. Nat Rev Drug Discov 2005; 4(11): 881-2.
[http://dx.doi.org/10.1038/nrd1881] [PMID: 16299918]

[69]   Hoyer D, Allen A, Jacobson LH. Hypnotics with novel modes of action. Br J Clin Pharmacol 2020; 86(2): 244-9.
[http://dx.doi.org/10.1111/bcp.14180] [PMID: 31756268]

[70]   https://dailymed.nlm.nih.gov/dailymed/drugInfo.cfm?setid=e5b72731-1acb-45b7-9c13-290ad12d3951 2020.

[71]   https://www.accessdata.fda.gov/drugsatfdadocs/label/2019/212028s000lbl.pdf2020.

CHAPTER 6

Antiepileptic Drugs

Tamer E. Fandy[1], Michaela Leffler[2] and M. O. Faruk Khan[3,*]

[1] Department of Pharmaceutical and Administrative Sciences, University of Charleston School of Pharmacy, Charleston, WV 25304, USA

[2] Department of Pharmacy Practice, University of Charleston School of Pharmacy, Charleston, WV 25304, USA

[3] School of Pharmacy, University of Charleston, Charleston, WV 25304, USA

Abstract: This chapter is a comprehensive account of the medicinal chemistry of antiepileptic drugs. It provides the mechanism of drug action and detailed structure-activity relationships of the antiepileptic and related drugs and their clinical relevance to give the knowledge base for pharmacists. After a study of this chapter, students will be able to:

• Relate principles of gamma amino butyric acid (GABA) biosynthesis, storage, transport, and metabolism to the action of antiepileptic drugs.

• Define and differentiate among different types of seizures and epilepsy.

• Illustrate mechanism of action, SAR, metabolites, and clinical considerations of different classes of antiepileptic drugs including: barbiturates, hydantoins, oxazolidinediones, succinimides, amides, benzodiazepines, valproic acid and its derivatives, GABA-analogs, and miscellaneous compounds.

Keywords: Antiepileptic drugs, Agonists and Antagonists of GABA and different Ion Channels, Clinical use of Antiepileptic Drugs, Drug Receptor Interaction, GABA, Structure Activity Relationship.

HISTORICAL PERSPECTIVE

May 23, 1857, was the first time the use of potassium bromide was reported in the treatment of "hysterical epilepsy connected with the menstrual period" in young women and is considered the milestone for the modern antiepileptic drugs (AEDs). However, the serendipitous discovery of phenobarbital (Luminal®) by Alfred Hauptmann in 1912 began the pharmacological era of AEDs. F. Bayer &

---

* **Corresponding author M. O. Faruk Khan:** School of Pharmacy, University of Charleston, Charleston, WV 25304, USA; Tel: 304-357-4860; E-mail: mdomarkhan@ucwv.edu

M. O. Faruk Khan & Ashok E. Philip (Eds.)

Company marketed Luminal the previous year as a hypnotic agent, which Hauptmann used to sedate several epileptic patients in a ward where he worked as

a resident psychiatrist. To his surprise, those patients displayed fewer epileptic episodes overnight and did not seize the following day. In 1934, Boston City Hospital appointed Tracy Putman as the director to search for better AEDs, and with the help of Frederic Gibbs, they established the first electroencephalic laboratory for this purpose. Using a cat model, his team tested several non-sedative phenyl compounds by Parke, Davis, & Company; phenytoin proved to be the only effective, yet, less toxic, AED. In 1936, phenytoin was clinically evaluated and successfully marketed in 1938 as a therapeutic agent to treat patients with frequent seizures and is still possibly the most widely used AED in the US Later, trioxidone (1940s) and the less toxic ethosuximide (1958) were introduced for the treatment of petit mal seizures. Over time, carbamazepine (1965) and valproic acid (1967) were introduced as anticonvulsants. In 1965, Henry Gastaut reported diazepam as the first effective benzodiazepine in treating status epilepticus and was followed by the introduction of clobazam, lorazepam, and midazolam as antiepileptic benzodiazepines [1].

In 1975, the National Institute of Neurological Disorders and Stroke (NINDS) established the Anticonvulsant Drug Development Program in the US. Not only did NINDS screen many thousands of compounds to identify leads, they also conducted target-oriented design and led optimizations to discover the modern AEDs with unique mechanisms of action. Modulation of voltage-gated cation channels (*e.g.*, sodium and calcium channels), potentiation of GABA-ergic activity, inhibition of glutamatergic processes and modification of neurotransmitters are a few mechanisms by which these AEDs decrease neuronal excitation or increase neuronal inhibition to exhibit their pharmacological effects. Because of this systematic drug discovery program, many newer drugs have been licensed including: vigabatrin, zonisamide, oxcarbazepine, lamotrigine, felbamate, gabapentin, topiramate, tiagabine, levetiracetam, pregabalin and lacosamide.

AEDs are used to manage epileptic seizures that affect ~1% of the population leading to substantial disability, if left untreated. For several decades leading up to 1993, phenobarbital, phenytoin, carbamazepine and valproic acid were the primary medications used for the treatment of seizures. Since then, the US FDA has approved several newer AEDs for use in epilepsy including perampanel (modulates AMPA mediated neurotransmission) and brivaracetam (binds to SV2A protein and sodium channels) and some others with novel mechanisms of action are in the immediate horizon to reach the marketplace, such as retigabine (opens potassium channels). Today, there are several AEDs and structural/mechanistic relatives that appear in the frequently prescribed medications. (Fig. **1**) [1].

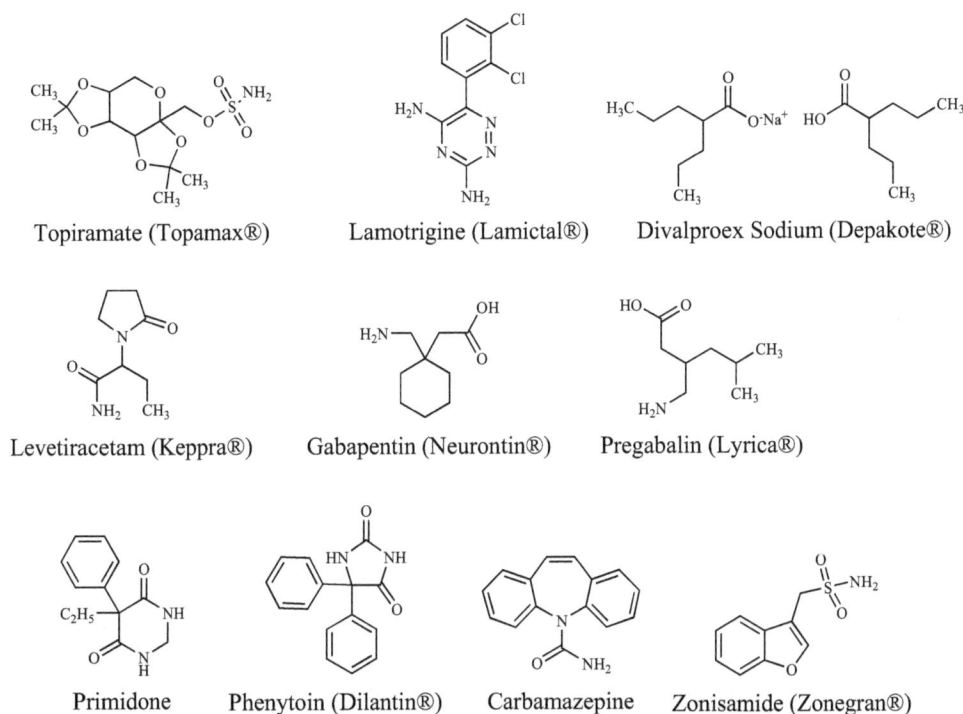

Topiramate (Topamax®)   Lamotrigine (Lamictal®)   Divalproex Sodium (Depakote®)

Levetiracetam (Keppra®)   Gabapentin (Neurontin®)   Pregabalin (Lyrica®)

Primidone   Phenytoin (Dilantin®)   Carbamazepine   Zonisamide (Zonegran®)

Fig. (1). Antiepileptic and structural/mechanistic relatives that are most frequently prescribed.

INTRODUCTORY CONCEPTS

Terminology

A *seizure* (Latin *sacire* meaning to take possession of) is caused by excessive neuronal excitation arising from disordered inhibition of a large population of cortical neurons. *Epilepsy* is a neurological disorder arising from disturbed electrical activities in the brain and defined by the International League Against Epilepsy (ILAE) as the occurrence of at least two unprovoked seizures separated by 24 hours. There are many etiological forms of epilepsy, 40 different forms are identified [2, 3]. An epileptic seizure is classified by the ILAE into three main types: partial, generalized, and unclassified seizures (Table **1**) [3].

Table 1. Classification of epileptic seizures [3].

Type of Seizure	Characteristics
Partial (focal): start on one side of the brain and may spread	a) simple: motor, sensory, autonomic, or psychic signs without impairment of consciousness; b) complex: with impaired consciousness; c) secondary to generalized seizures.
Generalized: Start on both sides of the brain	a) absence (petit mal; brief loss of consciousness with generalized epileptic discharges); b) myoclonic (sudden muscle jerks); c) tonic (stiffening of the body, upward deviation of the eyes, dilation of the pupils, and altered respiratory patterns); d) tonic–clonic (grand mal; the main seizure type); and e) atonic (abrupt falls from a brief loss of muscle tone and consciousness); f) clonic (rhythmic jerking of the body)
Unclassified: unknown onset	Seizures occurring in neonates and infants may result from differences in neuronal function due to the immature brain.

Pathophysiology of Epilepsy and Seizure

Epileptic syndrome is characterized by excessive neuronal excitation, reduced inhibitory neurotransmission, altered voltage-gated ion channels and ion concentration resulting in the *action potential* and *membrane depolarization*. This membrane depolarization induces the axon to release neurotransmitter glutamate, the main excitatory neurotransmitter acting through a variety of glutamate receptors causing epilepsy. There are several types of ionotropic glutamate receptors, such as alpha-amino-2,3-dihydro-5-methyl-3-oxo-4-isoxazolepropanoic acid (AMPA), kainate receptors, and N-methyl-D-aspartate (NMDA), with differential cation permeability and thus sensitivity to pharmacological agonists and antagonists. All these receptor subtypes are permeable to Na^+ and K^+. The influx of Na^+ and outflow of K^+ through these channels causes membrane depolarization and generation of the action potential. The NMDA receptor is also permeable to Ca^{++} ions that are normally blocked by Mg^{++} ions. However, when Mg^{++} is displaced under membrane depolarization state, the unhindered influx of Ca^{++} further depolarizes the membrane leading to neuronal injury and cell death (*excitotoxicity*). Inhibitors of these ionotropic receptors suppress seizure activity. Three subtypes of metabotropic glutamate receptors exist and differ in agonist potency, mechanism of signal transduction, and pre- versus post-synaptic localization [4].

Gamma amino butyric acid (GABA) is the major *inhibitory neurotransmitter*. The $GABA_A$ (postsynaptic) and $GABA_B$ (presynaptic) receptors are the two major subtypes of GABA receptors. Upon activation, the postsynaptic $GABA_A$ receptors allow Cl^- influx, hyperpolarizes the membrane and inhibits action potentials. Thus, barbiturates and benzodiazepines are $GABA_A$ receptor agonists that suppress seizure activity. $GABA_B$ receptors, on the other hand, open K^+ channels through second messenger systems and thus their agonists, such as baclofen, exacerbate hyperexcitability and seizures [4]. Fig. (**2**) shows the $GABA_A$ receptor diagram with binding sites of major AEDs [4].

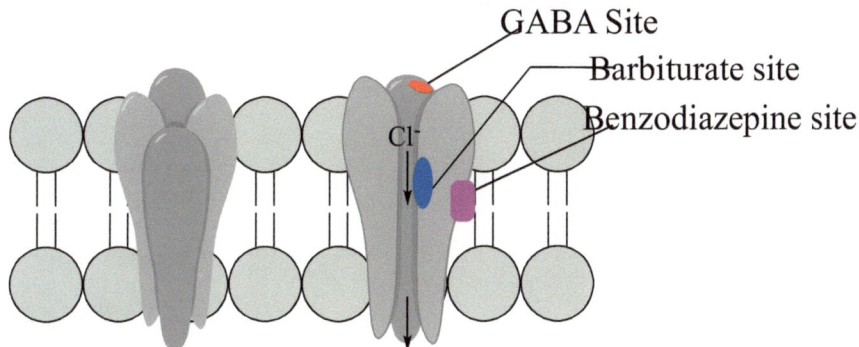

Fig. (2). $GABA_A$ receptor showing binding sites of major AEDs.

Intrinsic and Extrinsic Ionic Factors Modifying Neuronal Excitability [4]

• Voltage-gated Na^+ channels control the intrinsic excitability of CNS by rapid depolarization constituting the action potential. The GABA receptor complex mediates the inflow of Cl^- ions to repolarize and thereby decrease excitation.

• Ca^{+2} Channels maintain continuous firing of neurons resulting in increased excitability. The phosphorylation of the NMDA receptor increases permeability to Ca^{+2} ions. The T-Type Ca^{+2} channels are low-threshold, while L-, N-, P- and Q-Type Ca^{+2} channels are high-threshold type channels.

• K^+ channels utilize membrane repolarization thereby decreasing excitability. Activation of secondary messengers, cyclic GMP open the K^+ channels. Increased extracellular K^+ concentration resists the outflow of K^+ ions resulting in increased excitability.

Glutamate and GABA Biosynthesis and Metabolism

The synthesis, release, reuptake, and metabolism of glutamate and GABA are tightly controlled in astrocyte and neurons. In both GABAergic and glutamatergic neurons, glutaminase converts glutamine (Gln) to glutamate (Glu), which is converted to GABA by glutamic acid decarboxylase (GAD) in the GABAergic neurons. Glu is also formed from α-ketoglutarate (TCA Cycle member) by the action of α-ketoglutarate-linked aminotransferases. Glu and GABA are transported and stored into vesicles for release. High-affinity membrane transporters transport the released neurotransmitters into neurons and surrounding astrocytes for recycling or further metabolism. Gln is formed in the astrocytes by the incorporation of ammonia into Glu catalyzed by Gln synthetase. GABA from GABAergic neurons is transported into the astrocytes where it is converted to succinic semialdehyde (SSA) by the action of GABA-aminotransferase. SSA dehydrogenase converts SSA into succinic acid, which is incorporated into the TCA Cycle (Fig. **3**) [5].

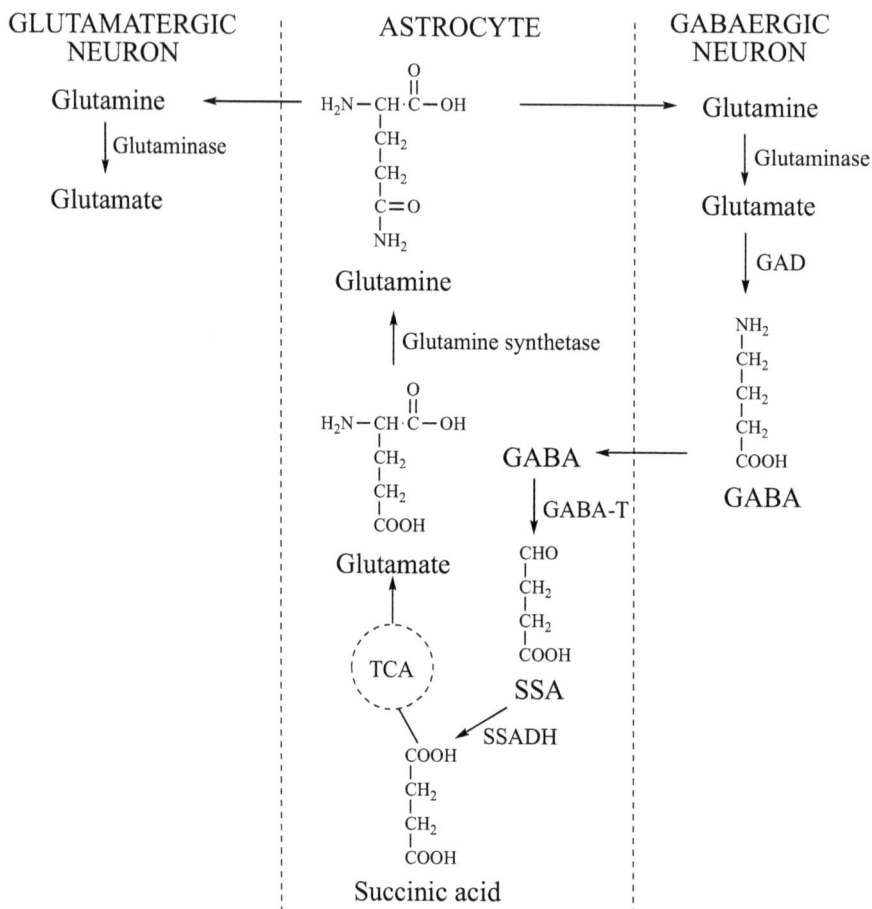

GLUTAMATERGIC NEURON — ASTROCYTE — GABAERGIC NEURON

Glutamine → (Glutaminase) → Glutamate

Glutamine (astrocyte)

Glutamine synthetase

Glutamate

TCA

GABA ← (from GABAergic neuron)

GABA-T

SSA

SSADH

Succinic acid

Glutamine → (Glutaminase) → Glutamate → (GAD) → GABA

Fig. (3). Illustration summarizing the synthesis, packaging, release, transport, and metabolism of glutamate and GABA. GAD, glutamic acid decarboxylase; GABA-T, GABA aminotransferase; SSA, succinic semialdehyde; SSADH, succinic semialdehyde dehydrogenase;

ANTIEPILEPTIC DRUGS IN CLINICAL PRACTICE

With the addition of modern AEDs over the past two decades, the treatment of seizures has broadened significantly. Many of the newer AEDs provide more predictable dose-response profiles, unique mechanisms of action and thus better clinical advantages over the first-generation AEDs. The first-generation AEDs reduce the neuronal discharge primarily through sodium channel blockade and GABA potentiation. Some of the newer agents act through targeting specific GABA subunits and synaptic vesicle inhibition. The specific targeting is advantageous in that these drugs exhibit fewer side effects and by increasing the variety of drug targets, they are more viable treatment options for the more refractory seizure types. The seizure type, clinical and side effect profiles of the AEDs and patient characteristics such as age and medication history govern the choice of AEDs. Table **2** and Fig. (**4**) provide a summary of the clinically used first-, second- and third-generation AEDs with their mechanism of action, effects on neuronal transmission and treatment choice [6 - 8].

Table 2. Summary of the clinically used antiepileptic drugs with their sites and mechanisms of action and recommended clinical uses [6 - 8].

Site and Mechanism of Action	1ˢᵗ-generation	2ⁿᵈ/3ʳᵈ-generation	Mono/(Adjunct) Therapy for Type of Seizure (Choice)
A. Presynaptic and glutamatergic neuron (excitatory neuron) sites			
Na⁺ channel blockade Fast inactivation Slow inactivation	Phenytoin Carbamazepine Valproate/divalproex	Fosphenytoin Topiramate Zonisamide Oxcarbazepine Lamotrigine Felbamate Rufinamide Lacosamide	Tonic-clonic, focal (adjunct) Focal/tonic-clonic (1st-line) Absence/myoclonic/tonic-clonic (1st-line), focal (2nd-line) Focal/tonic/tonic-clonic (adjunct) Focal (1st-line), absence/myoclonic(adjunct) Focal (1st-line), tonic-clonic (3rd-line) Focal/tonic-clonic(1st-line) Tonic-clonic/focal/myoclonic (1st-line) Tonic/atonic (adjunct) Focal (adjunct)
Ca²⁺ channel blockade	Ethosuximideᵃ Valproate/divalproex	Topiramate Zonisamideᵃ Gabapentin Lamotrigine Pregabalin	Absence (1st-line) See above for both See above Focal (1st-line) See above Focal (adjunct, 2nd-line)
NMDA receptor blockade		Felbamate	See above

(Table 2) cont.....

Site and Mechanism of Action	1st-generation	2nd/3rd-generation	Mono/(Adjunct) Therapy for Type of Seizure (Choice)
A. Presynaptic and glutamatergic neuron (excitatory neuron) sites			
AMPA receptor blockade		Topiramate	See above
SV2a vesicle inhibition		Levetiracetam	Focal/myoclonic (1st line), absence (adjunct)
B. GABAergic neuron (inhibitory neuron) sites			
GABA$_A$ agonism/ activation	Benzodiazepines Barbiturates Tiagabine[c] Valproate/divalproex	Felbamate Topiramate Vigabatrin[b] Stiripentol	Absence/tonic-clonic/myoclonic (adjunct) Focal (adjunct, 2nd-line) Focal (adjunct) See above for both See above Focal (adjunct, 2nd-line) Davet syndrome (adjunct)

[a] T-Type calcium channel; [b] exact mechanism is unknown, but possibly inhibit GABA-T; [c] GABA reuptake inhibitor by blocking GABA transporter 1.

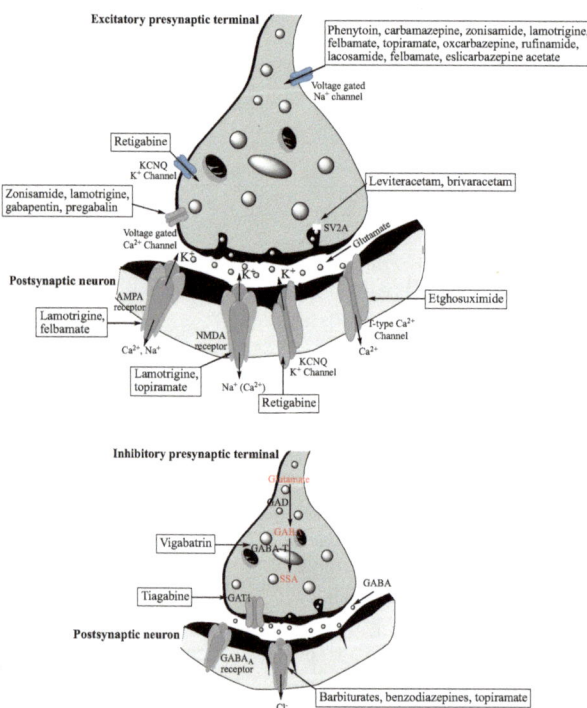

Fig. (4). Main sites and/or mechanism of action of current AEDs in excitatory (A) and inhibitory (B) synapses. AMPA, α-amino-3-hydroxy-5-methyl-4-isoxazolepropionic acid; GABA-T, GABA transaminase; GAT, GABA transporter; NMDA, N-methyl-D-aspartate. Adapted from [8].

MECHANISM OF ACTION OF ANTIEPILEPTIC DRUGS

The mechanism of action of the AEDs are not fully understood but are believed to act on diverse molecular targets. The AEDs act in both excitatory neurons (glutaminergic neurons) and inhibitory neurons (GABAergic neurons) as summarized in Table **2**. At the cellular levels, there are three major mechanistic considerations: a) blockade of ion channel (Na^+, Ca^{2+}, K^+) actions/kinetics, b) augmentation of GABA inhibitory neurotransmission, c) attenuation of excitatory glutamate neurotransmission. There are also several drugs that work either by multiple mechanisms or by unknown mechanisms. The major classes of antiepileptic drugs based on their mechanism of action include (Table **2** & Fig. **5**) [6 - 10]:

1) Voltage-gated (pre-synaptic) Na^+ channel blockers

a. Enhancers of fast inactivation

b. Enhancers of slow inactivation

2) Voltage-gated (pre-synaptic) Ca^{+2} channel blockers

3) NMDA receptor antagonists

4) AMPA/Kainate receptor antagonists

5) Synaptic Vesicle Protein 2A (SV2A) ligands

6) GABA agonists/activators

a. Positive allosteric modulators of $GABA_A$ (Cl^- channel) receptors

b. Potentiators of GABAergic neurotransmission

c. Inhibitors of GABA metabolism and re-uptake

The *fast inactivation voltage gated Na^+ channel blockade* is the most common-mechanism of the first-generation AEDs and a few second-generation AEDs (Table **2**). Phenytoin is the prototype, which by blocking voltage-gated Na^+ channels in the motor cortex, prevents repetitive firing of neurons (Fig. **5**). Thus, phenytoin reduces inward sodium movement in pronouncedly depolarized neurons by binding to inactivated voltage-gated channels after depolarization, resulting in an increase in the inactivation period of frequently firing neurons [6].

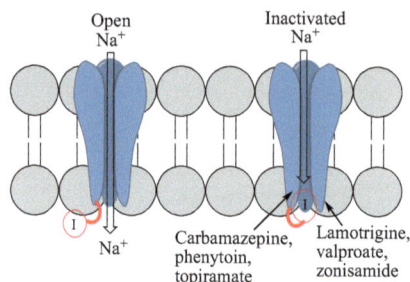

Fig. (5). Illustration of the active (open) and inactive (closed) sodium channel.

The *slow inactivation of voltage gated Na⁺ channel blockade* that blocks Na^+ influx in depolarized neurons is considered a separate, novel mechanism. Lacosamide is the prototype, which unlike fast inactivators, probably involves a structural alteration to the Na^+ channel over a prolonged period of time. Lacosamide is used to control patients with refractory partial (focal) epilepsy and status epilepticus [6].

The *Voltage-dependent Ca^{2+} channels* are homologues of the Na^+ channels and have low or high thresholds. The low threshold Ca^{2+} channels or T-type Ca^{2+} channels are expressed predominantly in thalamocortical relay neurons and are responsible for generating absence seizures. High-threshold Ca^{2+} channels are classified into L-, N-, P-, Q-, and R-types and are distributed throughout the nervous system. The antiepileptic effects of many AEDs, including gabapentin, are mediated through the blockade of voltage-dependent Ca^{2+} channels [6, 9].

The *N*-methyl-d-aspartate *(NMDA) receptor* coupled with glycine stimulates postsynaptic glutamate allowing Ca^{2+} influx into the neuron. During traumatic brain injury, (*e.g.* stroke and status epilepticus), this is a major mechanism for neurotoxicity. Several AEDs (e.g felbamate) inhibit NMDA receptor thereby the action of excitatory postsynaptic glutamate to reduce Ca^{2+} influx and excitatory potentials, thus imparting the antiepileptic effects. AMPA/Kainate receptors are also involved in postsynaptic Ca^{2+} and/or Na^+ influx. For example, topiramate modulates voltage-activated Na^+ channels and cation influx through AMPA/Kainate receptors, which is one mechanism among many others for its antiepileptic effects. It is considered that agents capable of inhibiting the AMPA receptor activity have the potential to confer neuroprotection [6, 9].

The inhibition of the presynaptic *vesicle protein 2a (SV2a)*, an integral part of neurotransmitter release into the synaptic cleft, will result in a broad-spectrum AED. Levetiracetam is the first of several agents acting by this mechanism. The recently approved AED brivaracetam is a more potent inhibitor of SV2a and provides a broader spectrum of antiepileptic efficacy over levetiracetam [6].

The first-generation AEDs are mostly *GABA potentiators/agonists*. Three types of GABA potentiators are: positive allosteric modulators of $GABA_A$ (Cl⁻ channel) receptors, potentiators of GABAergic neurotransmission and inhibitors of GABA metabolism and re-uptake. For example, benzodiazepines and barbiturates are $GABA_A$ agonists that open Cl- channels and push the neuron to hyperpolarization. Binding extracellularly between α_1 and γ_2 subunits of $GABA_A$, benzodiazepines open the Cl⁻ channel to permit its influx and subsequent hyperpolarization and decrease in the membrane potential, which is antiepileptic. Valproic acid is believed to work in part by promoting the formation and inhibiting the degradation of GABA [6].

CHEMISTRY OF ANTIEPILEPTIC DRUGS

Pharmacophore for Antiepileptic Drugs

A suggested pharmacophore model of AEDs identifying clonazepam's pharmacophore sites as an example is illustrated in Fig. (**6**) [11 - 13]. According to this model, four functional sites are critical for optimal antiepileptic effects, which are:

1. Site A, an aryl hydrophobic site.

2. Site B, a hydrogen bonding domain (HBD).

3. Site C, another hydrophobic-hydrophilic site controlling the pharmacokinetic properties.

4. Site D, an electron donor group.

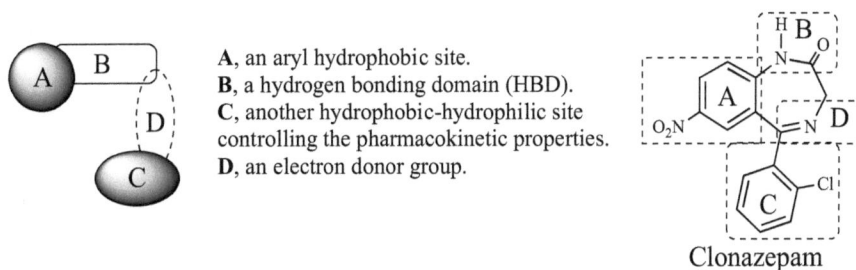

A, an aryl hydrophobic site.
B, a hydrogen bonding domain (HBD).
C, another hydrophobic-hydrophilic site controlling the pharmacokinetic properties.
D, an electron donor group.

Clonazepam

Fig. (6). a) The Proposed pharmacophore model contains four binding sites for interaction with a macromolecular complex *in vivo*; b) Clonazepam identifying the binding sites as an example.

Chemical Classes of Antiepileptics Drugs

The AEDs can be classified into the following groups according to the chemical structure: barbiturates, hydantoins, oxazolidinediones, succinimides, amides, benzodiazepines, valproic acid and its derivatives, GABA-analogs, and miscellaneous compounds (Fig. **7**).

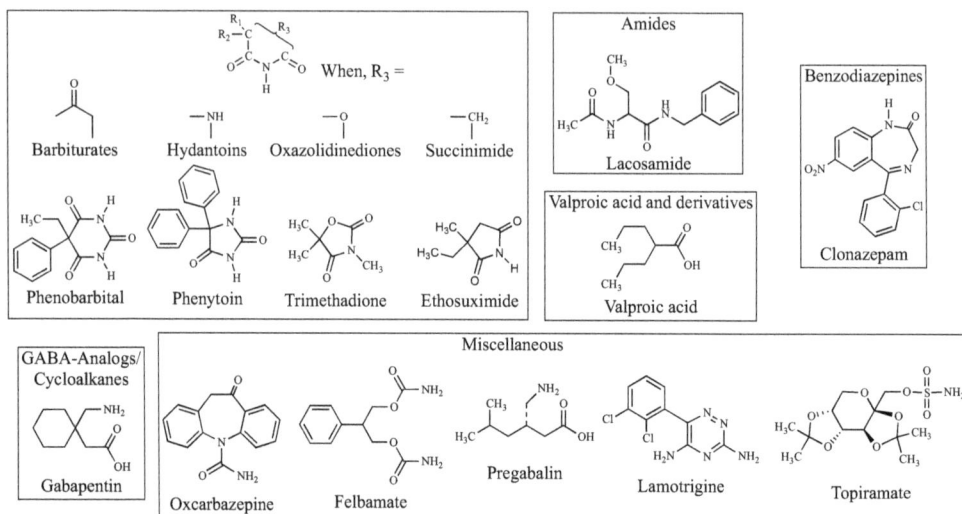

Fig. (7). Chemical classes of antiepileptic drugs with examples.

General Structure Activity Relationship

Barbiturates, hydantoins, oxazolidinediones, succinimides and amides (such as glutarimides) possess an imide, or acetyl ureas and cyclic (or acyclic) heteroatomic systems. Overall, R1 and R2 in these drug classes should be hydrocarbons. Lower alkyls, such as ethosuximide with methyl and ethyl substitution tend to be active against absence seizures. If one or both of the hydrocarbon substituents are aryl groups, such as phenytoin, the activity tends to be directed toward generalized tonic-clonic and partial seizures. When the imide *N* atom has a methyl or other small alkyl substitution, such as mephenytoin with a methyl on imide *N* atom of phenytoin, the drug is then useful in the treatment of tonic-clonic (grand mal) epilepsy. Phenacetamide, a phenylacetylurea is active against grand mal. The SAR of all the specific drug classes will be discussed in the individual drugs section as appropriate.

INDIVIDUAL ANTIEPILEPTIC DRUGS

Barbiturates and Related Drugs

In 1864, the German researcher and founder of Bayer Pharmaceuticals Company, Adolf von Baeyer, first synthesized barbituric acid (Fig. **8**) by combining urea with malonic acid. The name "barbiturate" came from amalgamating 'Barbara' with 'urea', possibly when von Baeyer and his colleagues were celebrating their discovery in a tavern during a Saint Barbara celebration by the patron saint of artillerists [14]. Barbituric acid itself is not pharmacologically active. However, in 1903, two German chemists working at Bayer, Emil Fischer and Joseph von Mering, discovered barbital, which was an effective sedative agent. The drug was marketed under the trade name, Veronal, after the most peaceful Italian city of Verona. In 1912, Bayer introduced phenobarbital (discovered by Emil Fischer), under the trade name Luminal, as a sedative-hypnotic. When the side effects and dependencies barbiturates were reported in the 1950s and 1960s, several barbiturates were designated as controlled substances under the Controlled Substances Act 1970 [14].

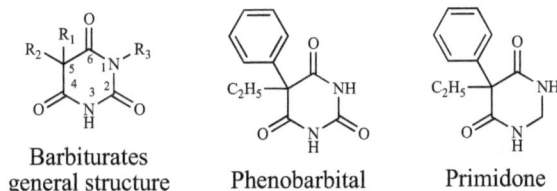

Barbiturates
general structure   Phenobarbital   Primidone

Fig. (8). Structures of barbiturates and related drugs.

Barbiturates are a broad class of sedative-hypnotics, which are largely replaced by the safer benzodiazepines (see later and chapter 13). Only the long-acting barbiturates, *phenobarbital* (5-ethyl, 5-phenyl barbituric acid) and *mephobarbital* (1-methyl phenobarbital) display enough anticonvulsant properties to be used as antiepileptic drugs. Note that N_1 and N_3 of barbiturates are not distinguishable. Both drugs being substituted with an aromatic ring at R_2 are effective against generalized tonic-clonic and partial seizures.

SAR of Barbiturates

Both hydrogen atoms at C_5 must be substituted. There is a decrease in onset time and a decrease in duration as C_5 alkyl chain length increases. The bulk on C_5 (*i.e.*, aromatic ring) is a common feature for drugs with activity for generalized seizures and also for partial seizures and status epilepticus, but not good for absence seizures. This increases the lipid solubility, and thus the rate of cell-penetration (including CNS). This leads to a shorter onset and increased susceptibility to microsomal metabolism [15].

Phenobarbital and Primidone

Phenobarbital (Luminal®) is a GABAergic agent that acts by binding to $GABA_A$ receptors, thereby modulating Cl^- current and also inhibiting glutamate-induced depolarizations. Other effects include blockade of Na^+ conductance and Ca^{2+} currents at L and N type channels [16]. This renowned drug is cheap and effective in a single daily dose and is used as a 3rd and 4th line drug for focal/generalized seizures. It is also useful to treat neonatal seizures [17]. Sedation, thinking/memory problems, depression, long-term bone problems are its major side effects. It may be somewhat addictive requiring slow withdrawal and is thus a Controlled Substance category IV drug. It is a pregnancy risk category D drug that may cause a significant rate of birth defects.

Phenobarbital is a weak acid with pK_a 7-8. It is about 90-100% bioavailable after oral administration with peak plasma concentration within 6-18 hrs. and steady-state (SS) in 15-20 days. Its volume of distribution is 0.5-1 L/kg and 40-60% protein bound. The major metabolite of phenobarbital is the *p*-hydroxy (hepatic, CYP 2C9 mediated) and/or the *p*-hydroxy glucuronide. Very little of phenobarbital is metabolized, about 20-40% excreted unchanged in the urine. The half-life in adults is 40-135 hrs. and in children is 40-70 hrs. Increasing the pH of urine (alkalization) increases its rate of excretion. No known active metabolite of phenobarbital is known. *Mephobarbital* is *N*-dealkylated to phenobarbital, possibly the active drug, which makes it a prodrug (Fig. **9**) [18].

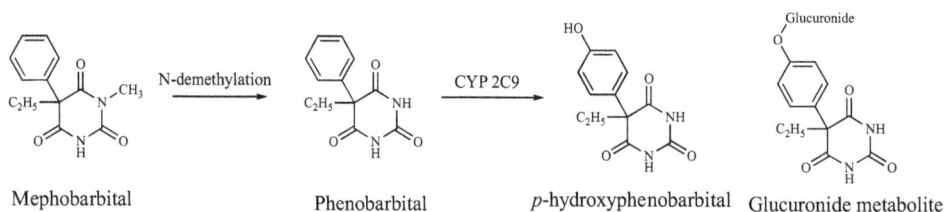

Fig. (9). Metabolism of phenobarbital and related drugs.

Primidone is a pyrimidinedione and not a barbiturate but is related, where C_2 oxidation leads to conversion into phenobarbital *in vivo*. Although phenobarbital is thought to be the active form, primidone is active in its own right. Note its structural similarity to barbiturates. This renowned drug is used as a 3rd and 4th line drug for focal/generalized seizures as well as benign essential tremors [19].

Primidone has a bioavailability of 90-100% with peak plasma concentration within 3-4 hrs. of oral administration. It reaches a steady state in 15-20 days. It has a volume of distribution of 0.6 L/kg and 20-30% protein bound. It is metabolized hepatically to phenobarbital and phenylethylmalonamide (PEMA). PEMA is an active metabolite, which may be more toxic than therapeutic. About 50-70% of primidone is excreted as PEMA and 40-60% parent unchanged in the urine. It has a half-life of 3-22 hours, decreases over time induced by phenobarbital and 17-30 hrs. by PEMA (Fig. **10**) [20].

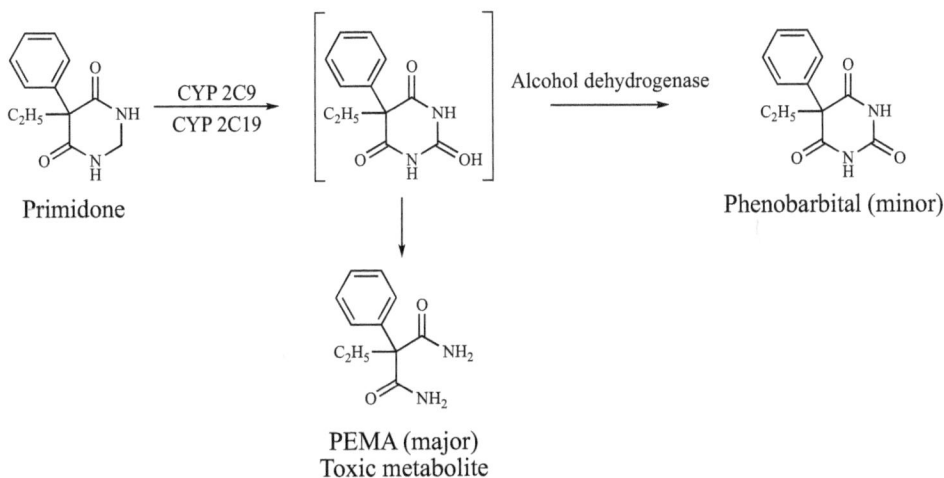

Fig. (**10**). Metabolism of primidone.

Hydantoins

Hydantoin was discovered in 1861 by Baeyer in the course of his study of uric acid. He obtained it through the hydrogenation (reduction) of allantoin and hence the name. Hydantoin is a weak acid. Nirvanol (5-ethyl-5-phenyl hydantoin) was the first 5,5-disubstituted hydantoin introduced as a hypnotic in 1916 by Wemecke with similar efficacy, but less toxicity than phenobarbital. However, its long-term use led to the detection of some toxicity and was replaced by better alternative phenytoin (5,5-diphenylhydantoin; Dilantin®). The use of phenytoin in the treatment of epilepsy was first recommended in 1938 after testing a number of phenyl derivatives for anticonvulsant action. The major advantage of this drug was noted to be a good antiepileptic activity, without the hypnotic action of the barbiturates [21]. A few clinically used hydantoins are shown in Fig. (**11**). Hydantoins are close structural relatives of barbiturates, only lacking the 6-oxo group. They are cyclic monoacylureas rather than diacylureas. As a consequence of losing a carbonyl group, they are weaker organic acids than barbiturates and thus, their sodium salt (*e.g.*, phenytoin sodium) generates a strong alkaline solution.

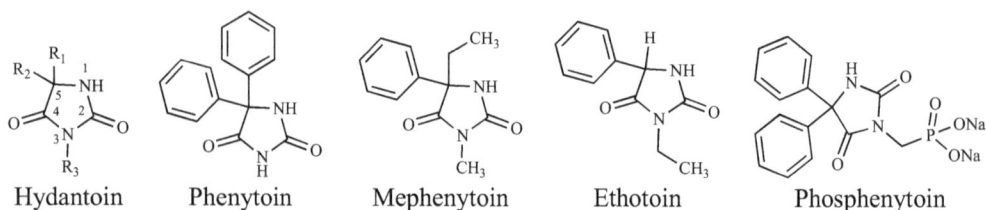

| Hydantoin | Phenytoin | Mephenytoin | Ethotoin | Phosphenytoin |

Fig. (11). Structures of hydantoinn and related drugs. Note how the numbering results in the major substitutions arising from C5 similar to the barbiturates.

SAR OF HYDANTOINS

• Bulk in position C_5 (aromatic ring) confers usefulness in generalized seizures, partial seizures and status epilepticus but not well for absence seizures.

• Among the phenylalkylhydantoins the ethyl and propyl are optimal for effective hypnotics, increasing the size of the alkyl chain decreases this activity. Among a variety of aromatic groups including: phenyl, naphthyl, phenanthryl, and substituted phenyl groups, or alicyclic groups, phenyl is the best. Phenytoin, the most generally used hydantoin AED, exhibits no narcotic effects. Thiohydantoins are either inactive or toxic.

• The N-3 methylation reduces toxicity as well as the hypnotic activity. However, mephenytoin (3-methyl-5-ethyl-5-phenylhydantoin; Mesantoin®) is nearly as effective as an anticonvulsant as phenytoin with very low toxicity.

• It has been shown in the case of phenytoin that the ability to form hydrogen bonds as well as a certain degree of motional freedom at the two phenyl groups are important features in the antiepileptic action of phenytoin and related drugs [22].

INDIVIDUAL DRUGS

Phenytoin

As mentioned before, free phenytoin is a *weak* acid (pKa is 8.06 - 8.33), with *poor* water solubility. Phenytoin sodium forms water-soluble *Na* salt. At pH > 11 (alkaline pH; ~3 units > pKa), phenytoin exists primarily in its ionized salt form, which is water-soluble. This is why IV phenytoin is dissolved in alkaline vehicle (pH 12) to avoid precipitations of its free unionized form. However, after injection, it may become turbid and less bioavailable at blood pH thus increasing the risk of breakthrough seizures. It is also advised to avoid IM administration due to the painful crystallization of insoluble free phenytoin, which is ineffective in status epilepticus.

Phenytoin is a voltage-dependent membrane Na^+ channels blocker. The Na^+ channel is responsible for the action potential. It binds and stabilizes inactivated state of Fast Na^+ channel leading to the obstruction of positive feedback of maximal seizure activity. The binding is affected through hydrogen bonding and hydrophobic interactions of aromatic rings (Fig. **12**). Its Na^+ channel blockade in Purkinje fibers is antiarrhythmic. It is indicated as an adjunct in the treatment of focal/generalized seizures [23].

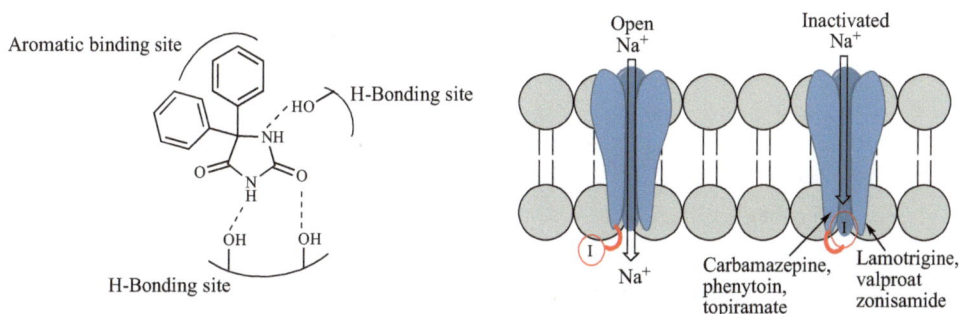

Fig. (12). Illustration of the binding mode of phenytoin to the membrane sodium channel.

Phenytoin is readily absorbed after oral administration and its bioavailability is about 70-100%. It is 90-95% protein-bound, especially to albumin, thus hypoalbuminemia caused by burns, hepatic cirrhosis, nephrotic syndrome, malnourishment, pregnancy, or cystic fibrosis that result in albumin concentration <3.5g/dL, may lead to adverse drug reactions. It has an onset of action 0.5-1h and a half-life of 10-34h. It is advisable not to change between generic phenytoin of different manufacturers or different dosage forms such as chewable tablets to extended-release (ER) capsules. The reason to avoid switching is to avoid fluctuations in phenytoin levels, as this medication has a very narrow therapeutic window. The ER capsules contain 8% less free phenytoin than chewable tablets and suspension forms. Switching requires dose adjustments. It is metabolized extensively by *p*-hydroxylation *via* CYP2C9/2C19 followed by methyl conjugation & excreted (<5% unchanged) in the urine (Fig. **13**). It shows genetic polymorphisms among ethnic groups (Asian populations) for CYP2C9/2C19 variants. Phenytoin is a potent inducer of CYP2C, CYP3A families and Uridine 5'-diphospho-glucuronosyltransferase (UGT) and p-glycoprotein leading to potential interactions with numerous drugs [23, 24]. Phenytoin is known for its high protein binding, Michaelis Menten kinetics and narrow therapeutic window.

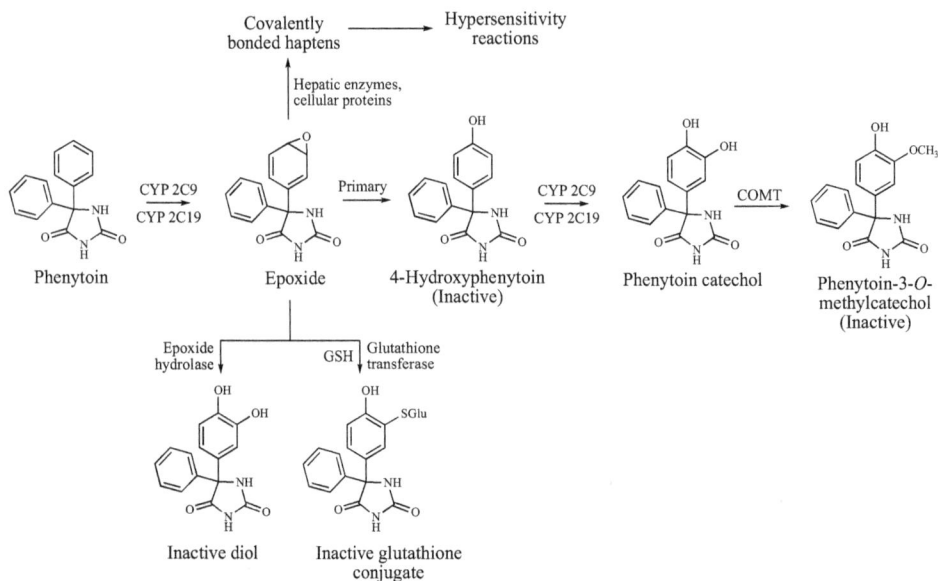

Fig. (13). Metabolism of phenytoin and its routes of hypersensitivity and toxicity.

Phenytoin's adverse drug reaction (ADRs) include rashes, which may be mild to life-threatening severe such as Stevens-Johnson syndrome and toxic epidermal necrolysis. Other ADRs may include osteomalacia, GI disturbances, blood dyscrasias, anemia, folic acid deficiency, hepatotoxicity, peripheral neuropathy (chronic), hypothyroidism, lupus-like syndrome, myasthenia gravis, peripheral neuropathy, pseudolymphoma, and heart block. It is a pregnancy category D drug due to potential teratogenicity. Special monitoring of the patient is needed if there are ADR symptoms such as rash, CNS symptoms, or ataxia and low serum albumin level. The patient should be counseled to be cautious in driving and handling machinery [23].

Fosphenytoin

Fosphenytoin (Cerebyx®) is a water-soluble phosphate ester prodrug of phenytoin, which is rapidly hydrolyzed to phenytoin *in vivo* (Fig. **14**). Phenytoin sodium must be buffered to an alkaline pH to maintain solubility and is very irritating when injected. Fosphenytoin leads to significantly less venous irritation & phlebitis than phenytoin sodium. When used IV, doses should not exceed 150 mg phenytoin sodium equivalents per minute (1.5 mg of fosphenytoin = 1 mg phenytoin). It exhibits rapid absorption *via* the IM route. Its pharmacokinetic parameters and ADRs are similar to phenytoin. It is indicated for the control of generalized convulsive status epilepticus.

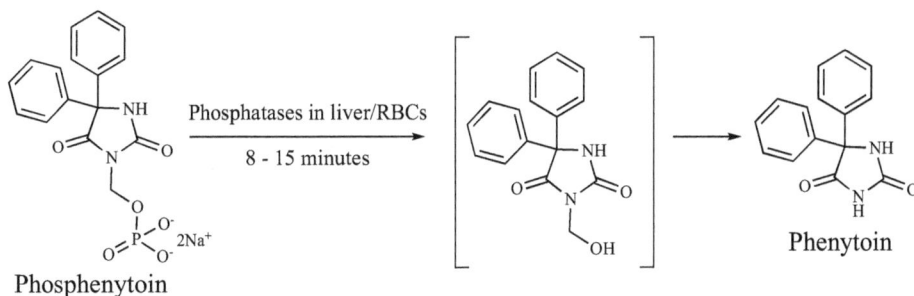

Fig. (14). Biotransformation of fosphenytoin to phenytoin.

Ethotoin

Ethotoin is ethyl phenyl hydantoin, dealkylated to the active drug. In this case, there is free hydrogen at C_5, which explains its significantly less efficacy as antiepileptic, but more sedating. It is metabolized by *p*-hydroxylation and then glucuronidation. This medication is not used clinically in the treatment of epilepsy.

Oxazolidinediones

Oxazolidinedione is an oxazolidine 2,4 dione (Fig. **15**). Replacement of the N-H group at position 1 of the hydantoin with an oxygen atom yields the oxazolidine-2,4-dione system. Trimethadione and paramethadione are two major drugs in this class.

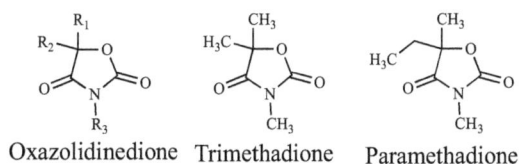

Oxazolidinedione   Trimethadione   Paramethadione

Fig. (15). General structure of oxazolidinedione and clinically used drug examples.

Drugs

Trimethadione (Tridione®), 3,5,5-trimethyl oxazolidine-2,4-dione, is indicated for use in the treatment of absence seizures. The absence of bulky substituents at the C_5 position exhibit activity against absence seizures. Trimethadione reduces T-type Ca^{2+} currents in the thalamus that increases the threshold for repetitive activities and thus decreases the abnormal thalamocortical rhythmicity, which is clinical in absence seizures [24]. It is metabolized to 5,5-dimethyl oxazolidine-2,4-dione (dimethadione), which is also active. Both trimethadione and dimethadione are excreted in the urine and are toxic. This is why trimethadione is reserved for use only when other seizure medicines are unsuccessful. Due to the toxicity of this medication and its relative, dimethadione, they are not commonly used in practice except when other commonly used medications are rendered ineffective.

Paramethadione (Paradione®), 3,5-dimethyl-5-ethyl oxazolidine-2,4-dione, acts in a similar mechanism like trimethadione. It is metabolized by *N*-dealkylation with a half-life of 12-24 hours. It is excreted to some extent through the kidney. The metabolite is active and probably accounts for most activity, the half-life of which is 14 days and is also excreted *via the* kidney. It is fairly toxic and is therefore not regularly used in clinical practice for the treatment of seizures [25].

Succinimides

When the dicarboxylic acid groups of succinic acid are cyclized through an imide (O=C-N-C=O) function, it is known as succinimide. This group of drugs resulted from a search for a less toxic version of the oxazolidinediones by replacing the "O" with CH_2 (Fig. **16**). Ethosuximide and methosuximide are clinically used drugs in this class that are used in clinical practice.

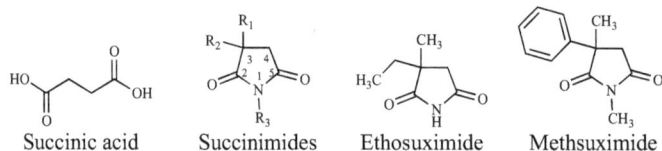

Fig. (**16**). General structure of succinimides and clinically used drug examples.

Ethosuximide and Methsuximide

Ethosuximide (Zarontin®) acts by blocking T-type Ca^{+2} channels in thalamocortical neurons [26]. Ethosuximide is lacking bulky groups attached at C_3 which corresponds to C_5 in the other related structures and thus is good for absence seizures. Indeed, it is the drug of choice for treating absence seizures [27]. It is absorbed completely after oral administration giving about 100% bioavailability with a peak in 1- 4 hrs. and steady-state in 6-12 days. It has a volume of distribution of 0.7 L/kg distributing throughout the tissues and CSF and little protein binding (<10%). The major metabolite is from oxidation of the ethyl group *via* CYP3A4/2E1 to hydroxyethyl [3-(1-hydroxyethyl) succinimide] and its conjugate, both are inactive (Fig. **17**). About 10-20% of the metabolites are excretion in the urine with a half-life of 20-60 hrs [28]. Common side effects of this medication include nausea, vomiting, abdominal discomfort, dizziness, and headache. Less common, but more serious, side effects include agranulocytosis, serious skin reactions, aplastic anemia, and depression.

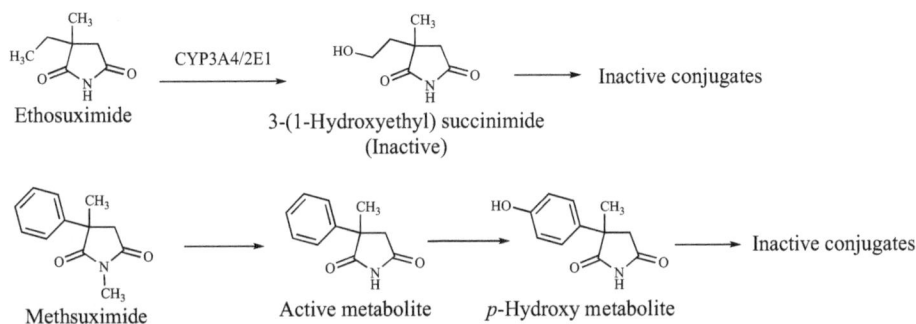

Fig. (17). Metabolism of ethosuximide and methsuximide.

Methsuximide (Celontin®) has a bulky group at C_3 (phenyl) which is good for the absence but also picks up some partial seizure activity. It is N-dealkylated to an active metabolite. The half-life of methsuximide is 1.4 h, while the N demethyl has a half-life of 38 h. So, most activities are due to metabolite, and the metabolism is followed by *p*-hydroxylation and conjugation (Fig. **17**) [29].

Benzodiazepines

All the antiepileptic benzodiazepines (BZDs) in clinical use are GABA agonists. The antiepileptic BZDs in clinical use are diazepam, clonazepam and clobazam. Lorazepam and midazolam are also introduced in the case of the need for emergency therapy. The BZDs are classified as first-generation AEDs with a wide-spectrum of antiepileptic action. The sedative effects and the high risk of development of tolerance and dependence are major limitations of BZDs in long term, prophylactic treatment of epilepsies. Diazepam, clonazepam and lorazepam are all considered first-line agents in the emergency management of acute seizures and status epilepticus [30]. See Chapter 5 for detailed SAR and pharmacokinetics of individual BZDs.

Dibenzazepines

These are dibenzazepines structurally related to the tricyclic antidepressants. The H_2NCO functional group is referred to as a carbamoyl or carboxamide. Since both of these drug structures have -N-CO-N-, structure, they are considered as urea derivatives or ureides.

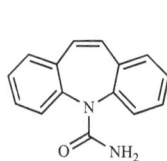

Carbamazepine   Oxcarbamazepine

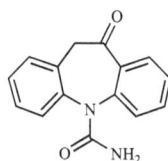

Carbamazepine (Tegretol®, Others)

Carbamazepine (CBZ) acts through sodium channel blockage during rapid sustained neuronal firing thus preventing post-tetanic potentiation [31]. It is indicated for the first, or second-line treatment of focal seizures, and tonic-clonic generalized seizures. However, if absence, myoclonic, or juvenile myoclonic generalized seizure types are suspected, carbamazepine should be avoided. Other uses include as a mood stabilizer in the treatment of bipolar disease pain reliever in trigeminal neuralgia, and prophylaxis of migraines [32]. It is highly lipophilic exhibiting low water solubility leading to slow erratic absorption, especially with intermediate release tablets. CBZ provides 70-85% bioavailability after oral administration with a peak in 4-12 hours and steady-state in 20-30 days. It is widely distributed in CSF, placenta and breast milk with a volume of distribution of 1-2 L/kg and 40-90% protein binding.

Carbamazepine undergoes CYP 3A4 mediated hepatic metabolism. It forms 25% or more 10,11-epoxide, which is responsible for both activity and toxicity. The epoxide formation is increased when it is induced, or auto-induced (Fig. **18**). Valproic acid inhibits epoxide hydrolase, which may increase the toxicity when used in combination with carbamazepine. The metabolites are excreted in the urine (~70%) along with <1% as parent drug. The half-life of the parent drug is 20-60 hrs and of epoxide metabolite is 6 hrs.

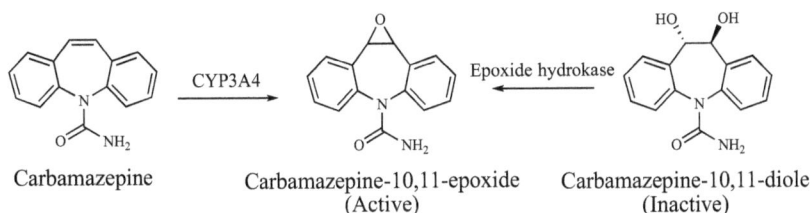

Fig. (18). Metabolism of carbamazepine.

Carbamazepine is a strong inducer of CYPs, P-glycoprotein, and UGT leading to a variety of drug interactions. In addition, it is an autoinducer at the liver enzyme CYP3A4. A secondary metabolic pathway of CBZ may lead to the formation of an iminoquinone metabolite that may form covalent adducts with proteins and enzymes leading to localized idiosyncratic toxicities (Fig. **19**) [32 - 34]. Some of the toxicities may include severe dermatologic reactions, which may be fatal, especially in those with Asian ancestry having the HLA-B*1502 allele. Thus, FDA recommends conducting pharmacogenomic testing before carbamazepine therapy to an Asian ancestry [34, 35]. It may also cause aplastic anemia and agranulocytosis. Some of the CNS side effects include alopecia, leukopenia (10% incidence), hypothyroidism, photosensitivity, and rash/pruritis. It is a pregnancy category D drug.

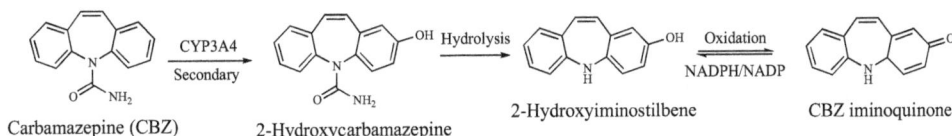

Fig. (19). Carbamazepine hypersensitivity and toxicity mechanism.

Oxcarbazepine (Trileptal®)

Oxcarbazepine (OXC; Trileptal®)) acts in a similar mechanism as carbamazepine blocking the fast Na$^+$ channels. It is indicated as monotherapy or adjunctive for focal seizures and monotherapy for pediatric epilepsy. It is also used as a mood stabilizer in bipolar disorder, and for pain in peripheral neuropathy and trigeminal neuralgias [36].

About 95% of OXC is metabolized to the active 10-monohydroxy derivative (MHD) that exhibits the majority of its pharmacological activity. Thus, it is considered a prodrug. The conjugated MHD (10-hydroxycarbazepine) is inactive (Fig. **20**) [37]. OXC has a bioavailability of 96-100% after oral administration, which may be increased in the presence of food. The peak concentration of OXC reaches in 1-2 hrs and of MHD in 4-6 hours. It is widely distributed and crosses the blood-brain barrier as well as placenta giving a volume of distribution of 0.7 L/kg. OXC is about 70% protein-bound, and that of MHD is 40%. The steady-state reaches in 2 - 3 days. The MHD or its conjugate, and < 1% of OXC are eliminated in urine. Since it undergoes MHD and conjugate formation without forming any epoxide, it is expected to be less toxic and has less serious drug interactions compared to CBZ. It is a pregnancy category C drug [36].

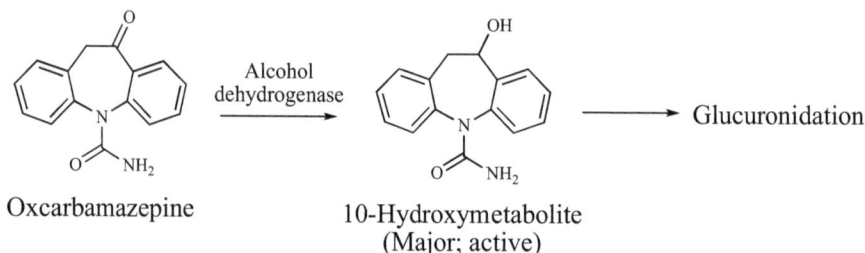

Fig. (20). Metabolism of oxcarbamazepine.

MISCELLANEOUS ANTIEPILEPTICS

Eslicarbazepine Acetate (Aptiom®)

Eslicarbazepine acetate (Aptiom®) is a prodrug of *eslicarbazepine* (*S*-licarbazepine), which is metabolized by glucuronidation and excreted in the urine (90%) with an elimination half-life of 13-20 hrs (Fig. **21**). Compared to R-isomer, the S-isomer crosses BBB more efficiently and more is thus more effective, with fewer ADRs. The FDA approved it under the brand name Aptiom® for the treatment of seizures. In clinical practice, it is a third option for the treatment of focal seizures.

Its mechanism of action is identical to that of oxcarbazepine with some pharmacokinetic differences that possibly confer improved tolerability. Like OXC and CBZ, it may be used to treat bipolar disorder and trigeminal neuralgia. Unlike CBZ, it is not converted to toxic epoxide metabolite, nor is it an autoinducer. However, it exhibits the potential for hyponatremia. It exhibits a bioavailability of 90% with or without food and is widely distributed throughout the tissues and organs with a Vd of 61 L and 40% protein binding [38]. Common side effects are dizziness, somnolence, nausea, headache, and double vision.

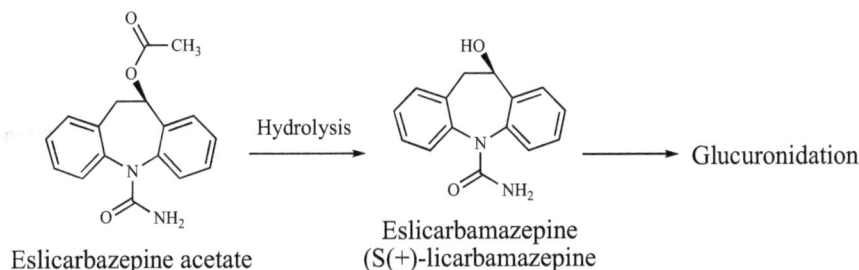

Fig. (21). Eslicarbazepine acetate prodrug and its metabolic activation to eslicarbazepine.

Valproic Acid/Valproate

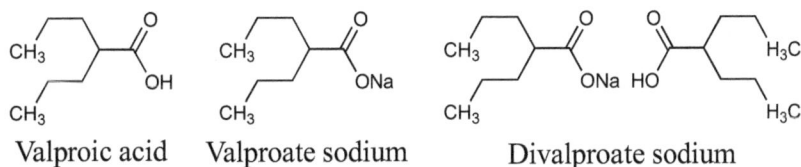

Valproic acid   Valproate sodium   Divalproate sodium

The anticonvulsant activity of Valproic acid (VPA; valproate; di-*n*-propylacetic acid, DPA; 2-propylpentanoic acid, or 2-propylvaleric acid) was serendipitously discovered by Pierre Eymard in France in 1962. It had been used as a lipophilic vehicle for a long time prior to its discovery as a medication to dissolve a bismuth salt. During his thesis work, Eymard along with his two other colleagues decided to use this for dissolving some of the khelline derivatives he synthesized in a seizure test. In this process, he discovered its antiepileptic activity [39].

Valproic acid is a liquid organic solvent and so is used as a liquid-filled capsule and not for intravenous use. Since it is a solvent, it causes GI irritation and being a liquid, it is not suitable to formulate into a sustained-release form. The development of valproate sodium salt solved the issue of water-solubility (thus intravenous use) and GI irritation, but it is too hygroscopic for solid oral dosage forms. However, divalproex sodium (Depakote®) is a stable salt for oral tablets and is less irritating to the stomach. It has also been formulated in extended-release forms (Depakote® ER).

Valproic acid blocks fast Na^+ channels and T-type Ca^{+2} channels. It is first-line therapy for several types of generalized seizures including myoclonic, tonic-clonic and absence seizures. It is also used in the prophylaxis of bipolar (mania) and migraine. For migraine prophylaxis, it is classified as a pregnancy category X due to teratogenicity and as category D for all other uses. It may cause hepatotoxicity and pancreatitis as well as nausea and vomiting. Other side effects include CNS effects, pruritis rashes and alopecia [40].

The bioavailability of VPA after oral administration is ~90%, food may delay the rate but not the extent of absorption. It is highly protein-bound (80-90%) and distributed with a Vd of 0.2 L/Kg. It may require dose adjustment in hypoalbuminemia(<3.5g/dL). The major metabolic pathway is glucuronidation (30-50% of dose) and to some extent β-oxidation. Genetic polymorphism may affect metabolism (Fig. **22**). It is excreted mostly through urine (50-70%) with an elimination half-life of 9-19 hrs [40].

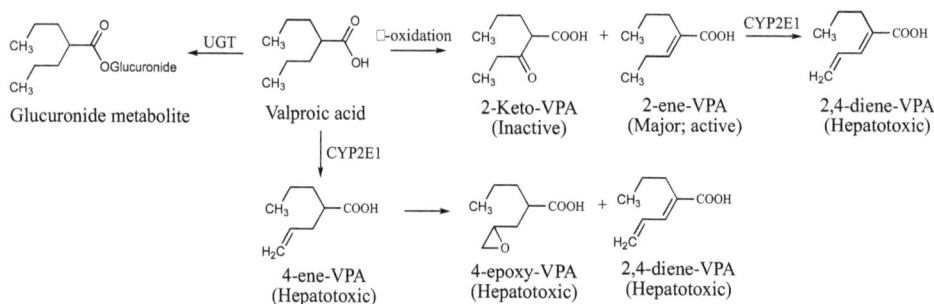

Fig. (22). Metabolism of valproic acid.

Felbamate (Felbatol)

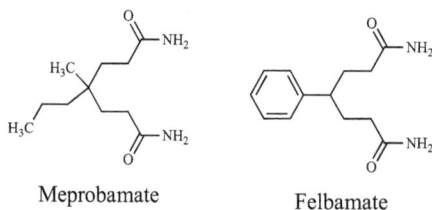

Meprobamate   Felbamate

Felbamate is a dicarbamate type anticonvulsant used to treat epilepsy. Carbamates are salts or esters of the hypothetical carbamic acid (H_2NCOOH), similar to meprobamate. But felbamate has a phenyl (fel-) instead of the methyl, propyl groups as in meprobamate. As monotherapy or adjunctive, it is indicated for the treatment of partial seizures in adults and adolescents 14 years and older. However, it is not indicated for use as a first-line treatment though. The mechanism of felbamate's anticonvulsant action is unknown. However, it is thought to modulate the strychnine-insensitive glycine receptor, which may be related to its antiepileptic effect by blocking the action of excitatory amino acids and suppressing seizure activity [41, 42].

Felbamate has an oral bioavailability of >80% and is 22-25% protein bound. Felbamate also has a volume of distribution of 0.73-0.85 L/kg in adults and an oral Tmax of 2-6 hours; as such, the half-life of felbamate is 20 to 23 hours. Felbamate undergoes hepatic metabolism *via* CYP2E1 and CYP3A4 and is excreted renally (90%, with 40-50% unchanged) and in the stool (<5%) [42].

Felbamate has a black box warning for the potential development of aplastic anemia, which can be fatal. Bone marrow suppression indicates the need to discontinue the medication. Patients with a history of liver dysfunction should not take this medication, and liver enzymes should be monitored throughout treatment. Other adverse effects include: loss of appetite, nausea, vomiting, dizziness, headache, somnolence and suicidal thoughts [42].

Gabapentin (Neurontin), Pregabalin (Lyrica) and Gabapentin Enacarbil (Horizant) [43]

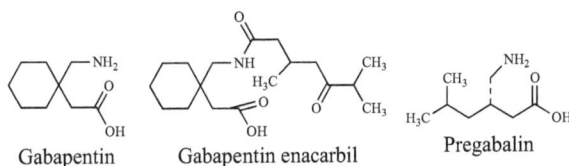

Gabapentin   Gabapentin enacarbil   Pregabalin

Gabapentin (GABA plus 5 carbons) is an anticonvulsant medication that was formulated with the idea of making GABA more lipid-soluble for better CNS penetration, but its actual mechanism of action is through a non-GABA agonist mechanism. Gabapentin does not bind to GABA (A) or GABA (B), nor does it influence the degradation or update of GABA; the true mechanism of its anticonvulsant and analgesic effects are currently unknown; however, it is thought to modulate Ca^{+2} influx at the nerve terminals by binding to α-2 -δ subunit of voltage-gated calcium channels within the CNS thus reducing excitatory neurotransmitter release [44, 45]. Gabapentin is widely used for the treatment of neuropathic pain.

Gabapentin has a bioavailability of 27-60% depending on dose and a T_{max} of 8 hours for once-daily formulations and 2 hours for immediate-release formulations. Taking gabapentin with food increases its rate and extent of absorption. Gabapentin is not protein-bound and has a large volume of distribution of 58 L in adults and 1.8-2.76 L/kg in children. Gabapentin is not metabolized, and as such, is excreted unchanged in the urine (76-81%) and in the stool (10-23%). The half-life of gabapentin is 5-7 hours in adults and ~4.5 hours in children.

Gabapentin has some noted adverse effects which include: peripheral edema, nausea and vomiting, ataxia, nystagmus, and fever. More serious adverse effects have also been documented. These include: Stevens-Johnson syndrome, hypoglycemia, anaphylaxis, dizziness, somnolence, and some psychiatric effects.

Pregabalin is a more potent *S*-isomer form of gabapentin, that is also used to treat neuropathic pain (fibromyalgia). It has similar pharmacodynamic and pharmacokinetic characteristics as gabapentin. It is a third-line option in the treatment of focal seizures and should be avoided in most types of generalized seizures including myoclonic, tonic-clonic, and absence seizures.

Gabapentin enacarbil was denied FDA approval in February 2010, citing concerns about possible increased cancer risk. Similar concerns had been raised about gabapentin itself in the past but were felt to be outweighed by its clinical utility as an anticonvulsant, whereas the treatment of restless legs syndrome was not seen to justify the same kind of risk. On April 6, 2011, Xenoport received FDA approval for Horizant (gabapentin enacarbil) for the treatment of moderate-to-severe restless legs syndrome.

Levetiracetam (Keppra) and Brivaracetam (Briviact®)

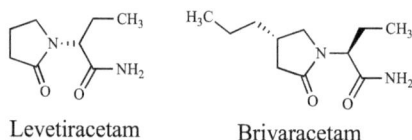

Levetiracetam   Brivaracetam

Levetiracetam is an N-methylpyrrolidin-2-one carboxamide derivative used to treat epilepsy, much like gabapentin. The mechanism of action of this drug is not currently known, but the stereoselective binding was found to be confined to synaptic plasma membranes in the CNS and not in peripheral tissues. The possible CNS effect may include: inhibition of voltage-dependent N-type calcium channels; facilitation of GABA-ergic inhibitory transmission through the displacement of negative modulators; reduction of delayed rectifier potassium current; and/or binding to synaptic proteins which modulate neurotransmitter release [46]. The *S*-enantiomer is responsible for the activity of the drug.

Levetiracetam is used in clinical practice as a first-line option for myoclonic seizures, an adjunctive option for tonic-clonic and myoclonic seizures, and a third line for absence type seizures.

Levetiracetam is rapidly absorbed orally and has a bioavailability of 100% in both immediate and extended-release oral formulations. Taking levetiracetam with food delays the T_{max} by 3 to 4.5 hours and increases the AUC by 21-25%. Levetiracetam is only 3.4% protein bound with a volume of distribution of 0.7 L/kg. This medication undergoes insignificant metabolism in the liver, primarily through enzymatic hydrolysis in the blood (24% of oral dose). Levetiracetam is renally excreted (66% unchanged) and has a half-life of 6 to 8 hours [46].

Some more common adverse effects related to levetiracetam include: loss of appetite, vomiting, increased risk of infectious disease, decreased bone mineral density, asthenia, dizziness, headache, abnormal behaviour, irritability, cough, and fatigue. More serious adverse effects to note include: Stevens-Johnson syndrome, toxic epidermal necolysis (TEN), decreased white and blood cell count, pancytopenia, thrombocytopenia, liver failure, anaphylaxis, somnolence, increased suicidal ideation, and angioedema [46]. Overall, it is considered one of the most well-tolerated antiepileptic medications.

Brivaracetam is a levetiracetam analog derived from an *L*-alpha-aminobutyric acid, in which 2-oxo-4-propylpyrrolidin-1-yl is substituted at position 2. It binds to synaptic vesicle protein 2A (SV2A) in the brain thus preventing the release of certain excitatory neurotransmitters. It is used as adjuvant therapy for partial seizures. It is readily absorbed with about 100% oral bioavailability. It is extensively metabolised by hydrolysis of the acetamide moiety to a carboxylic acid metabolite. The propyl side chain is also oxidized by CYP2C8, CYP3A4, CYP2C19, and CYP2B6. Glucuronidation and taurine conjugation are minor metabolic routes. The metabolites and some unchanged drug (<10%) are excreted primarily in the urine (>95%) and feces (<1%) [47].

Vigabatrin (Sabril) [48]

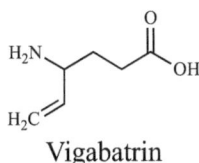

Vigabatrin

Vigabatrin is an anticonvulsant drug used as monotherapy for pediatric patients (1-24 months) with infantile spasms and as adjunctive therapy for adult patients with refractory complex partial seizures (CPS) who have inadequately responded to several alternative treatments. The structure of vigabatrin is (±)-4-amin--5-hexenoic acid. It is a GABA analog and is dosed as a racemic compound, with the S-enantiomer being the pharmacologically active form. The first and most notable chemical feature is the alkene group, which forms an irreversible, covalent bond with the gamma-aminobutyric acid transaminase (GABA-T) enzyme leading to its irreversible inhibition. GABA-T is responsible for the metabolism of the inhibitory neurotransmitter GABA and its blockade leads to increased levels of GABA in the central nervous system.

Vigabatrin is essentially completely orally absorbed and widely distributed throughout the body. It is not significantly metabolized (80% of a dose is recovered as parent drug), although it does induce CYP2C9, and it is eliminated primarily through renal excretion (95%). The half-life of vigabatrin is 10.5 hours in adults, 9.5 hours in children/adolescents 10-16 years of age, and 5.7 hours in infants/toddlers age 5 to 24 months.

Vigabatrin has a black box warning for the oral formulations (tablets, powder for solution) of potential permanent bilateral concentric visual field constriction (tunnel vision) and decreased visual acuity that is dose and exposure dependent. Accordingly, vision should be assessed at baseline and throughout therapy to monitor for changes in vision. Other serious adverse reactions include: liver failure, psychotic disorder and suicidal thoughts.

Lamotrigine (Lamictal®)

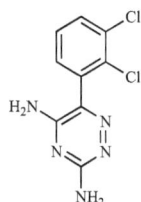

Lamotrigine

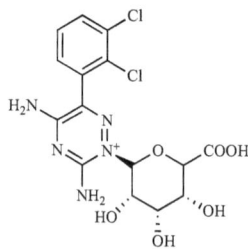

Lamotrigine
glucuronide metabolite

Lamotrigine (Lamictal) is one of the most effective and safest anticonvulsant drugs used to treat epilepsy including focal, tonic-clonic, and Lennox-Gastaut type seizures. Additionally, it is an effective and often used mood stabilizer for patients with bipolar disorder. Chemically it is a phenyl triazene derivative and mechanism of action is not fully understood. It inhibits the release of excitatory amino acid glutamate and voltage-sensitive sodium channels. It has also weak inhibitory effect on the $5\text{-}HT_3$ receptor. Sleepiness, headache, vomiting, trouble with coordination, and rash are common side effects. Reduced RBC count, increased risk of suicide, Stevens-Johnson syndrome, and allergic reactions are some of the serious side effects. It is a pregnancy category C drug [49]. It is rapidly and completely absorbed after oral administration. Lamotrigine is primarily metabolized *via* glucuronidation (UGT1A4 and 2B7) to an inactive metabolite, 2-N-glucuronide conjugate, which is mostly excreted in the urine [50]. Due to the very high risk of Stevens-Johnson syndrome, close attention must be paid to drug interactions and slow tapering of the dose at the beginning of therapy.

Tiagabine (Gabitril®)

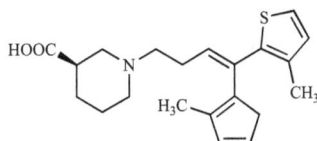

Tiagabine

Tiagabine (Gabitril) is an anticonvulsant drug indicated for the treatment of partial seizures as an adjunct therapy. By blocking the GABA transporter, it inhibits GABA reuptake thereby increasing the level of GABA in the CNS. This is how it exerts its antiepileptic action. Dizziness is the most common side effect, but can also cause nervousness, memory impairment, tremor, headache, diarrhea, and depression. At higher doses, it may cause confusion, aphasia and paresthesia.

It is rapidly and completely absorbed after oral administration (~90% bioavailability) with >95% protein binding. It is metabolized in the liver primarily by CYP3A4 and undergoes enterohepatic recirculation. Its metabolites are thus extensively excreted in the feces (63%) and also in the urine (25%), only about 2% is excreted unchanged.

Topiramate (Topamax®)

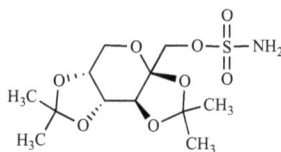

Topiramate

Structurally a sulfamate modified fructose diacetonide, topiramare (Topamax) is an anticonvulsant that is used prophylaxcally in migraine headaches in patients ≥12 years of age. It is also indicated as monotherapy or adjuvant therapy in the treatment of seizures including focal (partial) or primary generalized myoclonic seizures as well as Lennox-Gastaut syndrome. The major side effects include dizziness, weight loss, paraesthesia, nausea, diarrhea, and depression. A combination of several mechanisms has been proposed for its anticonvulsant activity, which is: blockade of voltage-gated Na^+ channels and high-voltag--activated Ca^{+2} channels; increasing GABA-A receptor activity; AMPA/kainate receptors antagonism; and carbonic anhydrase isoenzymes inhibition (weak) [51]. It is contraindicated in patients with sulfonamide sensitivity.

Topiramate is rapidly and well absorbed after oral administration, which is not affected by food. However, high-fat meal increases the rate and extent of its absorption from the sustained-release product. Due to high polarity, it is distributed mainly in the body water (0.6-0.8 L/Kg) and its metabolism is low. About 70% of the drug is excreted in the urine unchanged and the remainder is metabolized by hydroxylation, hydrolysis, and glucuronidation. It has a biological half-life of 19-23 hours [52].

Zonisamide (Zonegran®)

Like topiramate, zonisamide (Zonegran) is also a sulfonamide derivative (contraindicated in sulfa allergy). It is a new generation anticonvulsant used as adjuvant therapy for partial-onset seizures. The exact mechanism of action is unknown but may involve blocking Na^+ and Ca^{+2} channels and thereby stabilizing neuronal membranes and suppressing neuronal hyper-synchronization. It does not potentiate GABA activity despite showing an affinity for the receptor [52]. Drowsiness, dizziness, anorexia and headache are common side effects and it is categorized as pregnancy category C drug.

Zonisamide is rapidly absorbed after oral administration with a T_{max} of 2.8-3.9 hours. It is widely distributed in the body with a V_d of 1.45 L/kg. Zonisamide is excreted primarily in urine as parent drug as well as a glucuronide metabolite and slightly in feces (3%). The initial metabolite N-acetyl zonisamide (15% recovered in urine) undergoes a reduction by CYP3A4 to form the open ring metabolite, 2-sulfamoylacetyl phenol (SMAP), which is then glucuronidated and excreted in urine (50%) (Fig. **23**). It has a plasma elimination half-life of 63 hours [53].

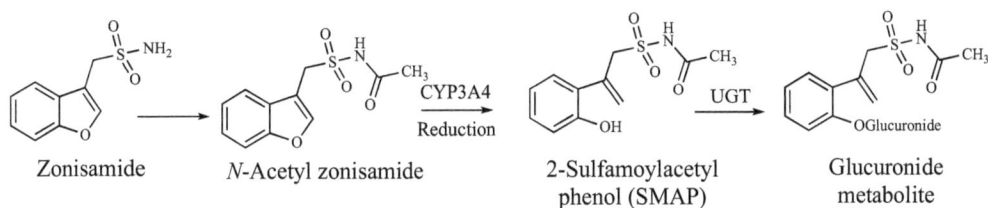

| Zonisamide | *N*-Acetyl zonisamide | 2-Sulfamoylacetyl phenol (SMAP) | Glucuronide metabolite |

Fig. (23). Metabolism of zonisamide.

Lacosamide (Vimpat®)

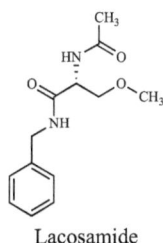

Lacosamide

Lacosamide is an amino acid derivative rationally designed as an anticonvulsant drug with antinociceptive and neuroprotective properties. It is used as adjuvant therapy for partial-onset seizures. It stabilizes hyperexcitable neuronal membranes by selectively enhancing slow inactivation of voltage-gated Na+ channels. Lacosamide has about 100% oral bioavailability with a T_{max} of 1-4 hours, which is unaffected by food. It is primarily distributed in body water (V_d is about 0.6 L/kg). Lacosamide is metabolized by CYP2C19 to inactive *O*-desmethyl metabolite (approximately 30%) and a structurally unknown polar compound (~20%). Approximately 40% of the dose is excreted in the urine unchanged [54].

Rufinamide (Banzel®)

Rufinamide, an aromatic amide, is a heteroarene comprising of benzylic and triazole rings. It is classified as an antiepileptic drug that works by prolonging the inactive state of voltage-gated sodium channels thus stabilizing membranes. It is used to treat childhood epilepsy like Lennox-Gastuat syndrome and in the treatment of partial seizures. Rufinamide is slowly, but almost completely absorbed after oral administration with a bioavailability of 70%-85% (decreased by the increase of dose) and T_{max} of 4-6 hours. Rufinamide is extensively metabolized *via* carboxyesterases mediated hydrolysis to an inactive carboxylic acid metabolite, CGP 47292 (Fig. **24**). A few minor acyl-glucuronides of CGP 47292 have also been detected in urine. The elimination half-life is 6-10 hours. Rufinamide is a weak inhibitor of CYP 2E1 and a weak inducer of CYP 3A4 enzymes thus leading to potential drug interactions. It is excreted renally (91%; 66% as CGP 47292, 2% as unchanged drug) and fecally (9%) [55].

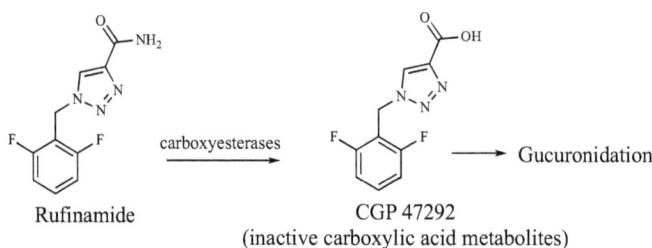

Rufinamide

CGP 47292
(inactive carboxylic acid metabolites)

Fig. (24). Metabolism of rufinamide.

Ezogabine (Potiga®)

Ezogabine, a carbamate ester, is a benzene-1,2,4-triamine derivative bearing ethoxycarbonyl and 4-fluorobenzyl substituents at positions N-1 and N-4 respectively. Ezogabine selectively activates potassium ion channels Kv 7.2-Kv7.5 but not cardiac Kv 7.1, thus avoiding cardiac side effects. It is useful in the treatment of pharmacoresistant epilepsy and is well tolerated.

It is rapidly absorbed orally, widely distributed (Vd 8.7 L/Kg) with high absolute bioavailability (60%) and a T_{max} of 30-120 minutes. It is eliminated by both urine (85%) and feces (14%) with a biological half-life of 7.5 hours. About 39% of the total dose is eliminated as unchanged drug. Hydrolysis and subsequent N-acetylation to form the N-acetyl metabolite (active) of ezogabine is the primary route of metabolism. Both ezogabine and N-acetyl metabolite are inactivated by N-glucuronidation, which is the predominant circulating metabolites (Fig. **25**). The N-acetylation is catalyzed by N-acetyltransferase 2 (NAT2), while glucuronidation is catalyzed by UGT1A4, with contributions by UGT1A1, UGT1A3, and UGT1A9 [56].

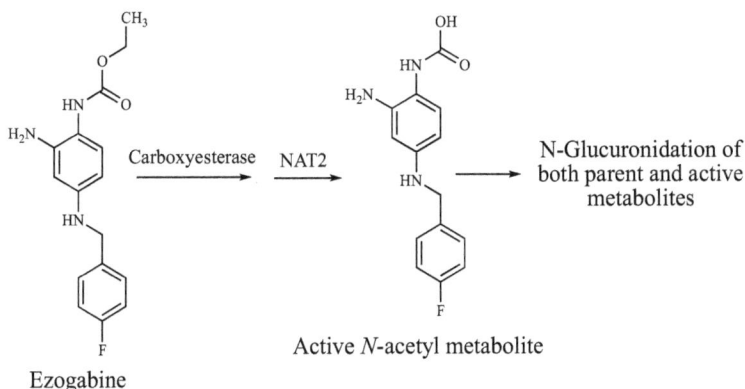

Fig. (25). Metabolism of ezogabine.

Perampanel (Fycompa®)

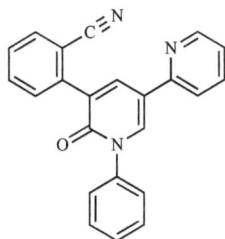

Perampanel

Perampanel is 2,3'-bipyridin-6'-one substituted at positions 1' and 5' by phenyl and 2-cyanophenyl groups respectively. It is used for the treatment of partial-onset seizures as an adjunct therapy. Its mechanism of antiepileptic action is not fully understood but may involve a non-competitive and selective antagonistic effect on the alpha-amino-3-hydroxy-5-methyl-4-isoxazolepropionic acid (AMPA) subtype of the excitatory glutamate receptor found on postsynaptic neurons in the CNS. It is rapidly and completely absorbed after oral administration. It is eliminated in the feces (48%) and to a lesser extent in the urine (22%). It is extensively metabolized by CYP3A4 and/or CYP3A5 and subsequent glucuronidation [57].

Cannabidiol (Epidiolex)

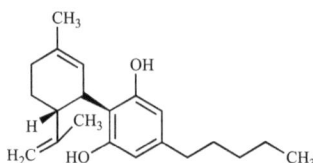

Cannabidiol

Cannabidiol (CBD) is a cannabinoid derived from marijuana which was approved in June 2018 by the FDA for the treatment of seizures associated with Dravet syndrome and Lennox-Gastaut syndrome for children aged 2 and older [58]. The mechanism of action of CBD in seizures is not clear and does not appear to be mediated through the cannabinoid receptors. The oral bioavailability of this drug is ~6% with significant first-pass metabolism. CBD has a volume of distribution of 32 L/kg and is rapidly distributed into the tissues, and may also accumulate in adipose tissue and contribute to its long half-life (56 - 61 hours). CBD undergoes extensive metabolism in the liver, primarily through hydroxylation to 7-O--Cannabidiol. This metabolite is further metabolized and excreted in the urine and feces. CBD is metabolized by several CYP enzymes, of which CYP3A4 and CYP2C19 are the primary isoforms. CBD is also metabolized by UGT1A7, UGT1A9, and UGT2B7 [59].

Epidiolex has been observed to cause dose-related elevations in liver enzymes (ALT and AST). Concomitant use of Epidiolex with Valproate or Clobazam can increase the risk of elevated liver enzymes. Liver function should be assessed prior to starting, and throughout the course of therapy. Hypersensitivity reactions, with pruritus, erythema, and angioedema, have been observed in patients taking cannabidiol. Other adverse reactions including sedation and suicidal behavior/ideation have also been observed [58].

CBD induces different pharmacological effects compared to tetrahydrocannabinol (THC), another active constituent found in the cannabis plant. CBD has several mechanisms of action independent on the endocannabinoid systems such as inhibiting adenosine uptake, enhancing the activity of 5-HT1A receptor and glycine receptor and blocking the orphan GPR55, which is a G-protein coupled receptor [59].

ANTIEPILEPTICS IN PEDIATRICS

The presentation of epilepsy and other seizure-related disorders in pediatrics typically varies from adults. Electroencephalogram patterns, seizure causes, and drug response can be vastly different in pediatric patients. Epilepsy occurs more frequently in infants (largest affected group) than in adults, and febrile seizures are the most commonly observed seizures. Levetiracetam has shown effectiveness in the management of focal seizures. The use of levetiracetam, valproate, lamotrigine, topiramate, and clobazam in treating generalized seizures in infants is not supported by strong evidence [60].

Genetic testing should be utilized in infants and children presenting with seizures [60]. Dravet syndrome, previously known as severe myoclonic epilepsy of infancy (SMEI), is a rare genetic dysfunction within the brain that causes epilepsy. This condition affects nearly 1 in 20,000-40,000 people and typically begins within the first year of life and remains lifelong. Children with this disorder have normal development, MRI and EEG are typical, prior to seizure onset; however, learning disabilities begin to develop as seizures continue to worsen. The number of seizures typically decreases with age, and the duration of seizures is often lower as the person gets older. Eight-out-of-ten cases of Dravet syndrome are due to genetic mutations in ion channels in the brain. This disorder is not typically inherited, but considered a de novo mutation in the *SCN1A* gene coding for sodium channels within the brain. Children with this syndrome may have different seizure types including: myoclonic, tonic-clonic, absence, atypical absence, atonic, focal, and status epilepticus seizures. Treatment is aimed at controlling seizures and preventing future seizures chronically through combination therapy. Typically, two or more medications are needed due to the multiple seizure types that may present. Sodium channel blockers, such as: phenytoin, carbamazepine, lamotrigine and rufinamide should be avoided due to exacerbation of seizures. Vigabatrin and tiagabine should also be avoided as they can increase the frequency of myoclonic seizures [61]. Cannabidiol (Epidiolex) was recently approved in June 2018 for the treatment of Dravet syndrome [62].

Recommendations for pediatric seizure management are still not complete for all etiologies, and more research is needed to improve the current guidelines. The FDA approved indications and dosages of several anticonvulsant medications are listed in Table **3**.

Table 3. Age Range for Antiepileptic Medications in Pediatrics [63].

Absence (petit mal)	Age Range (Years)
Divalproex ER	10+
Valproic Acid	10+
Ethosuximide	3+ and can be used in combination therapy

(Table 3) cont.....

Absence (petit mal)	Age Range (Years)
Methsuximide	1+ can be used in combination
Tonic-clonic (grand mal)	Age Range (Years)
Ethotoin	1+
Lamotrigine XR	13+
Levetiracetam	6+
Phenytoin	Age not specified, but commonly used in neonates and older
Complex partial	Age Range (Years)
Divalproex ER	10+
Valproic Acid	10+
Phenytoin	Age not specified, but commonly used in neonates and older
Ethotoin	1+
Partial	Age Range (Years)
Gabapentin	3+
Lacosamide	17+
Lamotrigine XR	13+
Levetiracetam	1 month and older
Levetiracetam XR	16+
Oxcarbazepine	2-3 as adjunctive therapy, 4-16 monotherapy
Perampanel	12+
Tiagabine	12+
Zonisamide	16+
Myoclonic	Age Range (Years)
Levetiracetam	12+
Epilepsy	Age Range (Years)
Carbamazepine	1+, (listed as children under 6)
Carbamazepine XR	6+
Lamotrigine	2+
Topiramate	2+
Lennox-Gastaut syndrome (LGS)	Age Range (Years)
Felbamate	2+
Rufinamide	4+

THERAPEUTIC DRUG MONITORING IN ANTIEPILEPTIC DRUGS

Some antiepileptic drugs are among the list of drugs that require therapeutic drug monitoring (TDM) to ensure safety and efficacy. TDM improves clinical outcomes by adjusting the dose of the medication within the therapeutic range. TDM is essential for drugs with a narrow therapeutic index, drugs that are subject to substantial interindividual variability due to pharmacokinetic differences, drugs that show a good correlation between clinical effect and plasma concentration and drugs with no laboratory biomarkers for clinical efficacy or toxicity [64].

Age can greatly affect the pharmacologic profile of antiepileptics. Body composition typically has great variation in extreme age ranges, particularly in the elderly and infants. TDM is valuable in preventing under-dosing, overdosing and toxicity in elderly patients. Pediatric patients may require a 2-3 times larger weight for weight dose than needed in adults as their plasma clearance is significantly higher than adults. Moreover, the dose-response is often less predictable in children [63]. Accordingly, several antiepileptic drugs require plasma level monitoring for safety in pediatrics. Carbamazepine has a therapeutic level of 4-12 mcg/mL, 40-100 mcg/mL for Ethosuximide, 10-20 mcg/mL for Phenytoin, and 50-100 mcg/mL for Valproic acid [63]. Table **4** lists individual antiepileptic drugs and their plasma reference ranges.

Table 4. Common antiepileptics drugs with plasma reference range [64].

Antiepileptic Drugs	Plasma Reference Range (mcg/mL)
Brivaracetam	0.2-2
Carbamazepine	4-12
Clobazam	0.03-0.3
Clonazepam	0.02-0.07
Eslicarbazpine acetate	3-35
Ethosuximide	40-100
Felbamate	30-60
Gabapentin	2-20
Lacosamide	10-20
Lamotrigine	2.5-15
Levetiracetam	12-46
Oxcarbazepine	3-35
Perampanel	0.18-0.98
Phenobarbital	10-40
Phenytoin	10-20
Pregabalin	2-8
Primidone	5-10

(Table 4) cont.....

Antiepileptic Drugs	Plasma Reference Range (mcg/mL)
Rufinamide	30-40
Stiripentol	4-22
Tiagabine	0.02-0.2
Topiramate	5-20
Valproic acid	50-100
Vigabatrin	0.8-36
Zonisamide	10-40

COMPARATIVE SAFETY OF ANTIEPILEPTIC DRUGS DURING PREGNANCY

Most seizures during pregnancy occur in women who already have epilepsy. Epilepsy in pregnancy is often managed with antiepileptics. The risk of congenital malformations (CMs) was meta analyzed in infants/children who were exposed to antiepileptics in utero through a systematic review. Most antiepileptics were associated with a higher risk of major CMs. For instance, drugs like ethosuximide, valproate, topiramate, phenobarbital, phenytoin, carbamazepine, and polytherapies were found to cause major CMs. On the other hand, lamotrigine and levetiracetam were found to be relatively safe and not associated with significantly increased risks of CMs [65].

CASE STUDIES

Case 1

BP is a 28-month-old male brought to the emergency department three days ago with seizure activity per his parents. He was started on medication to stop the seizures when he presented to the hospital. A neurologist was consulted and an electroencephalogram was completed. The results of the testing show that BP is experiencing partial seizures. He must be started on an antiepileptic for outpatient therapy. You have the following drug structures to select from.

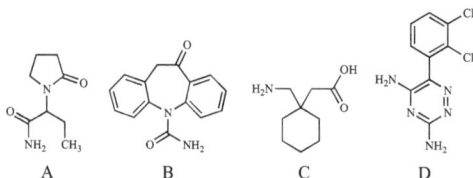

Questions

1. Which of the following drug(s) would be an appropriate therapy for the patient?

2. Why did you not choose the other structures?

3. How would your recommendation change if the patient's age was 5 years old?

4. What other medication would be useful to send home with the patient's parents in case of BP experiences status epilepticus at home?

Case 2

KJ is a 28-year-old female who presents to an outpatient neurologist appointment. She presents to the clinic to discuss medication options with her physician and pharmacist. KJ explains that she and her husband are considering becoming pregnant in the next six months and that she is concerned her current medication regimen is unsafe for pregnancy. KJ was diagnosed at 15 years old with grand mal seizures. She has been on phenytoin (A) therapy ever since and has only experienced two seizures since. Her neurologist has been pleased with her response to therapy. A phenytoin level today measures 8.6mg/L. You are given the following drug structures (A-D) as options for therapy:

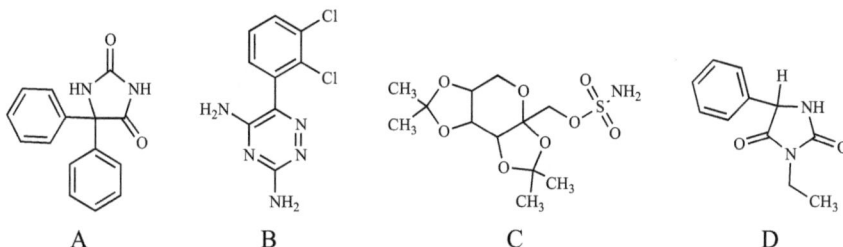

| A | B | C | D |

Questions

1. What additional information do you need to assess the patient's phenytoin level?

2. Is the patient's current medication safe to continue at this time?

3. Which of the medication structures are safe for use in pregnancy?

4. Which of the following medication structures are efficacious for patients with KJ's seizure type?

Case 3

BM is a 17-year-old male recently diagnosed with absence seizures. His mother brings him into a neurologist appointment for a first visit. He was started on a medication by his primary care provider two months ago. The patient's mother does not think that the medication is working because both she and the patient have not noticed a decrease in the patient's seizure frequency. Additionally, his mother expresses that he's had very abnormal behavior since starting the medication and has been very irritable with some near-violent events. You are given the following medication structures:

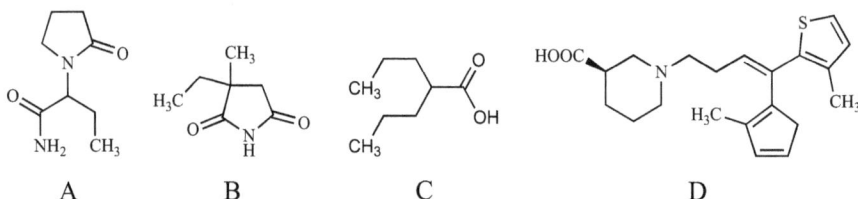

A   B   C   D

Questions

1. Which medication do you think the patient is currently on? How do you know?

2. Is this current medication appropriate therapy for the patient? Why?

3. Which medication(s) would be appropriate for the patient?

4. Would you recommend changes if the patient's age changed to 6 years old?

DRUG DISCOVERY CASE STUDIES

Discovery of Beclofen and Other GABA Analogues

The discovery of GABA in CNS and its role as an inhibitory neurotransmitter in the 1960s led Ciba chemists to synthesize its analogs, notably baclofen as a specific spinal GABA$_B$ receptor agonist. Baclofen found to relax skeletal muscles, making it a useful antispastic agent in multiple sclerosis or spinal disease. Following a similar concept, Parke, Davis and Company researchers designed and synthesized gabapentin to ease delivery in the brain. However, its 3-D structure does not correspond to GABA and thus it acts in a non-GABA mechanism. The other analog vigabatrin chemically reacts with and irreversibly inactivate GABA transaminase and exerts antiepileptic action as a GABAergic compound (Fig. **26**) [66].

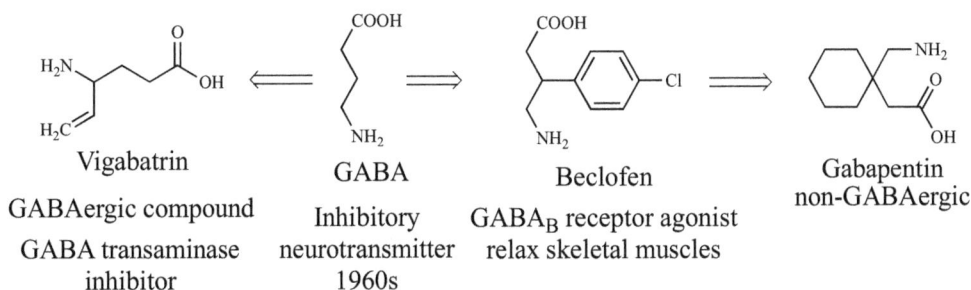

Fig. (26). Discovery of a few GABA analogs as antiepileptic agents.

Discovery of Brivaracetam

As mentioned in the previous case study, the discovery of GABA in the 1960s led the scientists to synthesize numerous GABA analogues in search of new sedative-hypnotic agents. Brivaracetam is an example of a success story of rationally designed AED in this area (Fig. **27**).

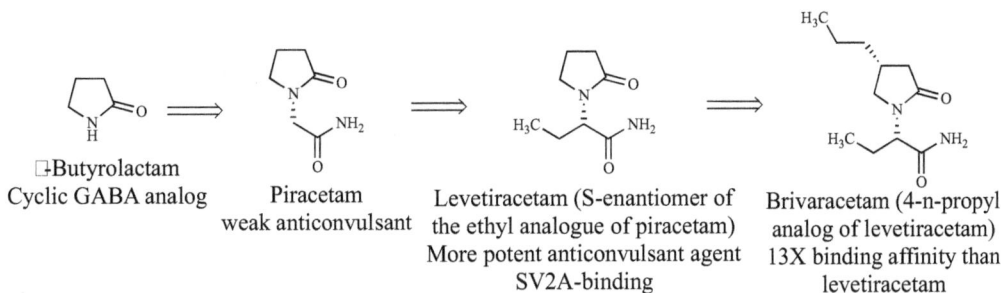

Fig. (27). Discovery of brivaracetam from γ-butyrolactam.

In the synthesis of the GABA derivatives, γ-butyrolactam (2-oxopyrrolidine) was used as a cyclic GABA analog. Some of these analogs, including the 2-oxo-1-pyrrolidine acetamide (piracetam), were found to improve memory in rodents through a non-GABAergic, unknown mechanism. Piracetam was later found to have weak anticonvulsant actions. The routine screening of piracetam derivatives by Alma Gower led to the discovery of levetiracetam, the (S)-enantiomer of the ethyl analogue of piracetam, in 1992 as a more potent anticonvulsant agent. This successful discovery of levetiracetam using audiogenic seizure-susceptible mice as a novel AED in the treatment of partial seizures prompted researchers to identify better therapeutic alternatives. Levetiracetam showed a high degree of stereospecificity suggesting the involvement of a specific protein target, which was soon identified to be a ubiquitous synaptic vesicle membrane protein, SV2A. Further studies revealed that SV2A is the molecular target for the anticonvulsant activity that facilitates low-frequency neurotransmission. Then, the development of a high-throughput binding assay utilizing this molecular target allowed the screening of ~13,000 compounds. From this assay brivaracetam, a 4-n-propyl analog of levetiracetam was discovered that has 13-fold greater binding affinity than levetiracetam. Positive preliminary results from stage III trials were recorded in 2008. The European Commission approved it in January 2016 and the Food and Drug Administration [15] approved it in May 2016 under the trade name Briviact. Effective on Mar 09, 2017, it is classified by the DEA as a schedule V drug under the Control Substance Act [67].

STUDENT SELF-STUDY GUIDE

1. What are the classifications of epileptic seizures and how do they differ in their characteristics?

2. Know the pathophysiologic characteristics of Epilepsy and seizure.

3. Explain the role of sodium, potassium, calcium, and magnesium cations in epilepsy and seizures.

4. Know the benefits that the newer AEDs provide versus first-generation AEDs

5. Understand what the four functional sites are that are critical for optimal antiepileptic effect.

6. Understand the SAR of each antiepileptic medication

7. Understand the role of GABAa and GABAb receptors in drug development for seizures and epilepsy

8. Explain why phenytoin must be adjusted in hypoalbuminemia

9. Understand why the structural differences of trimethadione and paramethadione compare to ethotoin and how this relates to antiseizure activity.

10. Understand the structural differences between eslicarbazepine acetate enantiomers and how this affects drug action in seizures.

STUDENT SELF-ASSESSMENT QUESTIONS

1. Which of the following drugs should not be used in patients with epilepsy?

a. Baclofen

b. Levetiracetam

c. Phenytoin

d. Carbamazepine

2. Which of the following is a first-generation AED?

a. ethosuximide

b. vigabatrin

c. lamotrigine

d. oxcarbazepine

3. The structure shown below is a:

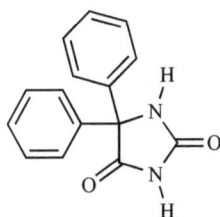

a. Barbiturate

b. Succinimide

c. Oxazolidinedione

d. Hydantoin

4. Which of the following medications is a voltage-dependent sodium channel blocker?

a. Ethosuximide

b. Phenytoin

c. Levetiracetam

d. Ezogabine

5. Which of the following is suitable for use in a 3-year-old child with partial seizures?

a. Levetiracetam XR

b. Lamotrigine

c. Levetiracetam

d. Zonisamide

6. Which of the following is safest for use in pregnancy?

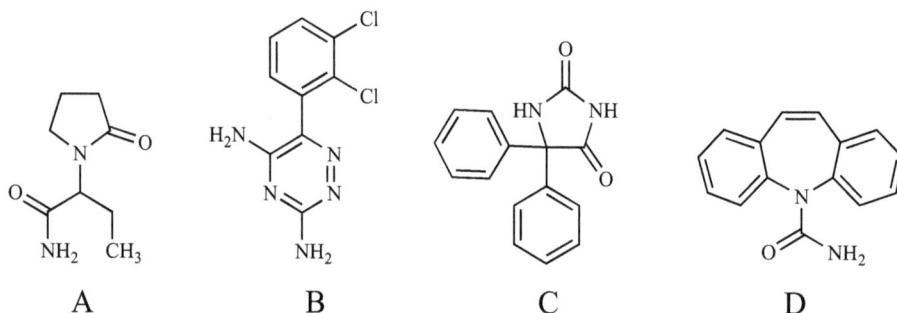

A   B   C   D

a. A

b. B

c. C

d. D

7. Which of the following is a medication structurally related to phenobarbital and indicated in essential tremor?

a. Phenytoin

b. Primidone

c. Barbital

d. Lacosamide

8. Which of the following is indicated in Lennox-Gastaut Syndrome?

a. Felbamate

b. Valproic acid

c. Levetiracetam

d. Perampanel

9. All of the following are common mechanisms of action of antiepileptic medications except (select all that apply):

a. NMDA receptor blockade

b. AMPA receptor activation

c. Sodium channel blockade

d. Calcium channel activation

10. Which of the following are precursors of GABA (select all that apply)?

a. Barbital

b. Glutamine

c. Glutamate

d. AMPA

11. Which of the following is a prodrug to phenytoin?

a. Fosphenytoin

b. Prophenytoin

c. Valproic acid

d. Trimethadione

CONSENT FOR PUBLICATION

Not applicable.

CONFLICT OF INTEREST

The author(s) confirms that there is no conflict of interest.

ACKNOWLEDGEMENTS

The authors would like to thank Leonard David Hilley for careful reading of the manuscript and insightful comments

REFERENCES

[1] Brodie MJ. Antiepileptic drug therapy the story so far. Seizure 2010; 19(10): 650-5.
[http://dx.doi.org/10.1016/j.seizure.2010.10.027] [PMID: 21075011]

[2] Fisher RS, Acevedo C, Arzimanoglou A, *et al.* ILAE official report: a practical clinical definition of epilepsy. Epilepsia 2014; 55(4): 475-82.
[http://dx.doi.org/10.1111/epi.12550] [PMID: 24730690]

[3] Goldenberg MM. Overview of drugs used for epilepsy and seizures: etiology, diagnosis, and treatment. P&T 2010; 35(7): 392-415.
[PMID: 20689626]

[4] Bromfield EB, Cavazos JE, Sirven JI. Basic Mechanisms Underlying Seizures and Epilepsy.An Introduction to Epilepsy. West Hartford, CT: American Epilepsy Society 2006.

[5] Cooper AJL, Jeitner TM. Central Role of Glutamate Metabolism in the maintenance of nitrogen homeostasis in normal and hyperammonemic brain. Biomolecules 2016; 6(2): 16.
[http://dx.doi.org/10.3390/biom6020016] [PMID: 27023624]

[6] Cook AMK, Bensalem-Owen M. Mechanisms of action of antiepileptic drugs. Therapy 2011; 8(3): 307-13.
[http://dx.doi.org/10.2217/thy.11.19]

[7] Fauci AS, Kasper DL, Eds. Harrison's principles of internal medicine. 17th ed. New York: McGraw-Hill 2008; pp. 2498-512.

[8] Bialer M, White HS. Key factors in the discovery and development of new antiepileptic drugs. Nat Rev Drug Discov 2010; 9(1): 68-82.
[http://dx.doi.org/10.1038/nrd2997] [PMID: 20043029]

[9] Deshmukh R, Thakur AS, Dewangan D. Mechanism of action of anticonvulsant drugs: a review. Int J Pharm Sci Res 2011; 2(2): 225-36.

[10] Leppik IE, Kelly KM, deToledo-Morrell L, *et al.* Basic research in epilepsy and aging. Epilepsy Res 2006; 68 (Suppl. 1): S21-37.
[http://dx.doi.org/10.1016/j.eplepsyres.2005.07.014] [PMID: 16384687]

[11] Pandeya SN, Raja AS, Stables JP. Synthesis of isatin semicarbazones as novel anticonvulsants--role of hydrogen bonding. J Pharm Pharm Sci 2002; 5(3): 266-71.
[PMID: 12553895]

[12] Khatoon Y, Shaquiquzzaman M, Singh V, Sarafroz M. Synthesis, Characterization and Anticonvulsant Activity of Some Novel 4, 5-Disubstituted-1, 2, 4-Triazole Derivatives. J Appl Pharm Sci 2017; 7(7): 158-67.

[13] Kumar R, Singh T, Singh H, Jain S, Roy RK. Design, synthesis and anticonvulsant activity of some new 6,8-halo-substituted-2h-[1,2,4]triazino[5,6-b]indole-3(5h)-one/-thione and 6,8-halo-substituted 5-methyl-2h-[1,2,4]triazino[5,6-b]indol-3(5h)-one/-thione. EXCLI J 2014; 13: 225-40.
[PMID: 26417257]

[14] Dundee JW, McIlroy PDA. The history of barbiturates. Anaesthesia 1982; 37(7): 726-34.
[http://dx.doi.org/10.1111/j.1365-2044.1982.tb01310.x] [PMID: 7048989]

[15] Hansch C, Steward AR, Anderson SM, Bentley D. The parabolic dependence of drug action upon lipophilic character as revealed by a study of hypnotics. J Med Chem 1968; 11(1): 1-11.
https://www.ncbi.nlm.nih.gov/pubmed/5637185

[http://dx.doi.org/10.1021/jm00307a001] [PMID: 5637185]

[16]   Phenobarbital. Wishart DS, Knox C, Guo AC, Cheng D, Shrivastava S, Tzur D, Gautam B, Hassanali M. DrugBank: a knowledgebase for drugs, drug actions and drug targets. Nucleic Acids Res 2019; 36(Database issue): D901-6.

[17]   Slaughter LA, Patel AD, Slaughter JL. Pharmacological treatment of neonatal seizures: a systematic review. J Child Neurol 2013; 28(3): 351-64.
[http://dx.doi.org/10.1177/0883073812470734] [PMID: 23318696]

[18]   Phenobarbital. Drug Facts and Comparisons. Facts & Comparisons [database online] St Louis, MO: Wolters Kluwer Health, Inc; March 2005. Accessed May 17, 2019.

[19]   Primidone. Drug Facts and Comparisons. Facts & Comparisons [database online] St Louis, MO: Wolters Kluwer Health, Inc; March 2005. Accessed May 17, 2019.

[20]   RHONEY. 2015. accesspharmacy.mhmedical.com/content.aspx?aid=1112258493

[21]   Ware E. The chemistry of the hydantoins. Chem Rev 1950; 46(3): 403-70.
[http://dx.doi.org/10.1021/cr60145a001] [PMID: 24537833]

[22]   Poupaert JH, Vandervorst D, Guiot P, Moustafa MM, Dumont P. Structure-activity relationships of phenytoin-like anticonvulsant drugs. J Med Chem 27(1): 76-8.
[http://dx.doi.org/10.1021/jm00367a015]

[23]   Phenytoin. Drug Facts and Comparisons. Facts & Comparisons [database online] St Louis, MO: Wolters Kluwer Health, Inc; March 2005. Accessed May 18, 2019.

[24]   Holbrook AM, Pereira JA, Labiris R, *et al.* Systematic overview of warfarin and its drug and food interactions. Arch Intern Med 2005; 165(10): 1095-106.
[http://dx.doi.org/10.1001/archinte.165.10.1095] [PMID: 15911722]

[25]   National Center for Biotechnology Information. PubChem Database. Calcium, CID=5460341. https://pubchem.ncbi.nlm.nih.gov/compound/5460341 accessed on May 18, 2019.

[26]   Coulter DA, Huguenard JR, Prince DA. Specific petit mal anticonvulsants reduce calcium currents in thalamic neurons. Neurosci Lett 1989; 98(1): 74-8.
[http://dx.doi.org/10.1016/0304-3940(89)90376-5] [PMID: 2710401]

[27]   Ethosuximide. Pfizer, Park-Davis. FDA access data. https://www.accessdata.fda.gov/drugsatfda_docs/label/ 2009/ 012380s031lbl.pdf2009.

[28]   Ethosuximide. Drug Facts and Comparisons. Facts & Comparisons [database online]. St Louis, MO: Wolters Kluwer Health, Inc; March 2005.

[29]   Methosuximid. Drug Facts and Comparisons. Facts & Comparisons [database online]. St Louis, MO: Wolters Kluwer Health, Inc; March 2005.

[30]   Isojärvi JI, Tokola RA. Benzodiazepines in the treatment of epilepsy in people with intellectual disability. J Intellect Disabil Res 1998; 42(S1) (Suppl. 1): 80-92.
[PMID: 10030438]

[31]   Rogawski MA, Löscher W, Rho JM. Mechanisms of action of antiseizure drugs and the ketogenic diet. Cold Spring Harb Perspect Med 2016; 6(5)a022780
[http://dx.doi.org/10.1101/cshperspect.a022780] [PMID: 26801895]

[32]   Carbamazepine.   Retrieved   on   March   30   2019. https://www.drugs.com/monograph/carbamazepine.html

[33]   Amstutz U, Shear NH, Rieder MJ, *et al.* Recommendations for HLA-B*15:02 and HLA-A*31:01 genetic testing to reduce the risk of carbamazepine-induced hypersensitivity reactions. Epilepsia 2014; 55(4): 496-506.
[http://dx.doi.org/10.1111/epi.12564] [PMID: 24597466]

[34]   Ju C, Uetrecht JP. Detection of 2-hydroxyiminostilbene in the urine of patients taking carbamazepine

and its oxidation to a reactive iminoquinone intermediate. J Pharmacol Exp Ther 1999; 288(1): 51-6. [PMID: 9862752]

[35] Ozeki T, Mushiroda T, Yowang A, *et al.* Genome-wide association study identifies HLA-A*3101 allele as a genetic risk factor for carbamazepine-induced cutaneous adverse drug reactions in Japanese population. Hum Mol Genet 2011; 20(5): 1034-41. [http://dx.doi.org/10.1093/hmg/ddq537] [PMID: 21149285]

[36] Drug level information: Oxcarbazepine. Retrieved on March 30 2019. https://dailymed.nlm.nih.gov/ dailymed/ drugInfo.cfm?setid=17325a80-fb9c-4a83-b4b4-98e0b999d852

[37] Dulsat C, Mealy N, Castaner R, Bolos J. Eslicarbazepine acetate. Drugs Future 2009; 34(3): 189. [http://dx.doi.org/10.1358/dof.2009.034.03.1352675]

[38] Aptiom. FDA Professional Drug Information. Retrieved on March 30 2019. https://www.drugs.com/pro/aptiom.html

[39] Löscher W. The discovery of valproate.Valproate. Milestones in Drug Therapy, Birkhäuser, Basel. 1999. [http://dx.doi.org/10.1007/978-3-0348-8759-5_1]

[40] Valproic acid. Drug monographs on Drugs.com. retrieved on April 01 2019.https://www.drugs.com/monograph/valproic-acid.html

[41] White HS, Harmsworth WL, Sofia RD, Wolf HH. Felbamate modulates the strychnine-insensitive glycine receptor. Epilepsy Res 1995; 20(1): 41-8. [http://dx.doi.org/10.1016/0920-1211(94)00066-6] [PMID: 7713059]

[42] Felbamate. Drug Facts and Comparisons. Facts & Comparisons [database online]. St Louis, MO: Wolters Kluwer Health, Inc; March 2005.

[43] Gabapentin and Pregabalin. Drug Facts and Comparisons Facts & Comparisons [database online] St Louis, MO: Wolters Kluwer Health, Inc; March 2005.

[44] McKeage K, Keam SJ. Pregabalin: in the treatment of postherpetic neuralgia. Drugs Aging 2009; 26(10): 883-92. [http://dx.doi.org/10.2165/11203750-000000000-00000] [PMID: 19761281]

[45] Levetiracetam. Drug Facts And Comparisons. Facts & Comparisons [database online]. St Louis, MO: Wolters Kluwer Health, Inc; March 2005.

[46] Brivaracetam. US National Library of Medicine. Accessed on June 27 2019.https://pubchem.ncbi.nlm.nih.gov/compound/9837243

[47] Vigabatrin. Drug Facts And Comparisons. Facts & Comparisons [database online]. St Louis, MO: Wolters Kluwer Health, Inc; March 2005.

[48] Lamotrigine. The American Society of Health-System Pharmacists. Retrieved 27 June 2005.

[49] Goa KL, Ross SR, Chrisp P. Lamotrigine. A review of its pharmacological properties and clinical efficacy in epilepsy. Drugs 1993; 46(1): 152-76. [http://dx.doi.org/10.2165/00003495-199346010-00009] [PMID: 7691504]

[50] Pollack MH, Roy-Byrne PP, Van Ameringen M, *et al.* The selective GABA reuptake inhibitor tiagabine for the treatment of generalized anxiety disorder: results of a placebo-controlled study. J Clin Psychiatry 2005; 66(11): 1401-8. [http://dx.doi.org/10.4088/JCP.v66n1109] [PMID: 16420077]

[51] Porter RJ, Dhir A, Macdonald RL, Rogawski MA. Mechanisms of action of antiseizure drugs. Handb Clin Neurol 2012; 108: 663-81. [http://dx.doi.org/10.1016/B978-0-444-52899-5.00021-6] [PMID: 22939059]

[52] https://pubchem.ncbi.nlm.nih.gov/compound/Topiramate

[53] https://pubchem.ncbi.nlm.nih.gov/compound/5734

[54]   https://pubchem.ncbi.nlm.nih.gov/compound/219078

[55]   https://pubchem.ncbi.nlm.nih.gov/compound/129228

[56]   https://pubchem.ncbi.nlm.nih.gov/compound/Retigabine

[57]   https://pubchem.ncbi.nlm.nih.gov/compound/9924495

[58]   https://www.accessdata.fda.gov/drugsatfda_docs/label/2018/210365lbl.pdf2018.

[59]   Report CP-R. Expert Committee on Drug Dependence https://www.who.int/ medicines/ access/controlled-substances/5.2_CBD.pdf2017.

[60]   Wilmshurst JM, Gaillard WD, Vinayan KP, *et al.* Summary of recommendations for the management of infantile seizures: Task Force Report for the ILAE Commission of Pediatrics. Epilepsia 2015; 56(8): 1185-97.
[http://dx.doi.org/10.1111/epi.13057] [PMID: 26122601]

[61]   2019.Dravet Syndrome https://www.ninds.nih.gov/Disorders/All-Disorders/Dravet-Syndro-e-Information-Page

[62]   Shafer P, Kiriakopoulos E. 2018.Dravet Syndrome https://www.epilepsy.com/learn/types-epileps--syndromes/dravet-syndrome

[63]   Medications A. Use in Pediatric Patients https://www.cms.gov/Medicare-Medicai--Coordination/Fraud-Prevention/Medicaid-Integrity-Education/Pharmacy-Educ-tion-Materials/Downloads/ac-pediatric-factsheet.pdf2013.

[64]   Patsalos PN, Spencer EP, Berry DJ. Therapeutic Drug Monitoring of Antiepileptic Drugs in Epilepsy: A 2018 Update. Ther Drug Monit 2018; 40(5): 526-48.https://journals.lww.com/drug-monitoring/Fulltext/2018/10000/Therapeutic_Drug_Monitoring_of_Antiepileptic_Drugs.2.aspx
[http://dx.doi.org/10.1097/FTD.0000000000000546] [PMID: 29957667]

[65]   Veroniki AA, Cogo E, Rios P, *et al.* Comparative safety of anti-epileptic drugs during pregnancy: a systematic review and network meta-analysis of congenital malformations and prenatal outcomes. BMC Med 2017; 15(1): 95-114.
[http://dx.doi.org/10.1186/s12916-017-0845-1] [PMID: 28472982]

[66]   Sneader W. Hormone analogues.Drug Discovery A History. West Sussex, England: John Wiley & Sons Ltd 2005.
[http://dx.doi.org/10.1002/0470015535]

[67]   Rogawski MA. Brivaracetam: a rational drug discovery success story. Br J Pharmacol 2008; 154(8): 1555-7.
[http://dx.doi.org/10.1038/bjp.2008.221] [PMID: 18552880]

CHAPTER 7

General and Local Anesthetic Agents

Carolyn J. Friel[*]

School of Pharmacy, Massachusetts College of Pharmacy and Health Sciences, Worcester, MA, USA

Abstract: This chapter is a comprehensive account of the medicinal chemistry of general and local anesthetic drugs. It provides the mechanism of drug action and details about structure-activity relationships of these drugs for pharmacists. After the study of this chapter, students will be able to:

• Select appropriate intravenous general anesthetic therapy based on patient-specific contraindications regarding cardiac and septic status.

• Evaluate inhaled general anesthetics about therapeutic regimens based on individual patient characteristics and medical procedures.

• Compare and contrast the potency, onset of action, and recovery time of the inhaled anesthetic based on MAC, blood: gas partition coefficients and oil:gas partition coefficients.

• Identify chemical metabolites of the inhaled anesthetics that increase the risk of nephron and hepatotoxicity.

• Identify the chemical classification to which a local anesthetic belongs based on drug structure.

• Select an appropriate local anesthetic for a patient with a specific allergy to PABA.

• Communicate the chemical rationale for local anesthetic buffering to health professionals.

Keywords: Drug-Receptor Interaction, General Anesthetics, Injectable Anesthetics, Inhaled Anesthetics, Local Anesthetics, Structure-Activity Relationship, The Clinical Use of Anesthetic Drugs.

---

[*] **Corresponding author Carolyn J. Friel:** School of Pharmacy, Massachusetts College of Pharmacy and Health Sciences, Worcester, MA, USA; Tel: 508-373-5612; E-mail: carolyn.friel@mcphs.edu

M. O. Faruk Khan & Ashok E. Philip (Eds.)
All rights reserved-© 2020 Bentham Science Publishers

HISTORICAL BACKGROUND

Indigenous populations have used plant and marine-based compounds to alleviate local pain presumably since before written records were kept. Local anesthetic use is initially reported in Homer's Iliad, which describes removing a shaft of an arrow and then putting a "bitter root" on the wound to take away the pain [1]. Electricity, in the form of electric eels and battery powered devices, refrigeration, ice and nerve compression were also used with minimal efficacy to produce local anesthesia [1]. The isolation of cocaine from Peruvian coca leaves was accomplished, in 1860 and it is considered as the first local anesthetic with widespread use and efficacy. Cocaine has inherent vasoconstrictor properties and is used today predominantly as a topical anesthetic in the nose and throat. The addictive properties of cocaine were realized early on and led to the development of procaine and other ester anesthetics.

The first demonstration of an inhaled anesthetic for surgery was performed by William Morton at the Massachusetts General Hospital, in Boston, in 1846. The agent used was ether and the successful demonstration and subsequent publication of its anesthetic properties led to its widespread acceptance as an inhaled anesthetic [2]. Other inhaled anesthetics used in the 1800s included chloroform and nitrous oxide. The first modern inhaled anesthetic developed was halothane, introduced in 1956. Today, there are fifteen local anesthetics available, two of which are available over-the-counter, and eight general anesthetics. All general anesthetics are used only in a clinical setting. No anesthetic is found in the top 200 drug list of drugs for 2017 [3].

INTRODUCTORY CONCEPTS

Mechanism of Action of General Anesthetics

The mechanism of action of the inhaled general anesthetics is not fully elucidated. The independent work by Meyer and Overton in the 1880s showed that anesthetic potency increased in direct proportion to lipid solubility [4, 5]. When the cell membrane was discovered to be composed of a lipid bilayer, the mechanism of action of the anesthetic drugs was hypothesized to be due to a disruption of the nerve cell membrane. This "lipid hypothesis" held favor for a hundred years until advanced pharmacological testing could identify specific receptor interactions. The inhaled anesthetics have been found to interact with ion channels such as the gamma-aminobutyric acid A ($GABA_A$) receptor, N-methyl-D-aspartate (NMDA) receptor, α-amino-3-hydroxy-5-methyl-4-isoxazolepropionic acid (AMPA) receptor, nicotinic receptor, sodium channels, potassium channels, calcium channels and ryanodine receptors [5]. The exact role that each of these protein targets plays in the mechanism of action of the general anesthetics is the focus of intense research today [5 - 12]. Determining the mechanism of action of these compounds will greatly aid a rational drug discovery program and lead to improved anesthetic drugs of the future.

The injectable general anesthetics are all small lipophilic molecules that can penetrate the BBB quickly. The mechanism of action of the injectable general anesthetics is through the activation of CNS inhibitory receptors, such as $GABA_A$, in or through inactivation of excitatory receptors, such as the NMDA receptor. The individual mechanisms are discussed with the drug below.

Mechanism of Action of Local Anesthetics

The mechanism of action of the local anesthetics is more elucidated than the general anesthetics. The local anesthetics work on both efferent nerves, neurons that carry messages from the brain to the periphery and afferent nerves, neurons that transmit messages from the periphery to the central nervous system (CNS). Neurons transmit messages of "pain" to the brain *via* an action potential. The action potential is initiated by the opening of sodium channels that allow an influx of positively charged sodium ions, thus depolarizing the cell and initiating the action potential sequence. The local anesthetic drugs bind to a specific binding site on sodium channels and block the passage of sodium into the cell and thus inhibit the action potential. Local anesthetics have varying effects on neurons depending on the diameter of the nerve fiber, myelination status, firing rate, and location of the nerve. In general, small nerve fibers that mediate temperature and pain sensation are more susceptible to local anesthetics than larger myelinated fibers that mediate pressure, touch and motor information [13].

The mechanism of action of the local anesthetics is *via* binding to the sodium channel and preventing further influx of sodium ions. They are believed to bind to a specific pocket deep inside the channel in their cationic form. The local anesthetic drug can contact the binding site either by entering the neuron in its neutral lipophilic state and accessing the binding site directly from within the membrane (hydrophobic pathway) or by passing all the way through the membrane, equilibrating with its cationic species, and then accessing the binding site from the interior pore (hydrophilic pathway). The local anesthetics do not access the binding site by moving directly into the channel from the exterior of the neuron [14, 15].

CLASSES OF GENERAL ANESTHETICS AND THEIR DISCUSSION

The general anesthetics are divided into two classes based on their route of administration; the injectable general anesthetics and the inhaled general anesthetics.

The Injectable General Anesthetics

The four general anesthetics covered in this section are propofol, fospropofol ketamine and etomidate (Fig. **1**). All four injectable drugs are used for the induction and maintenance of anesthesia.

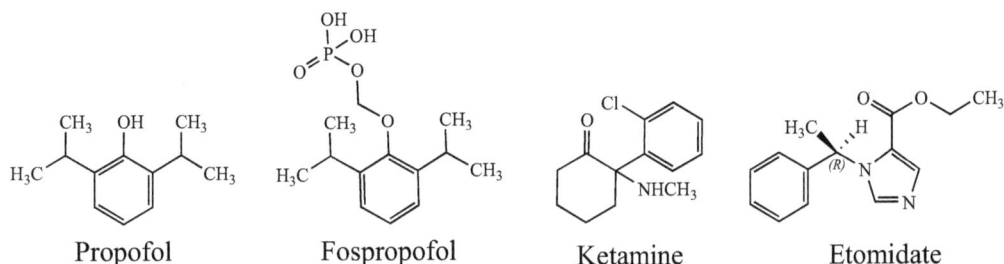

Fig. (1). The injectable general anesthetics.

Propofol is highly lipophilic with a log P of 4.15 [16]. The low water solubility necessitates its formulation in an oil-in-water emulsion using soybean oil, glycerol, and egg lecithin. Disodium edetate (0.005%) is added to retard the growth of microorganisms. Strict aseptic technique must be adhered to when handling propofol as the emulsion can support the development of microorganisms and lead to sepsis in a patient. Propofol quickly passes through the blood-brain-barrier (BBB) and produces a loss of consciousness within 40 seconds of administration [17]. Propofol is known to bind to the GABA$_A$ receptor and potentiates the effects of GABA, the major inhibitory neurotransmitter in the brain. Propofol is extensively metabolized *via* glucuronidation of the phenolic hydroxyl as well as Phase I oxidation of the para position followed by Phase II metabolism (Fig. **2**) [18, 19]. Rapid awakening of the patient occurs 10 to 15 minutes after the infusion is stopped. The most notable adverse reactions of propofol are respiratory depression, bradycardia hypotension and elevated triglycerides.

Fospropofol, a water soluble pro-drug of propofol, was approved by the United States Food and Drug Administration (FDA) in 2008. Fospropofol is quickly metabolized *via* endothelial alkaline phosphatase enzymes to yield propofol (Fig. **2**). The pro-drug does not need to be formulated in lipids and thus, avoids the hyperlipidemic concerns of propofol administration. The disadvantage of the pro-drug is that the onset of action is delayed compared to the onset of propofol (8 minutes for fospropfol *versus* 40 seconds for propofol).

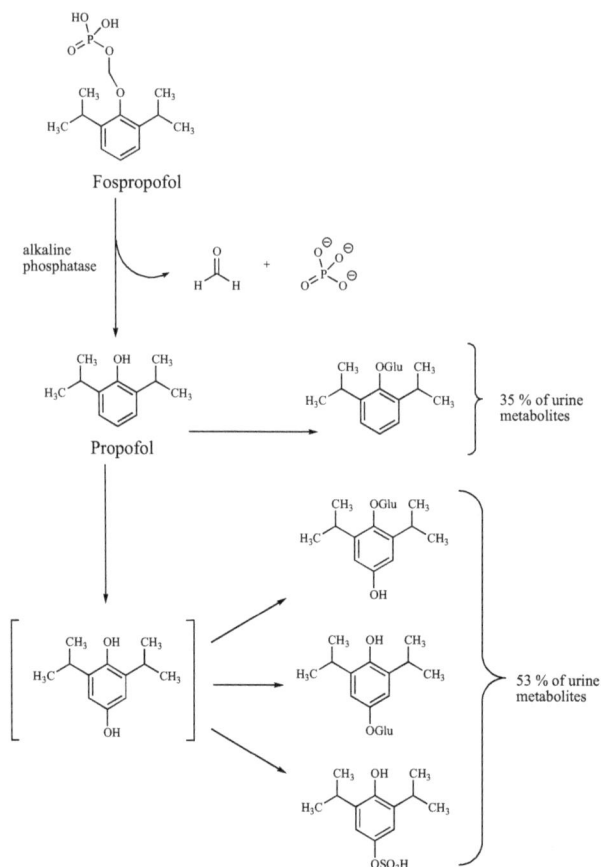

Fig. (2). Metabolism of fos/propofol.

Ketamine is marketed as the racemic mixture, although the S enantiomer is 3-4 times more potent as an anesthetic [20]. The proposed mechanism of action of ketamine is *via* binding to an allosteric site distinct from the glutamate-binding site on the NMDA receptor. By blocking the action of glutamate, ketamine prevents the flow of cations, such as calcium, sodium and potassium along their concentration gradients and prevents depolarization of the neuron [21]. Ketamine is classified as a "dissociative anesthetic" and as such, produces psychological side effects ranging from transient pleasant "dream-like" states to vivid hallucinations and delirium. Ketamine is metabolized in humans primarily *via* N-demethylation by CYP3A4 with minor contributions by CYP2B6 and CYP2C9 (Fig. **3**) [22, 23]. Patients must be monitored for increases in blood pressure, and ketamine is contraindicated in patients if transient increases in blood pressure are considered a serious hazard.

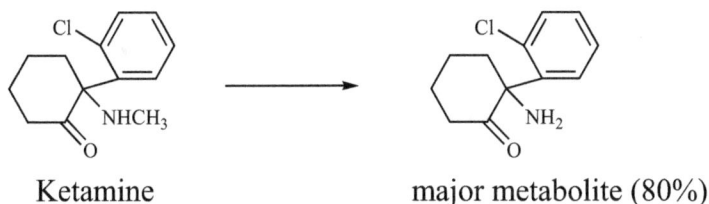

Fig. (3). Metabolism of ketamine.

Etomidate is a chiral compound marketed as the more potent R (+) enantiomer. The mechanism of action is believed to be similar to propofol's, namely, modulation of the GABA$_A$ receptor. Similar to propofol, etomidate is also poorly water-soluble and is marketed in the United States as a 2 mg/mL solution containing 35% v/v propylene glycol. The lipophilicity of the compound ensures distribution across the BBB and quick onset of action. Metabolism includes ester hydrolysis with 75% of the drug eliminated in the urine as the inactive carboxylic acid (Fig. **4**) [24].

Etomidate has lesser effect on cardiac output or blood pressure, but it does suppress the adrenal axis even after a single dose. Etomidate has been shown to inhibit 11β-hydroxylase and 11β/18 hydroxylase, two enzymes involved in the synthesis of cortisol and aldosterone, respectively [25]. The clinical significance of this adrenocortical suppression is unclear and the safety of etomidate in septic patients is under investigation [26].

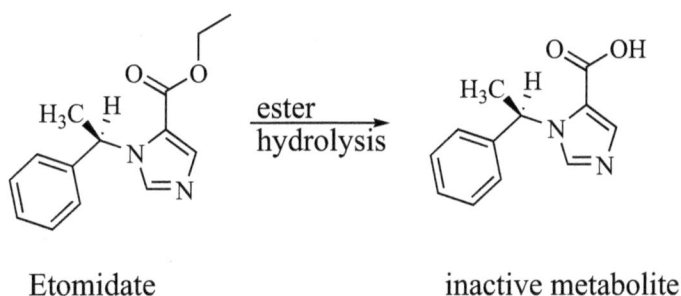

Fig. (4). Metabolism of etomidate.

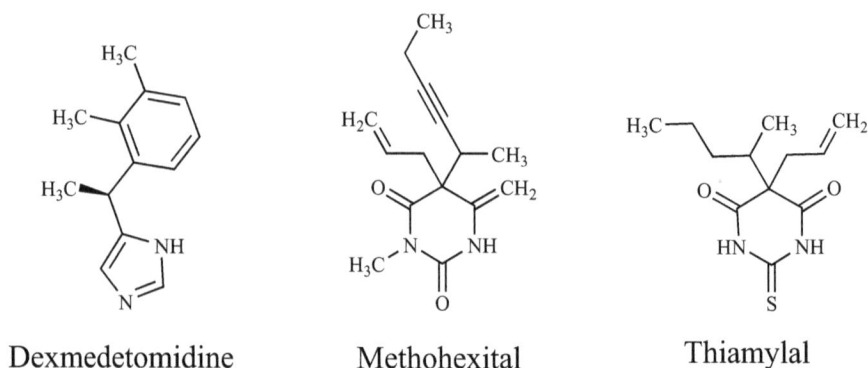

| Dexmedetomidine | Methohexital | Thiamylal |

Fig. (5). Adjuvant drugs used in General Anesthesia.

Adjuvant drugs used in General Anesthesia

Adjuvant drugs are often used during general anesthesia to aid in the induction of anesthesia or to decrease the required general anesthetic maintenance dose. Drugs classes used as adjuvants include the barbiturates, local anesthetics, opioids, benzodiazepines, α-2 adrenergic receptor agonists as well as neuromuscular blockers. The structures of some adjuvant drugs are seen in Fig. (**5**). Dexmedetomidine is a selective α-2-adrenoceptor agonist that has sedative and analgesic effects without respiratory depression [27]. Dexmedetomidine was approved in 1999 by the FDA as a short-term sedative for patients on ventilators in intensive care units. In 2008 the FDA expanded the use of dexmedetomidine to include sedation of non-intubated patients prior to and/or during surgical and other procedures. Dexmedetomidine is the S enantiomer of medetomidine and is frequently used when total intravenous anesthesia (TIVA) is employed for general anesthesia [28].

Currently, only two intravenous barbiturates are used as induction agents for general anesthesia. Both methohexital and thiamyl have quick onsets of action and ultra-short duration of action. Due to their respiratory depression, the use of barbiturates is declining in favor of newer, safer drugs [29]. Methohexital remains the induction agent of choice for electroconvulsive therapy [30].

The Inhaled General Anesthetics

The inhaled general anesthetics in use today are seen in Fig. (**6**). These gases or volatile liquid vapors are delivered to the patient *via* a mask over the mouth and nose or a tube inserted into the trachea. The anesthetic equipment is designed to allow the precise concentration of the drug, as a percentage of the total gas flow, to be inspired. The anesthetic agent must travel from the apparatus into the alveoli, then into the blood, and finally into the tissues, including the brain. Anesthetic action begins when the partial pressure of the anesthetic agent reaches the appropriate concentration in the brain. The choice of an inhaled anesthetic is based on side effect profile, cost, potency, duration of action, and recovery time.

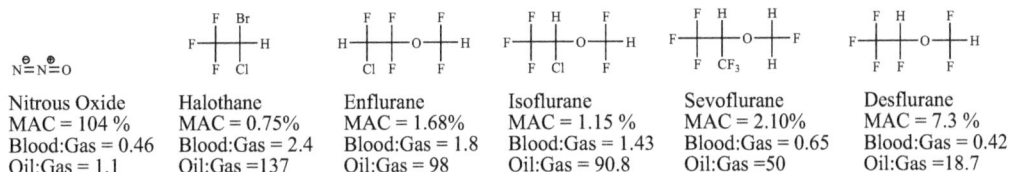

Fig. (6). The inhaled anesthetics and their properties.

The potency of an inhaled anesthetic is expressed as the minimum alveolar concentration (MAC). The MAC is recorded in one atmosphere and is defined as the mean concentration of the drug required to abolish movement in 50% of subjects in response to painful stimuli. The potency of the inhaled anesthetic has clinical importance as the gas is replacing oxygen in the inspired mixture. For example, nitrous oxide has the lowest potency, thus the highest MAC, and cannot be used alone to induce general anesthesia as it will lead to hypoxia and death.

The blood: gas partition coefficient is the ratio of the concentration of the drug in the blood to the concentration of the drug in the lungs at equilibrium (Fig. **6**). An ideal drug will have low blood solubility and thus quickly reach its equilibrium in the blood compartment before diffusing into the tissue and organ compartment. A drug with low blood: gas ratio would, therefore, have a quick onset of action as well as a quick recovery time. The other property of the anesthetic gases that can affect recovery time is the oil: gas partition coefficient. The oil: gas partition coefficient is directly related to the potency of the drug. The highly lipophilic compounds have lower MACs. The highly lipophilic compounds may accumulate in fat tissue compartments when used for greater than 5 hours, this may increase recovery time, especially in obese patients.

Elimination of the anesthetic drug occurs *via* the expiration of the agent as well as biotransformation. The inhaled anesthetics are metabolized to different extents in the liver and the kidneys. The degree to which they produce the nephrotoxic fluoride anion and hepatotoxic trifluoroacetic acid metabolite is important to know so that appropriate therapeutic choice can be made. Methoxyflurane, an inhaled agent, removed from the market due to nephrotoxicity, was associated with high plasma concentrations of fluoride anion. The amount of fluoride anion produced by all anesthetics and newly developed drugs is therefore monitored.

Both sevoflurane and enflurane have a higher production of the fluoride anion than the other inhaled anesthetics [31]. Another metabolite of concern is trifluoracetic acid. This can be generated by both halothane and isoflurane and can then acylate hepatic proteins. The loss of function of the hepatic protein can lead to toxicity as well as an immunogenic response to the conjugate [32]. The reader is referred to the individual drug monographs in the Textbook of Organic Medicinal and Pharmaceutical Chemistry for more information about their metabolic products [33].

CLASSES OF LOCAL ANESTHETICS AND THEIR DISCUSSION

The local anesthetics fall into two main classes, the amide anesthetics, and the ester anesthetics. The structure of the local anesthetics can be seen in Fig. (7). The majority of local anesthetics consist of three distinct parts. A substituted, lipophilic aromatic ring connected to either an ester or an amide linker group 3 to 4 atoms long, connected to tertiary nitrogen with a pK_a between 7.5 and 9.5. The tertiary nitrogen is predominantly charged at physiological pH. As discussed in the mechanism of action, only the uncharged drug molecule has the ability to penetrate the nerve cell and access the local anesthetic binding site. Due to the basic nature of the side chain, commercial supplies are often acidified to keep the compound in the protonated form and prevent the drug from crystallizing out in the vial. Unfortunately, the low pH of the solution is often painful upon injection. Careful buffering of the local anesthetic with sodium bicarbonate can minimize this pain [34].

Vasoconstrictors, such as epinephrine, levonordefrin and phenylephrine, are often used with local anesthetics to decrease the blood supply to the area the anesthetic is applied [35]. Decreasing blood flow keeps the anesthetic at the site of application resulting in less systemic absorption. The decreased blood flow to the area will also decrease the quantity of metabolizing enzymes present, which will also increase the duration of anesthetic action. The constricted capillaries and blanched tissue also make suturing and other manipulations easier to accomplish.

Local anesthetic overdose results in CNS stimulation (excitability, agitation, vomiting, tremors, and convulsions) followed by CNS and cardiac depression resulting in depressed blood pressure, depressed heart rate, coma and even death.[28] Treatment depends on the severity of the overdose. Mild cases may resolve upon withdrawal of the anesthetic. Severe overdoses may require oxygen, anticonvulsants, vasopressors and basic life support. Severe overdoses may also benefit from the infusion of a lipid emulsion [36 - 38]. There are multiple animal studies and human case reports that demonstrate the usefulness of using intralipid as an antidote for local anesthetic toxicity. The mechanism of antidotal action is theorized to be either a) a "lipid sink"; meaning that the infused lipid allows the lipophilic local anesthetic molecule to be absorbed into the lipid phase and then eliminated or b) to directly improve cardiac tissue function. Multiple theories exist on how lipids could improve cardiac tissue function. These include acting as a fatty acid source for mitochondrial respiration in the heart leading to increased ATP production or directly increasing calcium influx into myocardial cells enhancing contractility [38]. The American Heart Association includes the use of intralipids in the *Cardiac Arrests in Special Situations* section of the 2015 Guidelines for Cardiopulmonary Resuscitation [39]. Due to the lack of any comparative human studies the use of lipids is theoretically helpful and listed as a reasonable treatment option along with standard resuscitative care in patients with local anesthetic systemic toxicity.

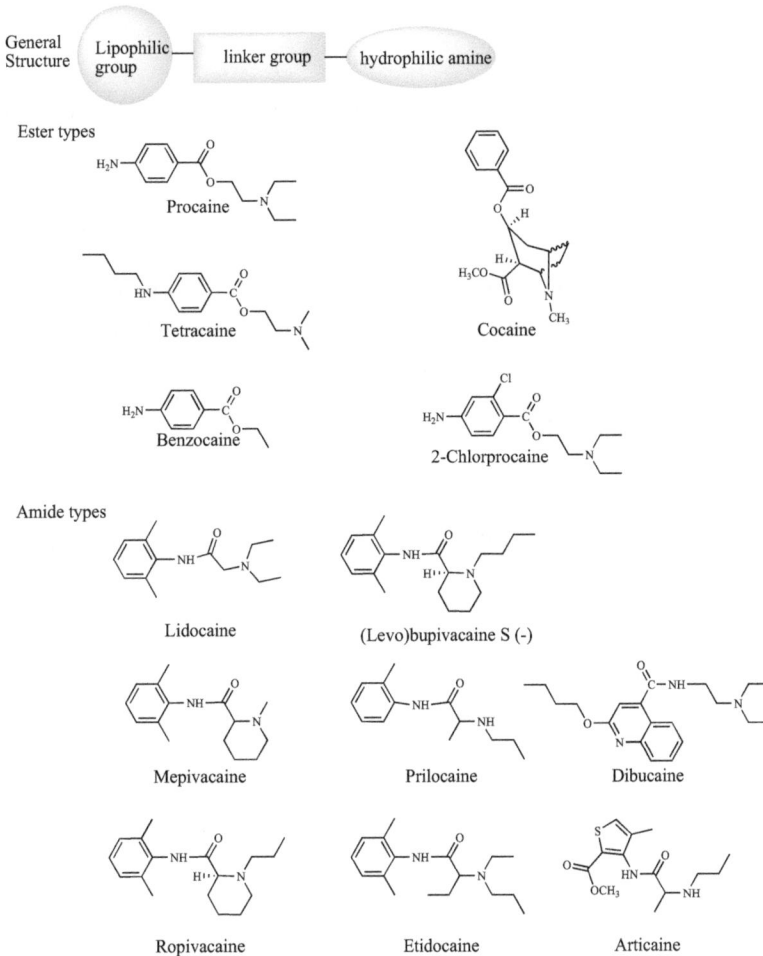

Fig. (7). Structure of local anesthetic drugs.

Another local anesthetic toxicity of concern is methemoglobinemia. Methemoglobinemia occurs when the ferrous iron (Fe^{2+}) found in hemoglobin has been oxidized by a drug or drug metabolite to ferric iron (Fe^{3+}). The oxidized form of iron cannot carry oxygen and as a result, the patient develops cyanosis, which does not respond to treatment with 100% oxygen. Case reports exist implicating lidocaine, prilocaine and benzocaine in causing methemoglobinemia. Treatment includes an intravenous infusion of a 1% methylene blue solution, 1 to 2 mg/kg, over 5 minutes [40]. Methylene blue is able to reduce the heme iron back to its oxygen carrying ferrous form. Rebound methemoglobinemia may occur up to 18 hours after a dose of methylene blue due to the local anesthetic redistributing out of the fat tissue. Repeat dosing with methylene blue may be necessary.

Ester Group Local Anesthetics

As seen in Fig. (**8**), when the "linker" group is an ester then the lipophilic aromatic ring is usually substituted with an electron donating group in the para position. This allows electron flow to the carbonyl group which enhances binding [41]. The ester functional group is metabolized by ubiquitous esterases, which inactivate the drug. The biological half-life of all local anesthetic drugs depends on the dose, route of administration, pH of the tissue, presence or absence of a vasoconstrictor and degree of protein binding [42]. Individual drug monographs should be consulted for specific pharmacokinetic information. Allergic reactions to the ester class are also more common due to the para amino benzoic acid (PABA) metabolite (Fig. **8a**). Allergies and photosensitivity reactions to PABA and similar "para" amine substituted aromatic rings, including sulfonamides, are commonly reported in the literature [43 - 47]. True immune-mediated reactions may result from the amine group directly participating in a nucleophilic reaction with a protein to form a hapten. Uptake of the hapten, antigen processing and T cell proliferation may be responsible for the allergic reaction. Alternatively, the amine group may undergo metabolic oxidation to form hydroxylamine and/or a nitroso group that can also covalently bind to proteins (Fig. **8b**) [48 - 50]. No PABA – protein hapten has been isolated from human serum, so this remains a theoretical explanation. Because the ester linked anesthetics have a higher potential for allergic reactions, current research is focused on the amide-type local anesthetics.

Amide Type Local Anesthetics

When the linker group is an amide, the aromatic ring is usually substituted in the meta position (mono or disubstituted) to decrease the rate of amide hydrolysis. Amide local anesthetics are not metabolized to PABA, but they may contain a paraben derived preservative. Patients that are allergic to PABA should receive a paraben free amide-type local anesthetic [51].

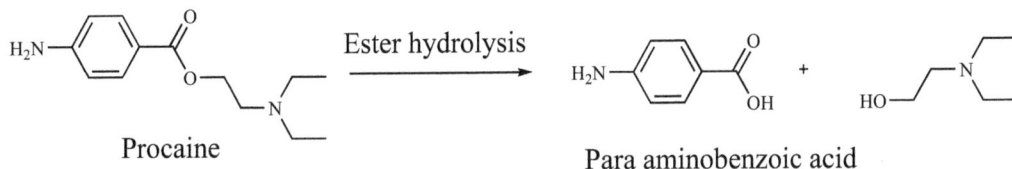

Fig. (8). (a) Metabolism of procaine to para aminobenzoic acid (b) PABA's theoretical role in allergic reactions.

CASE STUDIES

Case Study 1: A 28-year-old, 68 kg healthy women present at 38 weeks' gestation with elevated blood pressure for induction of labor. Her chart shows that she is pregnant with her first child and she has requested epidural analgesia as part of her birth plan. Her previous medical history is unremarkable, and she has allergies to penicillin and sulfonamides. Her blood pressure on admission was 150/90 and has remained stable; the fetal heart rate is stable. The anesthesiologist is called to start the epidural when she is 4 cm dilated. The epidural needle is placed, and the patient is started on a patient-controlled epidural analgesia regimen. The patient is started on a 10mL/hr epidural of 0.125% bupivacaine with a 5 mL patient-controlled bolus dose every 15 minutes as needed. Twenty minutes after the epidural begins, the patient develops slurred speech and quickly becomes incoherent. The anesthesiologist is paged and arrives within 3 minutes. Upon his arrival, the patient develops a tonic-clonic seizure. Oxygen is delivered *via* face mask and the epidural catheter is removed. The patient continues to decline, and the electrocardiogram shows a systole and no blood pressure is detected. Advanced cardiac life support is started, and the anesthesiologist requests the "antidote" from the obstetric code cart.

1. What is the presumed cause of the cardiac arrest?
2. What is the "antidote" for local anesthetic-induced toxicity is the anesthesiologist requesting?

Case study 2: The patient above is successfully resuscitated, and her baby delivered *via* emergency cesarean section. The patient and infant are dismissed post-op day 3 with prescriptions for Tylenol #3, 1 tablet every 6 hours as needed for pain, Senna 1 tablet every day and and Dermoplast® spray prn pain/itching on incision site. After two days of the appropriate use of all medications, the patient develops shortness of breath, cyanosis of the lips and fingertips and extreme exhaustion. She is brought to the emergency room by her husband. In the emergency room, she is administered 100% oxygen *via* nasal cannula, but her pulse oximeter remains at 78%.

1. What is the most likely diagnosis for this patient?
2. What medication is the most likely cause of her symptoms?
3. What medication should be used to treat this patient?

DRUG DISCOVERY CASE STUDIES

General Anesthetics: The development of Halothane

Halothane was the first compound specifically synthesized to be an inhaled general anesthetic. In 1950 the general anesthetics commonly used were ether, cyclopropane and chloroform. Ether and cyclopropane were not ideal due to their cardiotoxicity, flammability, and explosiveness. Chloroform was chemically stable but toxic to the liver.

In 1951, the Imperial Chemical Industries Ltd (ICI) embarked on a program to develop a new inhaled anesthetic [52]. The ICI was a large British company that produced chemicals, including explosives, paints and refrigerants. They also synthesized halogenated alkyl compounds to be used as propellants. These compounds were added under pressure to paint, shaving soap or perfumes and when the pressure was released through a valve the mixture was ejected as a spray and the halogenated compound would evaporate. The volatility of these compounds made them an easy starting point for pharmacologists looking for inhaled anesthetics. The ICI polled anesthetists for their requirements of an ideal drug and they chose to focus on compounds that were 1) nonflammable and non-explosive 2) had low toxicity and little metabolism 3) could be synthesized with at least 99.95% purity and 4) were volatile compounds for inhalation [52].

The early work by Booth and Bixby in the 1930s using $CFHCl_2$ and CF_3HCl on mice provided the starting point for their research [53, 54]. Unfortunately, this early work had been abandoned due to convulsions in mice. The ICI chemists and pharmacologists originally looked at compounds containing -CF_3 or =CF_2 groups to obtain stability and reduced toxicity compared to ether and chloroform. They also wanted to keep the hydrogen content low to reduce the compounds' flammability [55]. They found that compounds that contained no hydrogen atoms had a lower margin of safety and a lower potency compared with similar compounds containing at least one hydrogen. They also realized the importance that a low boiling point had on the saturated vapor pressure. One and two carbon halogenated compounds were prepared with H, F, Cl and Br in different ratios and tested for anesthetic potency in mice. Halothane was not one of the original ICI propellants and was specifically synthesized and tested because it had chemical stability, a boiling point that resulted in an ideal relative saturation for anesthesia and good anesthetic potency in mice.

Halothane proved to have ideal properties but provided a new problem, photochemical instability. Halothane evolves bromine when exposed to light. The addition of 0.01% thymol was found to prevent the free radical decomposition of halothane. Halothane was marketed in 1956 by ICI under the name Fluothane. Halothane has a limited role in anesthesia in the United States as it has been replaced by newer, safer inhaled anesthetics. Halothane is listed in the 2017 World Health Organization (WHO) Model List of Essential Medicines. This document serves a guide for countries employing a national formulary and considers safety, efficacy and cost of medications for inclusion on the list. Halothane, isoflurane and nitrous oxide are the only general inhalation anesthetics included on the list [56].

Amide Class Local Anesthetics: The Development of Ropivacaine

The last ester-type local anesthetic marketed was Chloroprocaine in 1955. Since that time the focus of local anesthetics has been on the amide-type structures. Focus turned to the amides because they have quicker onsets, higher potencies, increased chemical stability and a longer duration of action. Ropivacaine was first synthesized in 1957, but it was not marketed until 1996. Why was it marketed 40 years after the original synthesis? The development of ropivacaine is an example of a drug coming to market only after the different activity and toxicity of the stereoisomers was determined, and chemical separation became routinely available.

R	LD_{50} mice mg/kg	Chirality	Drug name	year marketed
CH_3	43.3	racemic	mepivacaine	1957
CH_2CH_3	24.5	racemic	not marketed	
$CH_2CH_2CH_3$	13.5	S	ropivacaine	1996
$CH_2CH_2CH_2CH_3$	12.7	racemic	bupivacaine	1963

Fig. (9). AB Bofors Nobelkrut amide anesthetics.

In 1957 the Swedish chemical company of AB Bofors Nobelkrut synthesized 35 aromatic amides of the N-alkyl pyrrolidine and N-alkyl piperidine carboxylic acid classes to test them for local anesthetic activity [57]. They determined that for high potency, the nitrogen containing ring should be attached to the carbonyl carbon of the amide at the ring carbon alpha to the nitrogen. Four of the compounds synthesized are shown in Fig. (9). The pharmacologic activity of these compounds was determined as was the lethal dose for 50% of the animals (LD_{50}). The LD_{50} dose was determined by intravenous injection in mice. Of the four compounds, the methyl substituted compound was found to have the lowest potency but also the lowest toxicity and thus it was chosen for further development. The R and S enantiomers of the methyl-substituted compound were resolved and no difference was seen in the LD_{50}. This compound, named mepivacaine, was marketed in 1957 as a racemate. It is notable that the drug was marketed the same year that it was first synthesized. Extensive pharmacological and toxicological studies were not conducted as they are today. Mepivacaine found success in the clinic but the search was still on for a longer-acting local anesthetic that could match the duration of the increasingly complicated procedures being conducted using local anesthesia. The N- butyl substituted compound was found to have a much longer duration of action and was marketed as racemic bupivacaine in Europe in 1963 and the United States in 1973 [58]. During the first ten years of clinical use in Europe most of the case reports involving bupivacaine reported deleterious CNS symptoms, common for all local anesthetics. The first case of a serious cardiac complication due to bupivacaine appeared in 1977. This was followed by multiple cases involving extrasystole, hypotension, bradycardia, ventricular fibrillation, cardiac arrest and death [58]. The cardiotoxicity of bupivacaine was recognized, and the search began for long acting local anesthetics that had a better cardiac profile than bupivacaine. The isomers of bupivacaine had been studied in vitro in 1972 and it was found that the S (-) enantiomer was less toxic. In the search for a novel anesthetic, the focus turned to the N-propyl substituted compound (Fig. **9**) that was overlooked in 1957 because it showed much greater toxicity than the methyl substituted compound. At this point, the differences in both activity and toxicity of the R and S isomers of the local anesthetics were recognized. The chiral separation of compounds had also become much more routine. The R and S isomers were resolved and underwent extensive in vitro and in vivo testing [59]. As with the N- butyl compound, the S enantiomer of the N-propyl compound showed less cardiotoxicity in pigs, pregnant sheep and human volunteers [59]. In 1996, Ropivacaine, the N-propyl derivative, was brought to the market as the S isomer by Astra Zeneca.

STUDENTS SELF-ASSESSMENT QUESTIONS

Use the information in Fig. (**5**) to answer the following four questions:

1) Which inhaled anesthetic has the quickest onset of action?

a. Nitrous Oxide

b. Isoflurane

c. Desflurane

d. Halothane

e. Enflurane

f. Sevoflurane

2) Which inhaled anesthetic should not be used alone to produce general anesthesia?

a. Nitrous Oxide

b. Isoflurane

c. Desflurane

d. Halothane

e. Enflurane

f. Sevoflurane

3) Which inhaled anesthetic would have the longest recovery time in a morbidly obese patient undergoing a seven-hour surgery?

a. Nitrous Oxide

b. Isoflurane

c. Desflurane

d. Halothane

e. Enflurane

f. Sevoflurane

4) Which inhaled anesthetic has the highest potency?

a. Nitrous Oxide

b. Isoflurane

c. Desflurane

d. Halothane

e. Enflurane

f. Sevoflurane

5) Which local anesthetics below should not be used in a patient with an allergy to PABA?

a. Benzocaine

b. Cocaine

c. Lidocaine

d. Prilocaine

e. Articaine

6) Which local anesthetic does not contain a chiral carbon?

a. Bupivacaine

b. Dibucaine

c. Etidocaine

d. Ropivacaine

e. Prilocaine

7) Which injectable general anesthetic is known to suppress the adrenal axis?

a. Propofol

b. Ketamine

c. Etomidate

8) Which injectable general anesthetic is a dissociative anesthetic?

a. Propofol

b. Ketamine

c. Etomidate

CONSENT FOR PUBLICATION

Not applicable.

CONFLICT OF INTEREST

The authors confirm that the contents of this chapter have no conflict of interest.

ACKNOWLEDGEMENTS

Declare none.

REFERENCES

[1]   Ring ME. The history of local anesthesia. J Calif Dent Assoc 2007; 35(4): 275-82.
        [PMID: 17612366]

[2]   Morton WTG, Ed. Remarks on the Proper Mode of Administering Sulphuric Ether by Inhalation.
        Boston, MA: Dutton and Wentworth 1847.

[3]   Kane SP. https://clincalc.com/DrugStats2018.

[4]   Kleinzeller A. Membrane Permeability: 100 Years Since Ernest Overton: 100 Years Since Ernest
        Overton. Charles Ernest Overton' s Concept of a Cell Membrane Academic Press 1999; 21(May): 1.

[5]   Franks NP. Molecular targets underlying general anaesthesia. Br J Pharmacol 2006; 147 (Suppl. 1):
        S72-81.
        [http://dx.doi.org/10.1038/sj.bjp.0706441] [PMID: 16402123]

[6]   Oakes V, Domene C. Capturing the Molecular Mechanism of Anesthetic Action by Simulation
        Methods. Chem Rev 2018.
        [http://dx.doi.org/10.1021/acs.chemrev.8b00366] [PMID: 30358391]

[7]   Eger EI II, Koblin DD, Harris RA, *et al.* Hypothesis: inhaled anesthetics produce immobility and
        amnesia by different mechanisms at different sites. Anesth Analg 1997; 84(4): 915-8.
        [http://dx.doi.org/10.1213/00000539-199704000-00039] [PMID: 9085981]

[8]   Eckenhoff RG. Promiscuous ligands and attractive cavities: how do the inhaled anesthetics work? Mol
        Interv 2001; 1(5): 258-68.
        [PMID: 14993365]

[9]   Barber AF, Liang Q, Amaral C, Treptow W, Covarrubias M. Molecular mapping of general anesthetic
        sites in a voltage-gated ion channel. Biophys J 2011; 101(7): 1613-22.
        [http://dx.doi.org/10.1016/j.bpj.2011.08.026] [PMID: 21961587]

[10]   Conway KE, Cotten JF. Covalent modification of a volatile anesthetic regulatory site activates TASK-
        3 (KCNK9) tandem-pore potassium channels. Mol Pharmacol 2012; 81(3): 393-400.
        [http://dx.doi.org/10.1124/mol.111.076281] [PMID: 22147752]

[11]   Brannigan G, LeBard DN, Hénin J, Eckenhoff RG, Klein ML. Multiple binding sites for the general
        anesthetic isoflurane identified in the nicotinic acetylcholine receptor transmembrane domain. Proc
        Natl Acad Sci USA 2010; 107(32): 14122-7.
        [http://dx.doi.org/10.1073/pnas.1008534107] [PMID: 20660787]

[12]   Vemparala S, Domene C, Klein ML. Computational studies on the interactions of inhalational
        anesthetics with proteins. Acc Chem Res 2010; 43(1): 103-10.
        [http://dx.doi.org/10.1021/ar900149j] [PMID: 19788306]

[13]   Catterall WA. From ionic currents to molecular mechanisms: the structure and function of voltage-

gated sodium channels. Neuron 2000; 26(1): 13-25.
[http://dx.doi.org/10.1016/S0896-6273(00)81133-2] [PMID: 10798388]

[14] Strichartz GR. The inhibition of sodium currents in myelinated nerve by quaternary derivatives of lidocaine. J Gen Physiol 1973; 62(1): 37-57.
[http://dx.doi.org/10.1085/jgp.62.1.37] [PMID: 4541340]

[15] Fozzard HA, Sheets MF, Hanck DA. The sodium channel as a target for local anesthetic drugs. Front Pharmacol 2011; 2: 68.
[http://dx.doi.org/10.3389/fphar.2011.00068] [PMID: 22053156]

[16] Krasowski MD, Jenkins A, Flood P, Kung AY, Hopfinger AJ, Harrison NL. General anesthetic potencies of a series of propofol analogs correlate with potency for potentiation of gamma-aminobutyric acid (GABA) current at the GABA(A) receptor but not with lipid solubility. J Pharmacol Exp Ther 2001; 297(1): 338-51.
[PMID: 11259561]

[17] Insert P, Ed. Diprivan (Propofol) Injectable Emulsion. Wilmington, DE: AstraZeneca 2005.

[18] Trapani G, Altomare C, Liso G, Sanna E, Biggio G. Propofol in anesthesia. Mechanism of action, structure-activity relationships, and drug delivery. Curr Med Chem 2000; 7(2): 249-71.
[http://dx.doi.org/10.2174/0929867003375335] [PMID: 10637364]

[19] Lee SY, Park NH, Jeong EK, *et al.* Comparison of GC/MS and LC/MS methods for the analysis of propofol and its metabolites in urine. J Chromatogr B Analyt Technol Biomed Life Sci 2012; 900(0): 1-10.
[http://dx.doi.org/10.1016/j.jchromb.2012.05.011] [PMID: 22672847]

[20] Hustveit O, Maurset A, Oye I. Interaction of the chiral forms of ketamine with opioid, phencyclidine, sigma and muscarinic receptors. Pharmacol Toxicol 1995; 77(6): 355-9.
[http://dx.doi.org/10.1111/j.1600-0773.1995.tb01041.x] [PMID: 8835358]

[21] Tyler MW, Yourish HB, Ionescu DF, Haggarty SJ. Classics in chemical neuroscience: ketamine. ACS Chem Neurosci 2017; 8(6): 1122-34.
[http://dx.doi.org/10.1021/acschemneuro.7b00074] [PMID: 28418641]

[22] Hijazi Y, Boulieu R. Contribution of CYP3A4, CYP2B6, and CYP2C9 isoforms to N-demethylation of ketamine in human liver microsomes. Drug Metab Dispos 2002; 30(7): 853-8.
[http://dx.doi.org/10.1124/dmd.30.7.853] [PMID: 12065445]

[23] Kharasch ED, Labroo R. Metabolism of ketamine stereoisomers by human liver microsomes. Anesthesiology 1992; 77(6): 1201-7.
[http://dx.doi.org/10.1097/00000542-199212000-00022] [PMID: 1466470]

[24] Giese JL, Stanley TH. Etomidate: a new intravenous anesthetic induction agent. Pharmacotherapy 1983; 3(5): 251-8.
[http://dx.doi.org/10.1002/j.1875-9114.1983.tb03266.x] [PMID: 6359080]

[25] Kulstad EB, Kalimullah EA, Tekwani KL, Courtney DM. Etomidate as an induction agent in septic patients: red flags or false alarms? West J Emerg Med 2010; 11(2): 161-72.
[PMID: 20823967]

[26] Sunshine J, Deem S, Weiss N, *et al.* Etomidate, adrenal function and mortality in critically ill patients. Respir Care 2012.
[http://dx.doi.org/10.4187/respcare.01956] [PMID: 22906838]

[27] 2013.https://www.accessdata.fda.gov/drugsatfda_docs/label/2013/021038s021lbl.pdf

[28] Ramsay MAE, Luterman DL. Dexmedetomidine as a total intravenous anesthetic agent. Anesthesiology 2004; 101(3): 787-90.
[http://dx.doi.org/10.1097/00000542-200409000-00028] [PMID: 15329604]

[29] López-Muñoz F, Ucha-Udabe R, Alamo C. The history of barbiturates a century after their clinical

introduction. Neuropsychiatr Dis Treat 2005; 1(4): 329-43.
[PMID: 18568113]

[30] Vaidya PV, Anderson EL, Bobb A, Pulia K, Jayaram G, Reti I. A within-subject comparison of propofol and methohexital anesthesia for electroconvulsive therapy. J ECT 2012; 28(1): 14-9.
[http://dx.doi.org/10.1097/YCT.0b013e31823a4220] [PMID: 22330701]

[31] Kharasch ED, Hankins DC, Thummel KE. Human kidney methoxyflurane and sevoflurane metabolism. Intrarenal fluoride production as a possible mechanism of methoxyflurane nephrotoxicity. Anesthesiology 1995; 82(3): 689-99.
[http://dx.doi.org/10.1097/00000542-199503000-00011] [PMID: 7879937]

[32] Martin JL, Keegan MT, Vasdev GMS, *et al.* Fatal hepatitis associated with isoflurane exposure and CYP2A6 autoantibodies. Anesthesiology 2001; 95(2): 551-3.
[http://dx.doi.org/10.1097/00000542-200108000-00043] [PMID: 11506133]

[33] Friel CJ. Anesthetics.Wilson and Gisvold's Textbook of Organic Medicinal and Pharmaceutical Chemistry. 12th ed. New York: Wolters Kluwer Lippincott Williams and Wilkins 2011; pp. 711-32.

[34] Xia Y, Chen E, Tibbits DL, Reilley TE, McSweeney TD. Comparison of effects of lidocaine hydrochloride, buffered lidocaine, diphenhydramine, and normal saline after intradermal injection. J Clin Anesth 2002; 14(5): 339-43.
[http://dx.doi.org/10.1016/S0952-8180(02)00369-0] [PMID: 12208437]

[35] Friel CJ, Eliadi C, Pesaturo K. Local anesthetic use in perioperative areas. Perioper Nurs Clin 2010; 5(2): 203-14.
[http://dx.doi.org/10.1016/j.cpen.2010.02.001]

[36] Weinberg GL. Treatment of local anesthetic systemic toxicity (LAST). Reg Anesth Pain Med 2010; 35(2): 188-93.
[http://dx.doi.org/10.1097/AAP.0b013e3181d246c3] [PMID: 20216036]

[37] Picard J, Meek T. Lipid emulsion to treat overdose of local anaesthetic: the gift of the glob. Anaesthesia 2006; 61(2): 107-9.
[http://dx.doi.org/10.1111/j.1365-2044.2005.04494.x] [PMID: 16430560]

[38] Ciechanowicz S, Patil V. Lipid emulsion for local anesthetic systemic toxicity. Anesthesiol Res Pract 2012; 2012131784
[http://dx.doi.org/10.1155/2012/131784] [PMID: 21969824]

[39] Lavonas EJ, Drennan IR, Gabrielli A, *et al.* Part 10: Special Circumstances of Resuscitation, 2015 American heart association guidelines update for cardiopulmonary resuscitation and emergency cardiovascular care. Circulation 2015; 132(18) (Suppl. 2): S501-18.
[http://dx.doi.org/10.1161/CIR.0000000000000264] [PMID: 26472998]

[40] Olson KR. Poisoning.Current Medical Diagnosis and Treatment. New York, NY: McGraw-Hill 2019.

[41] Buchi J, Perlia X. Design of local anesthetics.Drug Design. New York: Academic Press 1972; Vol. III: p. 243.
[http://dx.doi.org/10.1016/B978-0-12-060303-9.50012-4]

[42] Yagiela JA. Local anesthetics. Anesth Prog 1991; 38(4-5): 128-41.
[PMID: 1819966]

[43] Vu AT, Lockey RF. Benzocaine anaphylaxis. J Allergy Clin Immunol 2006; 118(2): 534-5.
[http://dx.doi.org/10.1016/j.jaci.2006.04.035] [PMID: 16890789]

[44] Kaidbey KH, Allen H. Photocontact allergy to benzocaine. Arch Dermatol 1981; 117(2): 77-9.
[http://dx.doi.org/10.1001/archderm.1981.01650020019016] [PMID: 6970547]

[45] Mackie BS, Mackie LE. The PABA story. Australas J Dermatol 1999; 40(1): 51-3.
[http://dx.doi.org/10.1046/j.1440-0960.1999.00319.x] [PMID: 10098293]

[46] Eggleston ST, Lush LW. Understanding allergic reactions to local anesthetics. Ann Pharmacother

1996; 30(7-8): 851-7.
[http://dx.doi.org/10.1177/106002809603000724] [PMID: 8826570]

[47]   Svensson CK, Cowen EW, Gaspari AA. Cutaneous drug reactions. Pharmacol Rev 2001; 53(3): 357-79.
[PMID: 11546834]

[48]   Bhole MV, Manson AL, Seneviratne SL, Misbah SA. IgE-mediated allergy to local anaesthetics: separating fact from perception: a UK perspective. Br J Anaesth 2012; 108(6): 903-11.
[http://dx.doi.org/10.1093/bja/aes162] [PMID: 22593127]

[49]   Cîrstea M, Suhaciu G, Cîrje M. Cross immunological reactions between three haptens of the "para" group and 4-aminoantipyrine. Physiologie 1979; 16(2): 103-8.
[PMID: 117463]

[50]   Winkler R, Hertweck C. Sequential enzymatic oxidation of aminoarenes to nitroarenes *via* hydroxylamines. Angew Chem Int Ed Engl 2005; 44(26): 4083-7.
[http://dx.doi.org/10.1002/anie.200500365] [PMID: 15929146]

[51]   Dance D, Basti S, Koch DD. Use of preservative-free lidocaine for cataract surgery in a patient allergic to "caines". J Cataract Refract Surg 2005; 31(4): 848-50.
[http://dx.doi.org/10.1016/j.jcrs.2004.09.059] [PMID: 15899466]

[52]   Suckling CW. Some chemical and physical factors in the development of fluothane. Br J Anaesth 1957; 29(10): 466-72.
[http://dx.doi.org/10.1093/bja/29.10.466] [PMID: 13471840]

[53]   Booth HS, Bixby EM. Fluorine derivatives of chloroform. Ind Eng Chem 1932; 24(6): 637-41.
[http://dx.doi.org/10.1021/ie50270a012]

[54]   Robbins BH. Preliminary studies of the anesthetic activity of fluorinated hydrocarbons. J Pharmacol Exp Ther 1946; 86: 197-204.
[PMID: 21018256]

[55]   Halsey MJ. A reassessment of the molecular structure-functional relationships of the inhaled general anaesthetics. Br J Anaesth 1984; 56 (Suppl. 1): 9S-25S.
[PMID: 6391531]

[56]   WHO.   http://apps.who.int/iris/bitstream/handle/10665/273826/EML-20-eng.pdf?ua=1   Accessed 8/29/2018.

[57]   Ba E, Egner B, Pettersson G. Local anaesthetics I. N-alkyl pyrrolidine and N-alkyl piperidine caboxylic acid amides. Acta Chem Scand 1957; 11(7): 1183-90.

[58]   Ruetsch YA, Böni T, Borgeat A. From cocaine to ropivacaine: the history of local anesthetic drugs. Curr Top Med Chem 2001; 1(3): 175-82.
[http://dx.doi.org/10.2174/1568026013395335] [PMID: 11895133]

[59]   McClure JH. Ropivacaine. Br J Anaesth 1996; 76(2): 300-7.
[http://dx.doi.org/10.1093/bja/76.2.300] [PMID: 8777115]

CHAPTER 8

Parkinson Disease and Antiparkinsonian Drugs

Ashok E. Philip[1,*], George DeMaagd[2] and M. O. Faruk Khan[3]

[1] *Department of Pharmaceutical Sciences, Union University School of Pharmacy, Jackson, TN38305, USA*

[2] *Department of Pharmacy Practice, Union University School of Pharmacy, Jackson, TN38305, USA*

[3] *School of Pharmacy, University of Charleston, Charleston, WV 25304, USA*

Abstract: This chapter is a comprehensive account of Parkinson's disease and the medicinal chemistry of antiparkinsonian drugs. It provides the mechanism of disease progression and drug action and detail structure-activity relationships of the antiparkinsonian drugs to give the knowledge base for pharmacists. After a study of this chapter, students will be able to:

• Discuss the epidemiology and etiology of Parkinson disease (PD)

• Describe the clinical features of idiopathic PD and differentiate between cardinal motor features and non-motor symptoms

• Discuss various risk factors and corresponding mechanisms responsible for the development of PD symptoms

• Review biosynthesis of dopamine, its metabolic outcomes, dopaminergic pathways, receptor distribution and corresponding signal transduction mechanisms

• Explain in detail the pathophysiologic mechanisms responsible for the clinical features of idiopathic PD

• Evaluate the clinical role of L-DOPA and discuss its mechanism of action, pharmacokinetics, adverse effects, motor complications, drug interactions, contraindications and precautions

• For each medication class listed below, discuss their mechanism of action, pharmacokinetics, adverse effects, motor complications, drug interactions, contraindications and precautions

   o Dopamine agonists

---

[*] **Corresponding author Ashok E. Philip**: Department of Pharmaceutical Sciences, Union University School of Pharmacy, Jackson, TN, USA; Tel: 731-661-5704; E-mail: aphilip@uu.edu

M. O. Faruk Khan & Ashok E. Philip (Eds.)

- ropinirole (Requip®, Requip® XL); pramipexole Mirapex®, Mirapex® ER); rotigotine transdermal patch (Neupro®), and apomorphine (Apokyn®)

  o Catechol-O-methyltransferase (COMT) inhibitors

  - entacapone (Comtan®) and tolcapone (Tasmar®)

  o Selective monoamine oxidase-B (MAO- B) inhibitors

  - selegiline (Eldepryl® and Zelapar® ODT) and rasagiline (Azilect®)

  - amantadine (Symmetrel®)

  o Anticholinergic agents (benztropine (Cogentin®) and trihexyphenidyl)

Keywords: Parkinson's disease (PD), Amantadine, Anticholinergic agents, Antiparkinsonian drugs, Apomorphine, Benztropine, Catechol--methyltransferase (COMT) inhibitors, Dopamine (DA), Entacapone, L-DOPA dopamine agonists, Muscarinic agents, Pramipexole, Rasagiline, Ropinirole, Rotigotine, Selective monoamine oxidase-B (MAO-B) inhibitors, Tolcapone, Selegiline, Structure-activity relationshipand drug-receptor.

HISTORICAL BACKGROUND

Parkinson's disease (PD) was first described by Dr. James Parkinson in 1817 as a "shaking palsy." PD is a chronic progressive neurodegenerative disease characterized by both motor as well as non-motor features. The cardinal motor features of the disease include resting tremor, bradykinesia, muscular rigidity and postural imbalance whereas non-motor symptoms include dementia, depression and others [1, 2]. Please refer to Table **1** for a description of motor and non-motor symptoms associated with PD.

In the United States, PD incidence is reported to be approximately 20 cases per 100,000 people per year (60,000 per year), with the mean age of onset close to 60 years. Overall, approximately 1 million Americans are currently affected by PD. The prevalence is reported to be approximately 1-2% in the 60 and > age group and increases to 1-3% in the 80 plus age group [3 - 6]. However, even though PD is primarily a disease of the elderly, reports indicate that patients may develop this disease in their 30s and 40s [4]. Also, the incidence of PD is reported as a ratio of 3:2 (male to female) with a recent study suggesting that the potential delayed onset in females could be related to interactions between gonadotropins and the nigrostriatal dopaminergic system [7, 8].

In 1867, Ordenstein introduced belladonna to treat Parkinson's disease. However, its use fell out of favor quickly. A series of discoveries of the basic etiology and histology of the disease led to the discovery of modern antiparkinsonian treatments. Levodopa, a dopamine precursor, was introduced in the 1960s after the milestone discovery of PD as a disorder of dopamine metabolism. Bromocriptine and deprenyl (selegiline) were introduced in the 1970s, followed by pergolide in the 1980s. In 1997, pramipexole and ropinirole were introduced as direct dopamine receptor agonists for the treatment of PD. The discovery of many genetic defects throughout the 1990s led to gene therapy for PD in 2005. Rasagiline, a selective MAO-B inhibitor, was approved in 2006 [9, 10].

INTRODUCTORY CONCEPTS

Clinical Overview, Etiology and Risk Factors

The cardinal motor symptoms of PD include:

- Resting tremor (usually resolves with voluntary movement and during sleep)
- Bradykinesia (slowness and decreased amplitude of movement)
- Muscular rigidity (resistance to passive movement of flexor and extensor muscles)
- Postural instability (loss of postural reflexes that lead to falling and gait disturbances)

The extrapyramidal system involves motor structures of basal ganglia and plays a prominent role in maintaining posture, muscle tone and regulating voluntary smooth muscle activity. From a neuropathology perspective, PD is a disorder of the extrapyramidal system with the etiology for motor symptoms attributed to the loss of pigmented dopaminergic neurons (symptoms are seen only at ~80% loss) in the pars compacta region of substantia nigra which project to striatum thereby resulting in depleted striatal dopamine (DA) levels. Also characteristic of PD is the presence of intraneuronal cytoplasmic protein/lipid aggregates referred to as Lewy bodies. It should be noted that even though reports highlight striatal dopamine depletion as the major cause of motor symptoms of PD, the presence of non-motor features supports the involvement of other neurotransmitters like norepinephrine [11 - 13].

Characteristic of PD is its variable and pronounced progression with end-stage disease resulting in serious complications that include pneumonia, often associated with mortality. Currently, with no treatments available to interfere with disease progression, pharmacological management of symptoms is the standard of care and must include a multidisciplinary approach [14, 15].

A number of risk factors attributed to the development of PD include: high caloric intake, elevated body mass index (BMI), elevated cholesterol, head trauma, medications and post-infection states (encephalitis), mitochondrial dysfunction, inflammation, oxidative stress, excitotoxicity, nitric oxide toxicity, signal mediated apoptosis, environmental toxins and genetic association [16 - 24].

Table 1. Motor and non-motor symptoms associated with PD [25 - 39].

Motor Symptoms	Non-motor Symptoms
Resting tremor: - Initial symptom in 70-90% of patients	Neuropsychiatric: - Depression - Dementia
- Resolves during sleep and voluntary movements - Primarily affects hands, may involve jaw, tongue, lips, chin and legs	- Anxiety/panic disorder - Psychosis (exacerbated by anticholinergics and DA agonists)
Bradykinesia: - Occurs in 80-90% of patients	Sensory: - Olfactory dysfunction
- Slow and decreased amplitude of movement	- Pain and Paraesthesia
Muscular rigidity: - Occurs in >90% patients	Sleep disorders: - Insomnia
- Resistance to passive movement of flexor and extensor muscles - Accompanied by cogwheel phenomenon Postural instability: - Occurs in late-stage PD - Loss of postural reflexes - Predisposes to falls and gait disturbances Other: - Dysarthria - Dystonia	- REM behavior disorder, daytime somnolence, sleep attacks, restless leg syndrome, sleep apnea Autonomic dysfunction: - Orthostatic Hypotension - Sexual dysfunction - Constipation - Sweating - Sialorrhea - Urinary retention Other: - Fatigue and Weight loss

MPTP-Induced Neuronal Cell Death

1-Methyl-4-phenyl-1,2,3,6-tetrahydropyridine (MPTP) is a pyridine analog recognized as a parkinsonism producing neurotoxin. MPTP is formed as a byproduct during the synthesis of the target 1-methyl-4-propiono-y-4-phenylpiperidine (MPPP), referred to as "synthetic or designer heroin". MPTP was consumed by illicit drug users in the 1970s-80s which resulted in the manifestation of clinical motor symptoms of PD. Evidence for MPTP-induced neurotoxicity came from the fact that patients who injected MPTP, either alone or as a main constituent, presented with motor symptoms of PD and had degeneration of DA neurons of the substantia nigra, a hallmark feature of PD.

Chemically, MPPP is a reverse ester analog of the opioid analgesic, meperidine. Studies have reported mechanisms involved in MPTP-induced neuronal cell death (Fig. **1**) [23, 40 - 50].

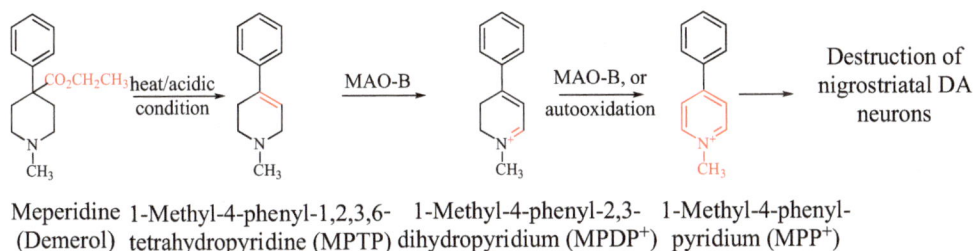

Meperidine (Demerol) | 1-Methyl-4-phenyl-1,2,3,6-tetrahydropyridine (MPTP) | 1-Methyl-4-phenyl-2,3-dihydropyridium (MPDP$^+$) | 1-Methyl-4-phenyl-pyridium (MPP$^+$)

Fig. (1). Mechanisms involved in MPTP-induced neuronal cell death. a) Under the influence of heat and acidic conditions, MPPP is first converted to MPTP. b) MPTP is then converted to 1-methyl-4-phenyl-2,3-dihydropyridinium (MPDP$^+$) species *via* two-electron oxidation at allylic α-carbon by MAO-B. It is postulated that the formation of MPDP$^+$ occurs in glial cells, which contain high concentrations of MAO-B, near striatal nerve terminals and nigral cell bodies. c) MPDP$^+$ is subsequently converted to the more stable 1-methyl-4-phenyl-pyridinium (MPP$^+$) species, either by MAO-B or *via* auto-oxidation. d) MPP$^+$ is taken up into the striatal dopaminergic nerve terminals *via* DA transporter. Once inside the neuron, MPP$^+$ concentrates on mitochondria and inhibits complex I of the electron transport chain and NADH oxidation thereby depleting ATP levels in nigrostriatal neuronal cells. Consequently, MPP$^+$ is recognized as the major neurotoxic metabolite of MPTP that selectively causes the destruction of nigrostriatal DA neurons.

Oxidative Stress

Other processes implicated in oxidative stress-driven neurotoxic effects that lead to neuronal cell death in substantia nigra include reactive products like epoxides, free radicals and quinones formed during DA synthesis and breakdown. Additionally, the oxidation-reduction cycle of iron in the substantia nigra pars compacta can also lead to the formation of free radicals and toxic metabolites that may contribute to the PD process. It should be noted that the effects of high oxidative stress could be secondary to an overwhelmed endogenous anti-oxidative molecule like glutathione [22, 23, 51 - 53]. A brief overview of the products and processes involved in oxidative stress-induced neurotoxicity is discussed in Fig. (**2**).

Environmental Toxins

Rotenone, Paraquat, Cyperquat, Dieldrin and Trichloroethylene are some of the pesticides and herbicides (Fig. **3**) implicated in the etiology of PD, with the risk being higher in rural farming communities [63 - 65].

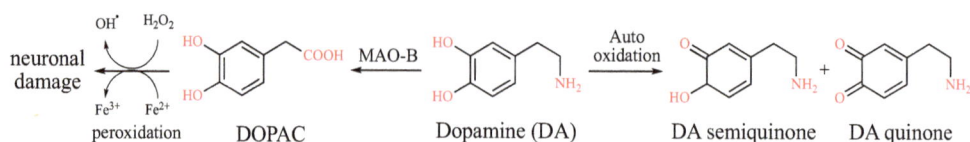

Fig. (2). DA products and related processes involved in oxidative stress [51 - 53]. Conversion of L-tyrosine to $_L$-DOPA could proceed *via* a direct insertion of one oxygen atom into L-tyrosine or proceed through an epoxide intermediate. It is postulated that during this conversion, an analogous epoxide formed could potentially alkylate nucleophilic groups of various proteins, DNA or RNA and precipitate neuronal cell death [54, 55]. DA catabolism *via* auto-oxidation results in the formation of electrophilic species semiquinone and quinone, as well as a neuromelanin pigment. The electrophilic species potentially alkylate sulfhydryl groups of glutathione, lead to diminished anti-oxidative actions of glutathione and precipitate oxidative stress. Additionally, the neuromelanin pigment exhibits the potential to accumulate in nigrostriatal neuronal cells and produce cell death [13, 56]. Based on evidence that mitochondrial complex I deficiency in substantia nigra was observed in post-mortem samples of PD patients, it is postulated that mitochondrial dysfunction leads to decreased ATP levels, disruption of hydrogen peroxide as well as cytotoxic hydroxyl radical homeostasis and contributes to neuronal cell death [57 - 61]. Hydrogen peroxide generated during MAO-catalyzed oxidation of DA has the potential to react with superoxide and form extremely cytotoxic hydroxyl radical [62].

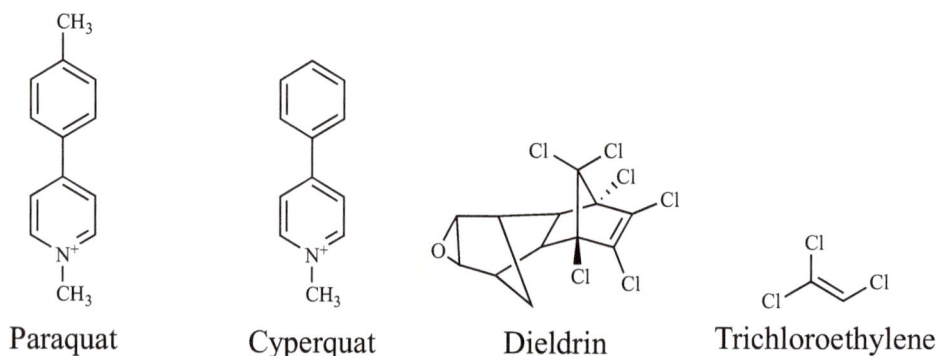

Fig. (3). Pesticides and herbicides implicated in etiology of PD [66].

Despite structural similarity between Paraquat, Cyperquat and MPTP or MPP$^+$, their mechanisms of neurotoxicity are not clear with earlier suggestions pertaining to mitochondrial complex I inhibition and uptake *via* DA transporter found to be physiologically improbable. Rotenone on the other hand is a lipophilic molecule with the ability to cross blood-brain barrier and suggested to act *via* inhibition of mitochondrial complex I and cause nigrostriatal DA neuronal degradation [66, 67]. Additional environmental toxins proposed to be involved include cyanide, carbon disulfide, methanol and organic solvents. Methocathinone, a psychostimulant, when injected, exposes neurons to manganese, and is considered as a possible risk factor. However, overall retrospective data is inconclusive, does not establish causality and suffers from an inability to quantify toxin exposure with PD related neurotoxicity [17 - 19, 68].

Interestingly, an inverse correlation exists between the risk of developing PD and cigarette smoking as well as caffeine intake [69].

- Epidemiological evidence highlights a lower frequency of PD incidence in cigarette smokers compared to non-smokers. It is proposed that the ability of components of cigarette smoke to inhibit MAO-B activity may be responsible for the decreased incidence of PD in smokers [69 - 73].
- PD related benefit, that is decreased incidence, associated with caffeine ingestion is attributed to its non-selective adenosine receptor antagonist activity, which results in attenuation of abnormal neuronal signaling mediated *via* intracellular kinase activation by A_{2A} receptors [74 - 76].

Genetic Association

Limited data supports genetic association with PD. Existing data is contentious with studies that examined the genetics of PDs conducted in small number of patients, displayed selection bias and presented conflicting results. Mutations in single genes linked to familial PD have been identified and involve the α-synuclein gene, DJ-1, PINK1, parkin, and LRRK-2 and suggests multiple gene involvement [77 - 85]. Mutations identified also include a recessively inherited early-onset PD gene which is involved in the maintenance of DA neuron integrity or survival. Overexpression of synuclein (Syn) proteins, especially α-Syn, in PD is a direct consequence of mutations. The abnormal aggregation of Syn proteins in PD, and in other neurodegenerative diseases like Alzheimer's, is toxic to neurons and is found in the histopathological component of PD Lewy bodies. Evidence also suggests that expression of alpha-Syn affects dopamine synthesis [86, 87].

PD-linked genes, DJ-1, PINK1, parkin, and LRRK-2, involved in the impairment of ubiquitin-proteasome system, autophagy-lysosome pathway, mitochondrial metabolic disturbances and alterations in kinase activity have also been studied and serve as potential targets for treatment [88]. The involvement of genes associated with detoxification of toxins and/or neurotransmitters, complicates the issue further and suggests a variable effect on mutations by the environment [89]. Also, the prevalence of PD throughout the world is inconsistent and highlights a converging role for environmental, genetic as well as ethnic differences in contributing to DA loss in PD [90, 91].

Dopamine: Biosynthesis, Metabolism and Receptor Function

DA Biosynthesis and Metabolism

Both phenylalanine and tyrosine serve as precursors for DA with dietary phenylalanine converted to tyrosine predominantly in the liver by phenylalanine hydroxylase (Fig. **4**). Once tyrosine is taken up into the brain, it is converted to L-DOPA (3,4-dihydroxy phenylalanine) by tyrosine hydroxylase which is the rate-limiting step. Subsequently, L-DOPA is rapidly converted to DA by L-aromatic amino acid decarboxylase (AADC) which is highly active both in the CNS and periphery.

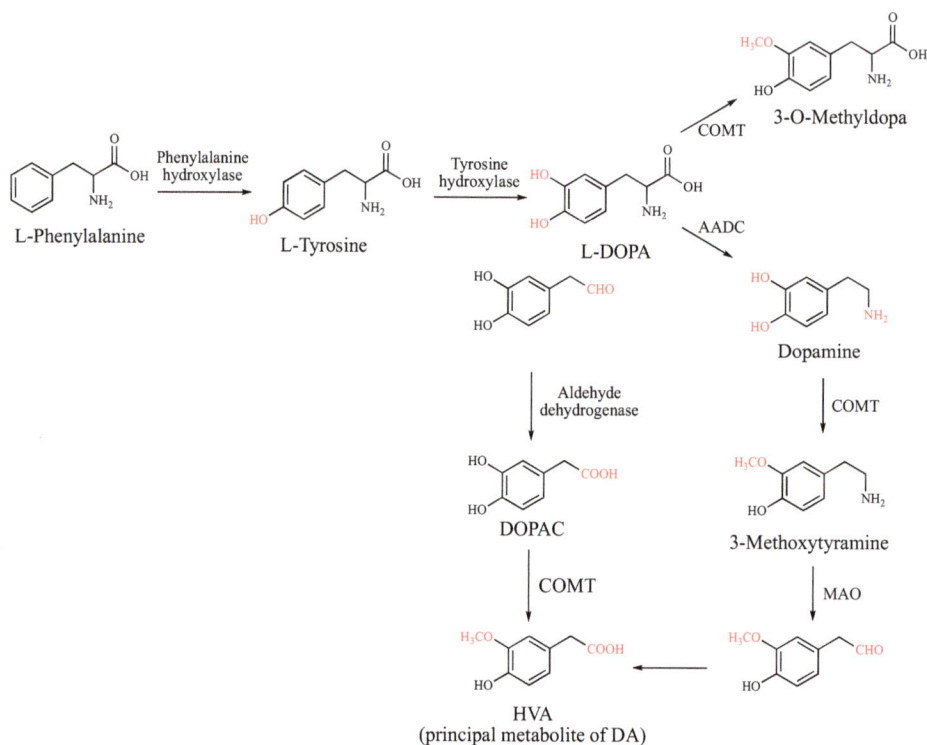

Fig. (4). Dopamine biosynthesis and metabolic pathways. L-DOPA, L-3,4-dihydroxyphenylalanine; AADC, Aromatic l-amino acid decarboxylase; COMT, catecholamine-O-methyl transferase; MAO, monoamine oxidase; DOPAC, 3,4-dihydroxyphenylacetic acid; DA, dopamine; HVA, homovanillic acid.

Termination of synaptic DA action is primarily mediated *via* its presynaptic reuptake by DA transporter (DAT) and/or norepinephrine transporter (NET). Once taken up, DA is metabolized primarily by MAO enzymes to an inactive aldehyde derivative which is further metabolized to 3,4-dihydroxyphenylacetic acid (DOPAC) by aldehyde dehydrogenase. DOPAC is subsequently metabolized to homovanillic acid (HVA) by catechol-O-methyltransferase (COMT) with HVA being the primary DA metabolite excreted in urine [92].

DA Receptors and Function

The DA receptors belong to the superfamily of G protein-coupled receptors (GPCRs) and are sub classified into "D_1 receptor family" and "D_2 receptor family" based on their effector coupling profile, signal transduction mechanisms, structural differences and anatomical distribution (Table **2**). The "D_1 receptor family" comprises subtypes D_1 and D_5 and considered to be *excitatory* owing to their ability to activate adenylyl cyclase *via* coupling to $G\alpha_s$ and stimulate formation of cellular cyclic adenosine monophosphate (cAMP). The "D_2 receptor family" on the other hand comprises subtypes D_2, D_3 and D_4 and considered to be *inhibitory* owing to their ability to inhibit adenylyl cyclase *via* coupling to $G_{i/o}$ and decrease production of intracellular cAMP, suppress Ca^{+2} currents in addition to activation of K^+ currents [92].

Table 2. DA receptors, distribution and signal transduction mechanisms [92].

Receptor Family Type	Distribution	Signal Transduction Mechanism
D_1 Receptor Family: **EXCITATORY** - D_1 Receptor	- substantia nigra pars reticulate (SNpr) - frontal cortex - nucleus accumbens, hypothalamus	couple to $G\alpha_s$ activate adenylyl cyclase ↑cAMP
- D_5 Receptor	- hypothalamus - striatum - nucleus accumbens	
D_2 Receptor Family: **INHIBITORY** - D_2 Receptor	- striatum - nucleus accumbens - olfactory tubercule - prefrontal cortex - amygdala - ventral tegmental area (VTA) - hippocampus - hypothalamus - substantia nigra pars compacta (SNpc)	couple to $G_{i/o}$ inhibit adenylyl cyclase ↓cAMP ↓Ca^{+2} currents ↑K^+ currents
- D3 Receptor	- nucleus accumbens - VTA and SNpc	
- D4 Receptor	- retina, hypothalamus prefrontal cortex, amygdala, hippocampus, pituitary	

The DA receptors are expressed presynaptically as well as postsynaptically. The presynaptic (auto) receptors belong to the D_2 family with D_2 subtype being the predominant autoreceptor type. In response to extracellular neurotransmitter levels, the presynaptic autoreceptors facilitate negative feedback response and consequently modulate rate of neuronal firing, neurotransmitter synthesis and release. Typically, activation of presynaptic D_2 family of autoreceptors leads to decreased DA release and attenuated locomotor activity whereas activation of postsynaptic receptors results in stimulation of locomotion [93].

Dopaminergic Pathways

Table **3** provides summary of DA actions on various physiological systems. The four major pathways of DA in the central nervous system (CNS) include [92]:

- *Nigrostriatal pathway*: Accounts for 75% of DA in brain and regulates movement. It consists of cell bodies that originate in substantia nigra with their corresponding axons terminating in striatum. This pathway is primarily impaired in PD and is also involved in movement related side effects, including tardive dyskinesia, associated with use of antipsychotic agents.
- *Mesolimbic pathway*: Originates in ventral tegmental area and project to nucleus accumbens. This pathway regulates reward behavior and its dysfunction is implicated in addiction, schizophrenia, psychoses as well as learning deficits.
- *Mesocortical pathway*: Originates in ventral tegmental area and projects to prefrontal cortex. This pathway regulates higher order cognitive functions like motivation, reward, emotion, and impulse control. Impairment of this pathway is implicated in schizophrenia as well as attention-deficit hyperactivity disorders.
- *Tuberoinfundibular pathway*: Originates in hypothalamus and projects to pituitary gland and median eminence of hypothalamus. DA released in this pathway is carried by hypophyseal blood supply to pituitary and regulates prolactin secretion.

Table 3. Physiological systems and corresponding DA actions [92].

Physiological System	DA Actions
Nigrostriatal pathway	Motor control (*via* D1 and D2 family)
Mesolimbic pathway	Reward behavior (*via* D1 and D2 family)
Mesocortical pathway	Cognitive functions like motivation, reward, emotion, and impulse control
Tuberoinfundibular pathway	Inhibition of prolactin release (*via* D2 receptors)
Kidney	Increased natriuresis (*via* D1 and D2 family)

(Table 3) cont.....

Physiological System	DA Actions
Heart and Vasculature	Low concentration - Vasodilation (*via* D1) High concentrations – vasoconstriction (*via* activation of α adrenergic receptors)
Pituitary gland	Inhibition of prolactin release (*via* D2
Sympathetic nerve terminals	Inhibition of norepinephrine release (*via* D2) Note: adrenal medulla - Tonic inhibition of epinephrine release (*via* D2)
Voltage-gated ion channels	Modulation of Na^+ and N-, P- and L-type Ca^{+2} currents

Pathophysiology

Currently, the two neuropathological features of PD include progressive loss of pigmented dopaminergic neurons in substantia nigra pars compacta (SNpc) that innervate striatum and presence of intracellular Lewy bodies (LBs) and neurites filled with abnormal α-synuclein [93, 94]. It should be noted that motor symptoms of PD do not manifest until ~80% of striatal dopaminergic neurons are lost. Additionally, as indicated earlier, appearance of non-motor symptoms (Table **1**), even during the earlier course of the disease, support the involvement of various neurotransmitters and neuromodulators. Especially, loss of adrenergic function, dysfunction within the glutamatergic, cholinergic, and serotonergic system as well as adenosine and enkephalins are all implicated in the pathophysiology associated with non-motor features of PD [95 - 98].

The striatum (caudate and putamen) is the primary input structure of basal ganglia and receives excitatory input *via* glutamatergic system from the cerebral cortex. The striatal neurons project to globus pallidus (GP) which in turn projects to ventroanterior (VA) and ventrolateral (VL) thalamus. Dopaminergic neurons that originate in substantia nigra pars compacta (SNpc) project to the striatum and synapse on two types of dopamine receptors D_1 (excitatory-type) and D_2 (inhibitory-type). They subsequently influence motor activity in the extrapyramidal system by modulating activity of the inhibitory γ-aminobutyric acid (GABA) neurons. Additionally, the striatum contains interneurons (local circuit neurons) that do not project beyond the striatum and rely on acetylcholine (ACh) and neuropeptides for neurotransmission [99].

There are two functionally distinct pathways, the *direct pathway* and *indirect pathway*, through which the striatal outflow reaches globus pallidus (GP). It should be noted that the overall effect of DA mediated stimulation of these two pathways is enhanced motor activity. ;The enhanced motor activity results from stimulation of direct pathway whereas stimulation of indirect pathway results in attenuated motor activity. Key features, function and differential effects of DA on these two pathways are summarized in Table **4**.

However, in PD, the net effect observed due to loss of dopaminergic neurons in substantia nigra pars compacta (SNpc) that innervate striatum results is enhanced activity of the *indirect pathway* which results in decreased motor activity. The net hypokinetic effect seen in PD is therefore attributed to increased activity of GPi/SNr neurons, subsequent enhanced inhibition of thalamus (VA/VL) and resultant decreased excitatory input from thalamus to motor cortex. Despite certain limitations, the basal ganglia model accounts for the characteristic hypokinetic symptoms associated with PD. It also provides a rational basis for the pharmacological management of PD, with clinical improvements seen in motor symptoms of PD due to restoration of dopaminergic activity in striatum *via* activation of D1 and D2 receptor types [99].

Additionally, the ACh interneurons worsen the decreased motor activity attributed to dopaminergic loss in SNPc by inhibiting striatal cells of the *direct pathway*. Normally, the ACh interneurons synapse on GABAergic striatal neurons that project to GPi and GPe and upon activation inhibit striatal cells of *direct pathway* while exciting striatal cells of *indirect pathway*. Therefore, the overall effect of activating the ACh interneurons is decreased motor activity. In PD, loss of dopaminergic function exacerbates ACh activity which leads to unopposed inhibition of the *direct pathway* and predominance of *indirect pathway* mediated diminished motor activity. Consequently, anticholinergic agents have found a place in the management of motor symptoms of PD [100].

Table 4. *Direct* and *Indirect* pathways and differential effects of DA [99].

Direct pathway	Indirect pathway
- Striatal neurons of *direct pathway* project directly to globus pallidus interna (GPi) and substantia nigra pars reticulate (SNpr) - Provides input to thalamus *via twosequentialinhibitoryGABA links* (striatum to GPi/SNpr and GPi/SNpr to VA/VL, respectively)	- Striatal neurons of *indirect pathway* project to globus pallidus externa (GPe) which innervates subthalamic nucleus (STN), which then project to GPi and SNpr. - Provides input to thalamus *via twosequential inhibitory* GABA links (striatum to GPe and GPe to STN respectively), followed by an *excitatory glutamatergic link* (STN to GPi/SNpr), which is then followed by an *inhibitory GABA link* to thalamus (GPi/SNpr to VA/VL)
- Primarily expresses *excitatory* D1-type receptors	- Primarily expresses *inhibitory* D2-type receptors

(Table 4) cont.....

Direct pathway	Indirect pathway
- Cortical signal excites striatal neurons *via* excitatory glutamate - Excited striatal cells *via* inhibitory GABA *inhibit (decrease)* GPi activity -*Inhibition* of GPi results in decreased inhibition of thalamus *i.e., dis-inhibition* - Decrease in inhibition signal from GPi results in increased firing from thalamus (VA/VL) to motor cortex (Fig. **5**)	- Cortical signal excites striatal neurons *via* excitatory glutamate - Excited striatal cells *via* inhibitory GABA *inhibit(decrease)* GPe activity -*Inhibition* of GPe results in decreased inhibition of STN *i.e., dis-inhibition* - Decrease in inhibitory signal from GPe results in increased activity of STN - Increased activity of STN results in increased activity of GPi *via* excitatory glutamate actions - Increased activity of GPi GABAergic neurons results in enhanced inhibition of thalamus (VA/VL) (Fig. **5**)
- DA released in striatum *enhances/excites* activity of direct pathway *via* D1-type	- DA released in striatum *reduces/inhibits* activity of indirect pathway *via* D2-type

- Net effect of *direct pathway stimulation*:
     - Increased excitatory thalamic input to motor cortex due to increased firing of VA/VL neurons
     - Enhanced motor activity
	- Net effect of *indirect pathway stimulation*:
	     - Decreased excitatory thalamic input to motor cortex, due to *increased inhibition* of thalamic (VA/VL) neurons
	     - Decreased motor activity

- In PD, loss of DA input to striatum from SNpc results in *decreased* activity of direct pathway	- In PD, loss of DA input to striatum from SNpc results in *increased* activity of indirect pathway and subsequent hypokinetic symptoms

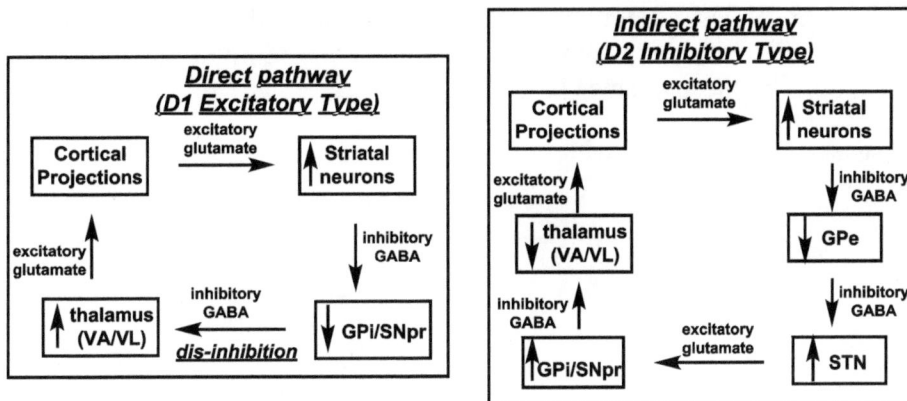

Fig. (5). Direct and Indirect pathways of Striatum - ↑ increased firing/excitation; ↓decreased firing/inhibition.

The histopathological hallmark of PD is the presence of intraneuronal protein and lipid aggregates referred to as Lewy bodies (LBs). The Lewy bodies found in dopaminergic neurons have defining characteristics that include round bodies with radiating fibrils and a core seen only on autopsies. Both the LBs and abnormal neurites are made up of aggregates of normal, misfolded and truncated proteins with α-synuclein being the primary component. Although associated with neuropathology and neurotoxicity of PD for many years, it is not clear how exactly these protein and lipid bodies originate [93]. Research supports the view that Lewy bodies may form secondary to refractory proteolytic processes involving abnormal breakdown or over production of proteins. Aggregation of αSyn protein due to genetic mutations is associated with formation of insoluble fibrils in the Lewy bodies associated with PDs with this protein being targeted for treatment of PD [101, 102]. Reports also indicate that decreased function or inhibition of the ubiquitin proteasome system (UPS) results in neurodegeneration along with formation of Lewy bodies [103, 104].

Recent data suggests that cerebrospinal fluid containing amyloid β 1-42 biomarker may predict cognitive decline associated with PD in addition to Alzheimer's disease pathology [19, 105]. Also, inflammatory responses secondary to loss of dopaminergic neurons may also contribute to the pathogenesis of PD with microglia and astrocyte activation supported by *in vitro* data [106 - 110].

Drug Induced Movement Disorders

A number of drugs cause drug induced movement disorders and must be included in the differential diagnosis to avoid inappropriate treatment of patients. Especially, elderly women, patients with co-morbidities (cognitive impairment) and those taking chronic high doses as well as multiple medications are at high risk. Table **5** provides a summary of drugs associated with drug induced parkinsonism (DIP) with the primary mechanism of action involving blockade of dopamine actions by these agents [111 - 119].

Table 5. Medications associated with movement disorders [111 - 119].

Medications	Associated Movement Disorder
Antipsychotics – Both Typical (I[st] Generation) and Atypical (IInd Generation)	Akathisia, acute dystonia, parkinsonism, Tardive Dyskinesia(TD), Neuroleptic Malignant Syndrome (NMS)
Antiemetics – metoclopramide, droperidol prochlorperazine	Akathisia, acute dystonia, parkinsonism, Tardive Dyskinesia, Neuroleptic Malignant Syndrome
Antidepressants	- Tremor and ataxia (with high doses of tricyclics) - Parkinsonism, TD and NMS (amoxapine) - Akathesia, Tremor and Serotonin Syndrome (SSRIs)

(Table 5) cont.....

Medications	Associated Movement Disorder
Sympathomimetics – amphetamine analogs, pseudophedrine, phenylephrine, demecarium, echothiophate	Tremor
Anticonvulsants – carbamazepine, phenytoin, lamotrigine and valproic acid	Tremor, Chorea
Miscellaneous – amiodarone, amphotericin B, lithium, levothyroxine, medoxyprogesterone, epinephrine, acyclovir, vidarabine, anti-HIV agents, verapamil, diltiazem, tacrolimus, tetrabenazine, cotrimoxazole	Tremor, Parkinsonism

PHARMACOLOGICAL AND NON-PHARMACOLOGICAL MANAGEMENT OF PARKINSON DISEASE (PD)

Currently, existing treatments and pharmacotherapies for PD are only effective for symptomatic management and have little, if any effect on disease progression. Restoration of dopaminergic activity in the striatum through various mechanisms [120] is the primary focus of pharmacological management of PD. These mechanisms include;

- Enhanced synthesis of DA in brain
- Decreased metabolism of DA, and
- Direct activation of DA receptors through use of DA agonists.

Additional mechanism involves use of anticholinergic agents to counteract the relative imbalance caused by DA loss and the resultant predominance of ACh actions. A summary of medication classes and their corresponding mechanisms is presented in Table **6** [99].

Combination of non-pharmacological strategies with appropriate pharmacological agents also provides patients with a level of symptomatic control necessary to maximize outcomes [121 - 124]. Numerous non-pharmacological management strategies utilized in the management of PD include physical and occupational therapy as well as some exercise programs. Also, patients who experience hypomimia of voice can work with speech-language pathologists to improve their voice articulation [125 - 129]. Deep brain stimulation (DBS) is a preferred neurological procedure for patients who continue to experience significant clinical features of PD like intractable motor fluctuations, tremor or dyskinesias [130 - 132].

Table 6. PD medication classes and corresponding mechanisms of action [99].

Medication Class	Mechanism of Action
Levodopa (LDOPA)/carbidopa Sinemet®, Sinemet CR®, Parcopa® ODT Lodosyn® - Carbidopa only Rytary® ER (carbidopa/levodopa) Duopa® (carbidopa/levodopa)[1] Inbrija® (levodopa)	Converted to DA in brain *via* decarboxylation primarily within presynaptic terminals of DA neurons in striatum

DA Agonists:
  - pramipexole (Mirapex®)
  - ropinirole (Requip®)
  - rotigotine (Neupro®)
  - apomorphine (Apokyn®)
Ergot-Class:
  - Bromocriptine
  - Cabergoline
  - Pergolide (Permax®)
	Direct agonists of striatal DA receptors

COMT Inhibitors:
  - entacapone (Comtan®)
  - tolcapone (Tasmar®)
	Inhibit COMT and block peripheral and central metabolism of levodopa

Selective MAO-B Inhibitors:
  - selegiline (Eldepryl®)
  - rasagiline (Azilect®)
  - Safinamide (Xadago®)
	Inhibit DA breakdown through selective irreversible inhibition of MAO-B in striatum. Also allow reduction of LDOPA dose

Anticholinergics:
  - benztropine
  - trihexyphenidyl
	Inhibit ACh interneuron function

Amantadine (Symmetrel®) Amantadine ER (Gocovri®) and Amantadine ER (Osmolex®)	Alters DA release in striatum, blocks DA reuptake into presynaptic neurons
Istradefylline (Nourianz®)	Selective adenosine A2A receptor antagonist

[1]4.63mg/20mg/1ml (100mg single-use cassettes) enteral suspension delivered *via* infusion pump into small intestine *via* Naso-jejunal tube for short-term use or percutaneous endoscopic tube gastrostomy (PEG-J) for long-term use.
[2]42 mg capsules, powder for inhalation. On demand use in patients on carbidopa/levodopa

Pharmacological Management of Parkinson Disease (PD)

Levodopa (LDOPA)

Since its introduction in the late 1960s, levodopa continues to be the mainstay therapeutic option for managing motor symptoms of PD [120, 133]. Even though it does not alter disease progression, it is highly effective for controlling motor symptoms of PD with mortality rate decreased by approximately 50%. It is available as Sinemet® (Immediate release), Sinemet® CR (Sustained release) and Parcopa® (Oral disintegrating tablet) forms.

However, the clinical response to chronic levodopa therapy (~5 years) deteriorates overtime due to its complex and variable pharmacokinetic and pharmacodynamic responses. As a result, motor complications observed include "wearing off" (loss of efficacy and rapid return of rigidity and akinesia at the end of dosing interval), "on/off phenomenon" (motor response fluctuations) and dyskinesias in 50-80% of patients on chronic therapy. As the disease progresses, the diminished ability of nigrostriatal system to synthesize, store and release endogenous dopamine as well as the inability of levodopa to restore normal striatal DA levels may be responsible for these motor complications [99, 133, 134].

Mechanism of Action

At physiologic pH, DA (NH_2 pka of 10.6) exists predominantly in its protonated form and does not cross blood-brain barrier (BBB). However, the less basic ₗ-DOPA (NH_2 pK_a of 8.72) exists predominantly in its polar form and is able to penetrate BBB [135 - 137].

Once in the brain, ₗ-DOPA is rapidly decarboxylated to DA by AADC (DOPA decarboxylase) (Fig. **4**) within presynaptic DA neurons in striatum. Consequently, ₗ-DOPA is referred to as DA pro-drug with therapeutic efficacy and associated adverse effects attributed to DA formed from ₗ-DOPA [99].

Pharmacokinetics [99, 134, 138, 139]

ₗ-DOPA is a large neutral/aromatic amino acid (LNAA) that undergoes rapid absorption from small intestine. This intestinal absorption, as well transport into the brain across the BBB is facilitated by an active transport system comprising large neutral/aromatic amino acid transporter. Factors that affect bioavailability of ₗ-DOPA (both rate and extent of absorption) include:

Rate of gastric emptying and pH of gastric juice: Delayed gastric emptying reduces levodopa absorption by slowing its movement into the proximal small intestine, site where majority of drug is absorbed. Also, food-induced delayed gastric emptying increases pre-systemic decarboxylation of ₗ-DOPA since DOPA decarboxylase is present in high concentration in gastric mucosa.[138] The net effect of both these processes is enhanced pre-systemic metabolism and consequent reduction of ₗ-DOPA's absorption and clinical response. Some medications like antacids promote gastric emptying by increasing the gastric pH as well.[136, 137]

Competition for absorption sites: Both ₗ-DOPA and dietary amino acids compete for LNAA transporter which results in marked reduction of $_L$DOPA absorption and reduced peak plasma concentrations. Therefore, it is recommended to avoid concurrent high protein diets with $_L$DOPA or reduce daily dietary protein intake to ~0.8 g/kg/body weight.[137] Similar competition exists for entry into brain between $_L$DOPA and dietary protein for LNAA transporter.[138]

Metabolism and Carbidopa

Majority of *exogenous*$_L$DOPA is rapidly decarboxylated to DA by AADC in the gut and other peripheral tissues (Fig. **4**). As a result of this extensive peripheral metabolism, only ~30% of administered dose reaches the systemic circulation with ~ <1% able to penetrate into the brain [99]. Therefore, clinically, $_L$DOPA is always administered with a peripheral decarboxylase inhibitor, carbidopa, to block this extensive peripheral metabolism (Fig. **6**). It should be noted that the *polar* carbidopa does not penetrate BBB effectively and therefore exhibits minimal inhibition of central decarboxylase. Overall, administration of $_L$DOPA in combination with carbidopa results in [141 - 143]: a) increased fraction of unmetabolized $_L$DOPA available to cross BBB, and b) reduced severity of dopamine induced nausea and cardiovascular effects (hypotension). $_L$DOPA is minimally bound to plasma proteins (20-30%) and exhibits a short elimination half-life (0.7 – 1.5 hours) [139, 140].

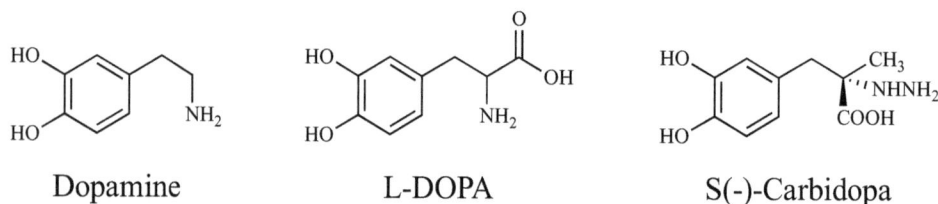

Dopamine   L-DOPA   S(-)-Carbidopa

Fig. (6). Carbidopa and $_L$DOPA.

Adverse Effects

Side effects commonly reported with levodopa/carbidopa include GI related nausea and vomiting (*due to stimulation of chemoreceptor trigger zone by DA formed from $_L$DOPA*), postural hypotension, sedation, vivid dreams, dizziness, dark urine/saliva/sweat, unusual sexual urges (hypersexuality), confusion and dyskinesias. The GI side effects are attributed to GI irritation as well as stimulation of chemo receptor trigger zone *via* D2 receptors. However, combining $_L$DOPA with carbidopa greatly decreases the incidence of GI related adverse effects caused by formation of excess DA from $_L$DOPA. Overall, occurrence of these side effects, especially the psychiatric disturbances are quite problematic in the elderly who constitute majority of PD patients. Additionally, the risk of falls in a PD patient, attributed to the motor features of the disease, is further complicated by levodopa induced *orthostatic hypotension*. This orthostatic hypotension observed with use of $_L$DOPA and other dopaminergic agents is typically explained by: a) presynaptic inhibition of norepinephrine release *via* D2 receptors [144] and b) activation of vascular D1 receptors by DA formed from peripheral decarboxylation of $_L$DOPA [92].

Drug withdrawal or abrupt discontinuation of levodopa precipitates a *neuroleptic malignant* like syndrome characterized by delirium, muscle rigidity, fever, and autonomic instability. Other adverse events that occur in majority of patients taking levodopa, usually within 3-5 years of treatment include onset of dyskinesias (chloreiform involuntary movements) and dystonias (abnormal muscle contractions). These complications which may be related to disease progression are contributed by $_L$DOPA [145, 146].

Motor Complications of $_L$DOPA

The initial clinical response to *exogenous*$_L$DOPA is highly effective which in part is complimented by the availability of endogenous central dopamine. However, as the disease progresses, the clinical response fades with the patient experiencing significant motor fluctuations with the use of long-term $_L$DOPA therapy [99]. The reduced or lack of clinical response typically presents as re-emergent clinical features of PD with the condition referred to as motor complications of $_L$DOPA therapy. These complications include:

- Loss of efficacy and rapid return of rigidity and akinesia at the end of dosing interval ("wearing off")
- Motor response fluctuations ("on/off phenomenon")
- Dyskinesias
- Dystonias

There is not a specific time frame for this reduction in clinical response, which varies from patient to patient, and may occur as early as 9 months or as late as 6 years with the prevalence of motor fluctuations as high as 60-90% in patients after 5-10 years of treatment [147 - 149].

As the disease progresses, development of motor fluctuations and dyskinesias occur due to progressive loss of presynaptic dopamine neurons and exposure of postsynaptic dopamine receptors to fluctuating concentrations of DA and pulsatile stimulation of DA receptors secondary to administration of multiple doses of short-acting $_L$DOPA. Desensitization of receptors due to chronic use of $_L$DOPA combined with loss of endogenous dopamine precipitates the reduction in clinical responses and subsequent motor complications. Additional factors that may contribute include changes in gastric motility, altered absorption and short half-life (0.7 – 1.5 hours) of $_L$DOPA, changes in intracellular signaling and firing patterns which cause further dysregulation of basal ganglia circuits [149 - 151].

"Wearing Off"

This is the most common $_L$DOPA induced motor complication, seen at the end of dosing interval. Quite often not reported due to their atypical and or subtle presentation, "wearing off" symptoms also include certain non-motor features like depression, restlessness, anxiety and fatigue [152 - 154].

"On/Off Phenomenon"

During later stages of PD, patients exhibit rapid fluctuation between an "off" period, which involves loss of therapeutic benefit from the medication, and "on" period which involves medication derived motor control [99].

Another complication that occurs during the later stages of PD (disease duration of five years or longer) is "freezing of gait" (FOG) which occurs in up to 60% of PD patients, and is more commonly seen in males and patients with akinetic-rigid PD type. It generally occurs during the "off" phase of "wearing off" complication but can also occur paradoxically during the "on" state. Triggers for FOG include anxiety and walking obstacles and occurs when patients are trying to turn, initiate a step, passing through a narrow passage, crossing a busy road prior to reaching a destination, duel tasking or when confronted with spatial restriction. The pathophysiology is unclear with imaging studies suggesting a dysfunction in parietal-lateral premotor circuits or loss of norepinephrine associated with locus ceruleus degeneration [155 - 157].

Dyskinesias

Hyperkinetic movements, dyskinesias, occur in patients as early as 2-4 years after initiation of therapy. They occur to varying degrees in approximately 40%-80% of patients treated with $_L$DOPA for 4-6 years [158]. Dyskinesias are abnormal involuntary movements involving the extremities, trunk and neck and include peak dose ("on" period) type and diphasic type. The peak dose dyskinesias are associated with high plasma levels of $_L$DOPA and present with choreic features involving the upper extremities, trunk and neck. Diphasic dyskinesias appear at the onset and offset of $_L$DOPA effect, and coincide with rising and falling $_L$DOPA levels. Retrospective evaluation of PD patient medical records reported that age at the time of PD onset was a predictor for development of dyskinesias, risk of dyskinesias being 70% in patients diagnosed at ages 40 – 49 and only 24%

in patients 70-79 years of age [159]. Other risk factors for developing dyskinesias include genetic factors, severity of PD and female sex, along with dose and duration of $_L$DOPA therapy [160, 161].

Dystonias

Occur in patients using dopaminergic agents within the same time frame as dyskinesias. Dystonias are alternative forms of "off" state characterized by involuntary sustained muscle contractions with twisting or squeezing movements. Additionally, patients develop abnormal posture which presents as fixed and painful positions, and occurs more commonly in the feet. Dystonias commonly occur in the morning as a result of end of dose "wearing off" or may also occur during the "on-state" associated with higher levels of levodopa [162, 163].

Drug Interactions [164]

Numerous drug interactions are reported with use of levodopa/carbidopa with monitoring and dose adjustments recommended.

- Concomitant use of antihypertensives potentiates postural hypotension observed with use of $_L$DOPA.
- Concomitant use of dopamine antagonists (antiemetics, metoclopramide, and antipsychotics) will result in loss of $_L$DOPA efficacy. An exception involves use of quetiapine in PD patients [117].
- Even though MAO inhibitors can be used concurrently with $_L$DOPA, caution should be exercised. However, use of non-selective MAO inhibitors (some antidepressants, phenelzine, tranylcypromine and linezolid is contraindicated.
- Tricylic antidepressants should be used with caution due to reports of hypertension and dyskinesias.
- Use of $_L$DOPA with general anesthetics like halothane results in cardiac arrhythmias and should be avoided [165, 166].
- Potential for decreased absorption of $_L$DOPA when given with iron salts exists even though the clinical relevance is unclear [164].

Contraindications and Precautions

Contraindications include documented hypersensitivity, uncompensated cardiovascular disease and narrow-angle glaucoma. Hepatic and renal impairment, severe pulmonary disease, hematologic, endocrine disease and patients with a history of melanoma are conditions which require careful use of $_L$DOPA. Particularly, risk of melanoma is attributed to the ability of dopaminergic agents to activate melanoma. It is therefore recommended to avoid use of dopaminergic agents in patients with undiagnosed skin lesions or a medical history of melanoma [164, 167].

Dopamine Receptor Agonists

Dopamine agonists through a direct action on postsynaptic dopamine receptors provide alternative pharmacotherapy option for the management of motor symptoms of PD. They are typically used as first-line agents in younger patients (<65) with mild to moderate motor features, or as adjunctive agents in more advanced disease [121, 122, 168, 169]. Despite being inferior to $_L$DOPA/carbidopa in terms of efficacy, they offer some distinct clinical advantages that are listed below.

• DA agonists do not require enzymatic conversion for activity and therefore do not rely on DA related synthesis, storage and release functional capabilities of the striatal neurons
• Lack competitive protein interactions with circulating amino acids
• Exhibit relatively longer duration of action than $_L$DOPA
• Associated with reduced incidence of motor complications like dyskinesias

The dopamine agonists are broadly classified into *ergot type* and *non-ergot type* which differ in their receptor affinities, which translates into considerable safety and tolerability issues.

Ergot Class

The ergot class which includes bromocriptine and cabergoline (Fig. **7**) are rarely used for PD, although may be used in hyperprolactinemia, acromegaly or neuroleptic malignant syndrome. These are non-selective agents that interact with both the inhibitory D_2 and excitatory D_1 receptors, as well as serotonin and adrenergic receptors [170]. Specifically, bromocriptine acts as a D_2/D_3 receptor partial agonist with minimal affinity for D_1 type/D_4 receptors whereas cabergoline acts as a D_2 full agonist and D_3/D_4 partial agonist with minimal affinity for D_1 type receptors [171, 172].

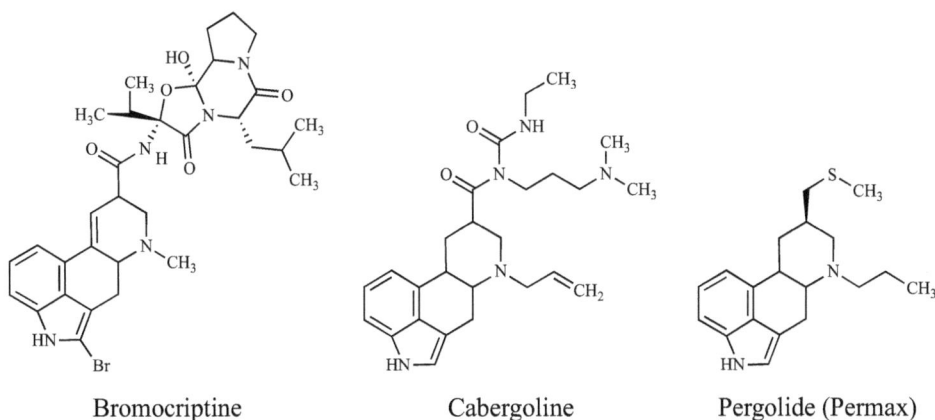

Fig. (7). Ergot dopamine agonists.

Primary safety concerns related to the ergot class include fibrotic changes like thickening, retraction and stiffening of heart valves, due to their strong affinity for and ability to activate 5-HT$_{2B}$ serotonin receptors expressed in the heart valves [173 - 176]. Pergolide (Permax®), a nonpeptide ergot derivative was withdrawn in 2007 due to its association with valvular heart disease [99]. However, the brand Prascend® is currently approved for control of clinical signs associated with Equine Cushing's Disease in horses. Moderate cardiac tricuspid valve regurgitation was more frequently observed with the use of high doses of cabergoline, although the risk is lower if used at low doses for treatment of hyperprolactinemia [177, 178]. Overall, patients taking ergot class of agents must be regularly monitored for signs and symptoms of cardiac problems.

Non-Ergot Class

The non-ergot derivatives (Fig. **8**) include ropinirole (Requip®, Requip® XL) and pramipexole (Mirapex®, Mirapex® ER), and rotigotine transdermal patch (Neupro®) along with apomorphine (Apokyn®).

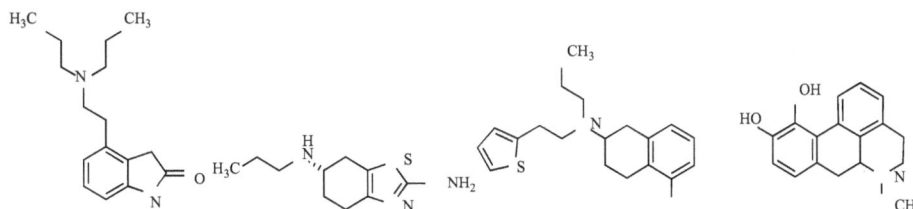

Fig. (8). Non-ergot dopamine agonists.

Mechanism of Action

These are direct DA receptor agonists that exhibit relatively higher receptor selectivity than the ergot class of agents. They exhibit selectivity for D_2 type receptors (D_2 and D_3) with minimal to no affinity for D_1 type receptors [99]. Activation of these receptors in the caudate-putamen region compensates for hypodopaminergic actions and is responsible for their clinical efficacy, improved safety and tolerability profile. *In vitro*, ropinirole was found to exhibit moderate affinity for opioid receptors and minimal affinity for D_1, $5\text{-}HT_1$, $5\text{-}HT_2$, benzodiazepine, GABA, muscarinic, alpha1-, alpha2-, and beta-adrenoreceptors [179]. Rotigotine, available as a transdermal patch, acts as D_1, D_2 and D_3 receptor agonist [180].

In addition to the clinical advantages offered by dopamine agonists, as described above, the non-ergot direct DA agonists exhibit:

- Low affinity for $5HT_{2B}$ and therefore the risk of fibrotic complications is less, although contribution cannot be completely ruled out with the use of ropinirole [179].
- Good oral absorption from GI tract and penetration across the blood-brai--barrier
- Relatively longer half-life relative than $_L$-DOPA (8-24 hours Vs 6-8 hours $_L$-DOPA) [99]
- Lack of potential for formation of neurotoxic reactive oxidation products from DA degradation relative to $_L$-DOPA [99]

A summary of FDA approved indications, pharmacokinetic profile and adverse effects related to the use of these agents is presented in Table **7** [121, 122, 168, 181 - 185]. In general, these DA agonists are dosed utilizing various regimens, initiated at low doses and are titrated slowly in order to minimize side effects and maximize clinical response [122, 168, 186]. Especially, the extended release formulations offer convenience, improved compliance and may avoid pulsatile receptor stimulation associated with dyskinesias [187, 188].

Rotigotine Transdermal Patch (Neupro®)

The patch was designed to release active drug *via* intact skin over 24 hours, and serves as an alternative option in patients with dysphagia, history of poor compliance or situations where oral therapy is restricted [189]. It is a highly lipophilic agent with an absolute bioavailability of ~37%. When applied to the trunk, the drug is detected in ~3 hours in plasma, with maximum levels reached at 15-27 hours, although peak concentration is not observed. Daily application results in predictable release and absorption of rotigotine, with steady-state concentrations reached within 1-2 days. It exhibits a large volume of distribution (84 L/kg), consistent with its wide tissue distribution along with 92% plasma protein binding. It undergoes extensive metabolism *via* conjugation and N-dealkylation catalyzed by numerous CYP isozymes and other systems involved with the metabolites primarily eliminated in urine. Its elimination half-life is reported to be in the 3-7 hours range [190, 191].

Table 7. Dopamine agonists: Indications, pharmacokinetics and adverse effects.

Dopamine Agonist	Pharmacokinetics	Adverse Effects/Comments
ropinirole (Requip®, Requip® XL) FDA Indication(s): Parkinson Disease and Restless Leg Syndrome	$\underline{A}$: IR 45-55% bioavailability $\underline{D}$:Vd 7.5L/Kg; 40% protein binding $\underline{M}$: CYP1A2 (major); inactive metabolites $\underline{E}$: Renal (<10% unchanged; $t_{1/2}$ ~6hrs	Sudden sleep attacks, somnolence, Orthostatic hypotension, nausea, dizziness, constipation, hallucinations, impulse control disorders, peripheral edema, dyskinesias - Monitor blood pressure, weight, day time alertness, heart rate - Take with food to reduce nausea
pramipexole (Mirapex®, Mirapex® ER) FDA Indication(s): Parkinson Disease and Restless Leg Syndrome	$\underline{A}$: >90% bioavailability $\underline{D}$: Vd 500 L; 15% protein binding $\underline{M}$: Minimal (<10%) $\underline{E}$: Renal 90% unchanged; $t_{1/2}$ 8hrs	Sudden sleep attacks, somnolence, Orthostatic hypotension, nausea, dizziness, constipation, hallucinations, impulse control disorders, peripheral edema, dyskinesias, vivid dreams - ↓ dose if CrCl < 60 mL/min - Monitor blood pressure, weight, day time alertness, heart rate - IR take with food to reduce gastric irritation
rotigotine transdermal patch (Neupro®) FDA Indication(s): Parkinson Disease and Restless Leg Syndrome	$\underline{A}$: transdermal $\underline{D}$: Vd 84L/kg; 89.5% protein binding $\underline{M}$: CYPs, UGT, sulfotransferases; inactive metabolites $\underline{E}$: renal; $t_{1/2}$ 3hrs initial	Sudden sleep attacks, somnolence, Orthostatic hypotension, peripheral edema, nausea, headache, application site reactions, hyperhidrosis, dizziness, constipation, dyskinesias, hallucinations, impulse control disorders, peripheral edema, vivid dreams - Apply to clean, dry, intact skin - Apply to new site each time - Do not apply heat over patch - Remove prior to MRI - Avoid if allergic to sulfites
apomorphine (Apokyn®) FDA Indication(s): acute, intermittent treatment of hypomobility ("off" episodes)	$\underline{A}$: SC $\underline{D}$: Vd 218L/kg $\underline{M}$: unknown $\underline{E}$: ~40mins	*Severe nausea,vomiting, hypotension,* peripheral edema, QT prolongation, somnolence, dizziness, dyskinesias, *yawning,* hallucinations, injection site reactions, nasal discharge - Avoid with 5HT3 antagonists - Pre-treat with trimethobenzamide - Monitor blood pressure

IR – immediate release; Vd – volume of distribution; SC – subcutaneous; $\underline{A}$ – absorption; $\underline{D}$ – distribution; $\underline{M}$ – metabolism; $\underline{E}$ - elimination

Apomorphine (Apokyn®)

Apomorphine, available as a subcutaneous (SQ) formulation is approved for acute, intermittent treatment of "off" episodes ("end-of-dose wearing off" and unpredictable "on/off" episodes associated with advanced PD. It exhibits high affinity for D_4 receptors, moderate affinity for $D_2/D_3/D_5$ and $\alpha_{1D}/\alpha_{2B}/\alpha_{2C}$ and low affinity for D_1 receptors [99].

The clinical benefits observed with apomorphine are limited by its short duration of action (mean terminal elimination half-life ~ 40 minutes), non-availability of oral formulations, extensive first pass metabolism, tolerance and side effect profile [192, 193].

When used for acute management of PD, pre- and post-treatment with an antiemetic (trimethobenzamide) is required to counter severe nausea observed with apomorphine use. Also, $5\text{-}HT_3$ receptor antagonists must be avoided due to risk of profound hypotension and loss of consciousness [194].

Adverse Effects

As discussed above, use of ergot class of agents is associated with serious fibrotic complications. Cases of retroperitoneal fibrosis, Raynaud's phenomena, pulmonary infiltrates, pleural thickening and effusions, cardiac valvulopathy, pericarditis, myocardial infarction, arrhythmias and hypertension have also been reported. Also, despite fibrotic complications associated with the ergot structure, monitoring is still recommended with the use of non-ergot DA agonists, especially ropinirole.

Side effects commonly seen with DA agonists include somnolence, sleep attacks, dizziness, vivid dreams, nausea and constipation, edema (ankles), chest pain, sweating, flushing, pallor, dyskinesia, rhinorrhea, and orthostatic hypotension. Of these, orthostatic hypotension, somnolence and nausea are particularly concerning in the elderly and due to their association with falls and fractures. The sudden irresistible sleep attacks are primarily associated with the use of ropinirole, pramipexole and rotigotine [184, 195].

Psychiatric side effects observed with dopamine agonists include confusion, cognitive changes, hallucinations, delusions and impulse control disorders. Management of severe delusions and hallucinations may require the use of atypical antipsychotic agents with clozapine and quetiapine being the most effective and well tolerated atypical antipsychotics [184, 185, 196]. Pimavanserin (Nuplazid®), an atypical antipsychotic was recently approved for the treatment of hallucinations and delusions associated with Parkinson's disease.

Impulse control disorders (ICDs) are unique psychiatric side effects more commonly observed with use of non-ergot DA agonists relative to $_L$-DOPA/carbidopa. These ICDs or compulsive behaviors associated with use of dopamine agonists include; hypersexuality, binge eating, excessive gambling or shopping, and pathological collecting. Proposed mechanism involves alteration or dysregulation of dopaminergic function in the striatum and other areas. Risk factors identified include dose, marital status, and patients <65 years of age with lower doses recommended in high risk patients [197, 200].

Rotigotine transdermal patch exhibits a systemic adverse reaction profile similar to oral agents with the most common treatment related adverse effects involving application-site reactions, somnolence, headache and gastrointestinal disturbances. The application-site reactions are attributed to sodium metabisulfite and its use should be avoided in patients with sulfite allergy. Additionally, the patch contains aluminum and when exposed to magnetic imaging or cardioversion procedures can cause skin burns [187, 188, 190, 191].

Drug Interactions

The dopamine agonists are associated with numerous drug interactions and should be used with caution with sympathomimetic decongestants and drugs with serotonergic properties (Table **8**) [222, 223]. Additionally, concomitant use of dopamine antagonists phenothiazines, butyrophenones, metoclopramide, and other agents like pimozide, amitriptyline, imipramine, methyldopa, reserpine and erythromycin decrease efficacy of these agents. Ropinirole undergoes metabolism *via* CYP1A2 and therefore concurrent use of CYP1A2 inhibitors like ciprofloxacin increases ropinirole levels [179].

An important drug interaction involves use of $5HT_3$ antagonists (ondansetron, dolasetron, granisetron, palonosetron and alosetron) to treat severe nausea associated with use of apomorphine. Due to the risk of severe hypotension, concurrent use of these $5HT_3$ receptor antagonists is contraindicated and pre-treatment with trimethobenzaminde is recommended. Also, the risk of arrhythmias is high when apomorphine is used along with drugs (thioridazine, quinidine, sotalol, erythromycin, and dofetilide) that prolong QT interval [194]. Additionally, use of entacapone may decrease elimination of apomorphine since it is metabolized by COMT [201].

Table 8. Dopamine agonists: drug interactions with serotonergic agents [222, 223].

Drug	Comments
MAO inhibitors: phenelzine/ isocarboxazid/ tranylcypromine	Contraindicated

(Table 8) cont.....

Drug	Comments
Antidepressants: TCAs, SNRIs, SSRIs	Use with caution
trazodone and nefazodone	Use with caution/monitor
St. John's Wort	Contraindicated
Buspirone	Use with caution/monitor
Meperidine, dextromethorphan, tramadol, methadone	Contraindicated
Cyclobenzaprine	Contraindicated

MAO: monoamine oxidase; SNRIs: Serotonin–norepinephrine reuptake inhibitor; SSRIs: Selective serotonin reuptake inhibitors

Contraindications and Precautions

Contraindications to dopamine agonists include use in patients with a history of hypersensitivity or true sulfite allergy. While the ergot derivatives are contraindicated in patients with cardiovascular disease, the non-ergots must be used with caution. Epidemiological studies have report that patients with PD have a 6-fold greater risk of developing melanoma, even though the etiology is unclear. It is generally recommended that patients and clinicians monitor for signs of melanoma on a regular basis with periodic evaluations conducted by dermatologists.

Common to all dopaminergic agents, abrupt withdrawal or rapid reduction in dose may precipitate neuroleptic malignant syndrome (NMS) which results in emergent hyperpyrexia, confusion, muscular rigidity and rhabdomylosis, along with akinetic crises [179, 194].

Precautions recommended with the use of dopamine agonists include complications related to their side effect profiles. Postural hypotension requires periodic monitoring while patients who drive while taking this class of medications must exercise caution. Patient should be monitored for gastrointestinal bleeding and ulceration. Recent studies have reported potential risk of heart failure with the use of pramipexole with FDA issuing a drug safety communication in September 2012 [202, 203].

Catechol-O-methyltransferase (COMT) Inhibitors

COMT metabolizes ₗDOPA both in the periphery and in the central nervous system to an inactive 3-methoxy-4-hydroxy-L-phenylalanine (3-OMD) as illustrated in Fig. **(5)**. As discussed earlier, since orally administered ₗDOPA is rapidly metabolized to DA by AADC in the periphery, carbidopa (a peripheral AADC inhibitor) is usually given in combination with ₗDOPA. However, even though use of ₗDOPA/carbidopa combination results in decreased peripheral conversion of $_L$DOPA to DA, consequently, the COMT pathway now becomes the major $_L$DOPA inactivating pathway and leads to increased formation of inactive 3-OMD. This led to research focused on use of COMT inhibitors in PD and the resultant marketing of entacapone (Comtan®) and tolcapone (Tasmar®) shown in Fig. **(9)** [99].

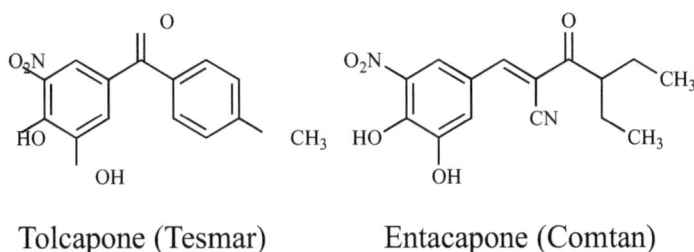

Tolcapone (Tesmar)   Entacapone (Comtan)

Fig. (9). Tolcapone and entacapone.

Mechanism of Action

The selective, reversible COMT inhibitors, by inhibiting inactivation of $_L$DOPA (both in the periphery and CNS) potentiate actions of $_L$DOPA. It should be noted that these agents are only indicated for adjunct use in combination with $_L$DOPA/carbidopa to treat PD patients experiencing signs and symptoms of end-of-dose "wearing off", and have no role as monotherapy [122, 14, 150, 204]. Corresponding clinical advantages include:

- Increased plasma half-life of $_L$DOPA,
- Increased fraction of $_L$DOPA dose that reaches the CNS and
- Increased amount of $_L$DOPA available for conversion to DA in CNS

Even though the clinical advantages observed by co-administering COMT inhibitor with $_L$DOPA/carbidopa are significant, it is important to reduce $_L$DOPA doses by 10-30% to avoid additive DA related adverse effects. Additional concern involves increase in severity and duration of dyskinesias. Tolcapone and entacapone are similar in terms of effectiveness but exhibit distinct pharmacokinetic and adverse effect profile, as discussed below.

Tolcapone (Tasmar®)

Tolcapone (Tasmar®) is a selective, central and peripheral, reversible COMT inhibitor with a longer duration of action (8-12 hours) and a reported elimination half-life of ~3 hours. It is primarily metabolized in the liver *via* glucuronidation and CYP2A6 and CYP3A4 enzymes with the metabolites eliminated in urine (60%) and feces (40%) [205].

Tolcapone has a limited role in management of PD due to its association with fatal hepatotoxicity (boxed warning included in drug label), and is contraindicated in patients with a history of hepatic disease. When used, appropriate monitoring of liver function and enzymes is recommended, especially during the first 6-8 months of therapy. Delayed onset (~6-12 weeks post initiation) of severe diarrhea and severe potentiation of $_L$DOPA/carbidopa effects also preclude its use and is considered as a last line treatment option [204].

Entacapone(Comtan®)

Entacapone is the COMT inhibitor primarily used in clinical practice and is marketed either alone as Comtan® or in combination with $_L$DOPA/carbidopa as Stalevo®. It is a selective, reversible COMT inhibitor and is primarily a peripheral inhibitor of COMT. It exhibits a short duration of action (2 hours) relative to tolcapone and is metabolized *via* isomerization to an active *cis*-isomer which undergoes glucuronidation, both the *cis*-isomer and the parent compound, to inactive conjugates. Majority (90%) of the drug is eliminated in feces.

Side effects associated with entacapone are primarily related to its potentiation of $_L$DOPA effects and can be reduced by making dose adjustments. Patient education with entacapone should include the potential for urine discoloration (to brownish orange) and occurrence of delayed onset diarrhea [204, 206 - 209].

Selective MAO-B Inhibitors

Both the isoforms of monoamine oxidase, type A and B are involved in the catabolism of DA and other monoamines *via* oxidative deamination. However, since MAO-B is the predominant isoform in the brain, it is the target for two selective MAO-B inhibitors approved for PD; selegiline (Eldepryl® and Zelapar® ODT with Emsam® Patch approved for treatment of major depressive disorder only) and rasagiline (Azilect®) [99].

Mechanism of Action

These agents inhibit MAO-B in a selective and irreversible manner with the propargylamine moiety required for irreversible inhibition. However, this selectivity is lost when doses greater than the recommended therapeutic doses are used [210].

Clinical advantages derived from selective inhibition of brain MAO-B include:

- Enhanced DA availability within the striatum and a resultant prolongation of dopaminergic activity
- Minimal inhibition of peripheral DA (and other monoamine) and consequently improved safety profile
- Clinical utility both as monotherapy and as adjuncts to $_L$-DOPA/carbidopa in advanced PD
- Lack of "cheese reaction" commonly seen with the use of non-selective MAO inhibitors
- Potential neuroprotective effect due to decreased formation of neurotoxic free radicals as a consequence of DA catabolism by MAO-B (Fig. **2**)

Selegiline (Eldepryl® and Zelapar® ODT)

Selegiline, earlier used as an effective monotherapy option for PD is currently relegated to adjunct use due to its association with CNS stimulant adverse effects like anxiety, insomnia, and agitation. These adverse effects are attributed to amphetamine and methamphetamine metabolites formed from selegiline *via* N-dealkylation, by the actions of CYP2B6 and CYP2C19 (Fig. **10**). The newer formulations, ODT and the transdermal patch, offer clinical advantages like improved bioavailability and minimal first-pass metabolism resulting in decreased formation of amphetamine metabolites [99].

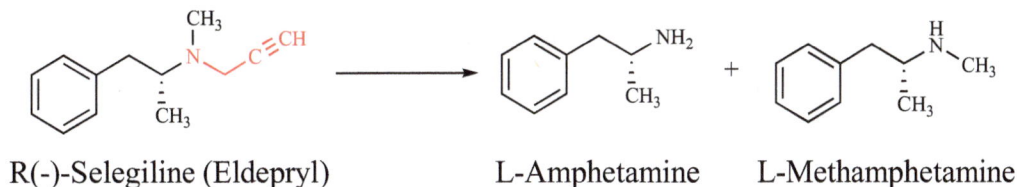

R(-)-Selegiline (Eldepryl)   L-Amphetamine   L-Methamphetamine

Fig. (10). Selegiline metabolism.

Rasagiline (Azilect®)

Rasagiline, also a selective irreversible MAO-B inhibitor is devoid of CNS adverse effects observed with use of selegiline. It primarily undergoes N-dealkylation *via* CYP1A2 to an inactive 1-aminoindan metabolite (Fig. **11**) [211].

Adverse Effects

Gastrointestinal side effects observed with use of MAO-B inhibitors include nausea, abdominal pain, anorexia, dyspepsia, dry mouth, stomatitis, dyspepsia, buccal mucosa irritation (with the ODT formulation), constipation and weight loss. CNS effects include confusion, hallucinations, compulsive behaviors, dizziness, fainting, abnormal dreams, depression, malaise, headache, paresthesia, insomnia and nervousness (typically seen with selegiline due to amphetamine metabolites). Extrapyramidal reactions reported include dyskinesias (seen with concurrent levodopa), ataxia and dystonia. Other side effects reported with these agents include orthostatic hypotension, rhinitis, conjunctivitis, rash, ecchymosis, melanoma, back pain, flu like syndrome, fever, arthralgia, arthritis, neck and back pain, dyspnea and sweating [212, 213].

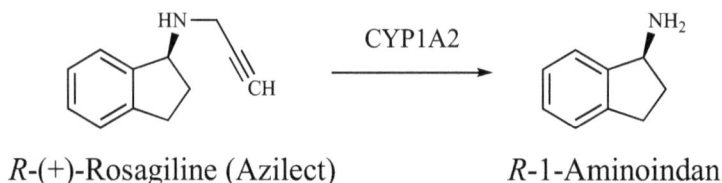

R-(+)-Rosagiline (Azilect)   *R*-1-Aminoindan

Fig. (11). Rasagiline metabolism.

"Cheese reaction", commonly associated with the use of non-selective MAO-A inhibitors (phenelzine, isocarboxazid, and tranylcypromine) are rarely seen with selective MAO-B inhibitors when used at recommended doses. However, the potential exists at high doses due to loss of MAO selectivity with several cases reported with use of selegiline. Rasagiline label highlights that consumption of tyramine at >150mg/day may increase the risk. Appropriate monitoring is therefore recommended for both these agents due to the potential for this interaction [213 - 215].

Drug Interactions and Contraindications

Owing to their mechanism of action, MAO-B inhibitors increase serotonin levels and consequently the risk of serotonin syndrome is high when used at high doses or if co-administered with other serotoninergic agents. Symptoms of serotonin syndrome include hyperpyrexia, myoclonus, hyperreflexia, diaphoresis, tremor, shivering, rigidity, agitation and hallucinations, and can be fatal if left untreated. Therefore, use of meperidine is contraindicated with both selegiline and rasagiline. Additionally, use of tramadol, methadone, and propoxyphene dextromethorphan, St. John's wort, and cyclobenzaprine is also contraindicated [213, 216]. Use of rasagiline is also contraindicated in patients with moderate to severe hepatic disease (Child-Pugh score > 6) [212].

Concurrent use of CYP1A2 inhibitor ciprofloxacin results in increased serum levels of rasagiline. Since selegiline and rasagiline can exacerbate levodopa side effects, appropriate levodopa dose adjustments are necessary when MAO-B inhibitors are added to therapy [216].

Safinamide (Xadago®)

Safinamide, approved in 2017, is the latest addition to the class of MAO inhibitors. In contrast to selegiline and rasagiline, it is a potent, selective, *reversible* inhibitor of MAO-B indicated as an adjunct to L-DOPA/carbidopa. Additionally, safinamide blocks Na^+ and Ca^{+2} channels, glutamate release and reuptake of dopamine. Safinamide exhibits good oral absorption (95%) with a terminal half-life of 20-26 hours. It is primarily metabolized by amidases and MAO-A with CYP3A4 playing a minor role. None of the metabolites of safinamide exhibit pharmacological activity. It is predominantly excreted in urine. Its use is contraindicated with other MAO inhibitors, opioids and serotonergic agents including dextromethorphan. Common side effects reported with use of safinamide include dyskinesia, fall, nausea, and insomnia [229].

Anticholinergic Agents

As discussed earlier in the pathophysiology section of the chapter, loss of dopaminergic function in striatum results in enhanced ACh activity, unopposed inhibition of the *direct pathway* and a predominance of *indirect pathway* mediated diminished motor activity. Based on this observation, anticholinergic agents have found a place in the management of PD motor symptoms [100]. Benztropine (Cogentin®) and trihexyphenidyl are the two agents primarily used in PD (Fig. **12**).

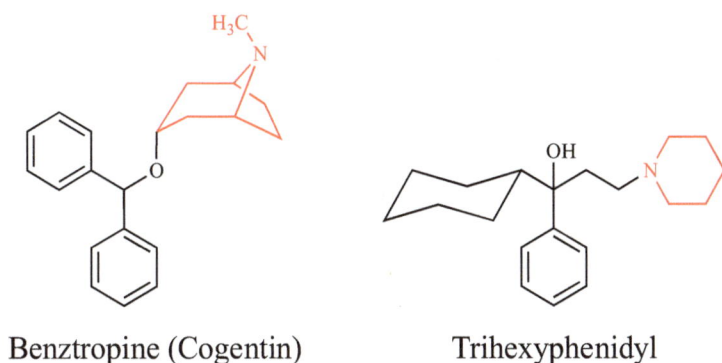

Benztropine (Cogentin)   Trihexyphenidyl

Fig. (12). Benztropine (Cogentin®) and trihexyphenidyl.

Currently, their clinical utility is restricted to management of mild tremors in younger patients (in their 60s) with no demonstrated benefit observed for the management of rigidity, bradykinesia and postural imbalance. More importantly, their severe adverse effect (Table **9**) profile stands out as their major clinical drawback [2, 100].

Table 9. Adverse Effect Profile of Anticholinergic Agents.

CNS Adverse Effects	Peripheral Adverse Effects
Sedation	Urinary retention
Blurred Vision	Constipation
Delirium	Dry mouth
Hallucinations	Postural hypotension
Confusion	Palpitations/tachycardia
Memory loss	

Amantadine

Amantadine (Symmetrel®), an antiviral agent, was identified to possess antiparkinsonism activity due to its ability to affect synaptic dopamine levels [217 - 219]. Currently, amantadine plays a minor role in the management of motor features of early PD, but is most beneficial when used for the management of dyskinesias secondary to dopaminergic therapy in advanced PD [219, 220].

Mechanism of Action

The probable mechanisms by which amantadine exhibits antiparkinsonism effects include:

- altered dopamine release from central neurons
- delayed reuptake of dopamine by neural cells
- anticholinergic effects, and
- blockade of N-methyl-d-aspartate (NMDA) receptors and excitatory neurotransmission which led to its role in the management of dyskinesias [221]

Similar to anticholinergics, the role of amantadine in PD is limited due to its side effect profile, especially in the elderly patients, that includes hallucinations, confusion, edema, and urinary retention. Especially, a reddish mottling of the skin referred to as livedo reticularis that affects upper or lower extremities is a unique adverse effect associated with amantadine. Additionally, since it primarily undergoes renal elimination, significant dose adjustments in elderly patients with renal impairment is recommended. Gocovri is an extended release formulation of amantadine approved for the treatment of dyskinesia in patients with Parkinson's disease receiving levodopa-based therapy. Osmolex is another extended release formulation approved the treatment of PD and drug-induced extrapyramidal reactions in adult patients.

Adenosine Receptor Antagonist

Istradefylline (Nourianz®) is a first in-class adenosine receptor antagonist indicated as adjunctive treatment to levodopa/carbidopa in adult patients with PD experiencing "off" episodes. It is a xanthine derivative that acts as an antagonist of the adenosine A2A receptor. It is primarily metabolized by primarily metabolized *via* CYP1A1 and CYP3A4 with a terminal half-life of ~83 hours. Common side effects observed with use of istradefyliine include dyskinesia, dizziness, constipation, nausea, hallucination, and insomnia [230].

CASE STUDIES

Case 1

GM is a 58 year-old male who sees his neurologist and complaints of unsteadiness in his right hand. His past medical history is significant for depression and constipation. On exam, it is noted that he lacks normal changes in facial expression, speaks in a monotone voice and has a strong body odor. Further examination reveals "ratchet like" rigidity in both arms, and a mild rest tremor of his right hand. His gait is notably slow, and his posture is slightly bent. GM also reports that he has noticed some loss in sense of smell which has affected his appetite. The remainder of his exam is within normal limits.

1. What are the motor and non-motor symptoms of PD seen in this patient?
2. Considering the age of this patient, discuss whether a dopamine agonist or $_L$-DOPA/carbidopa would be most appropriate to initiate in GM.
3. Based on the therapeutic option you recommend; how would you initiate therapy and monitor?

Case 2

LM is a 64 year old male who responded well to pramipexole titrated to 1mg tid over the last 18 months. He has experienced notable improvements in his ability to carry out activities of daily living. However, over the last few months he has noticed a gradual worsening of his symptoms and currently complains of feeling more "tied up", has difficulty getting out of a chair while his posture is more stooped.

1. What is the most appropriate therapeutic addition to LM's therapy at this time?
2. **Discuss the chemical basis of using *exogenous*$_L$-DOPA versus use of dopamine directly** (Fig. 6)
3. **What are the chemical and pharmacological reasons for co-administration**

of carbidopa with ₗ-DOPA (Fig. **6**)?

4. If LM develops further motor complications (*e.g.*, wearing off, freezing of gait), what are the options available to potentiate ₗ-DOPA actions?

5. What is the pharmacological basis for administration of COMT inhibitors with ₗ-DOPA?

6. **Explain the chemical basis for selecting rasagiline over selegiline as adjunct to ₗ-DOPA in this patient** (Figs. **9** and **10**)

7. What additional complication can arise from chronic use of ₗ-DOPA/carbidopa in advanced PD? How would you manage this complication?

DRUG DISCOVERY CASE STORY

Discovery of Pramipexole

The natural alkaloids (ergot alkaloids and their synthetic derivatives, such as pergolide and CQ 32-084) and apomorphine due to their dopamine agonist activities are used in the treatment of a wide variety of disease states including PD. Therefore, synthesis of new derivatives related to these alkaloids was pursued by scientists in the 1980s. It was hypothesized that the dopaminomimetic pharmacophore lies in a simplified ergoline structure or a rigid arylethylamine moiety, which lead to the synthesis of a variety of structures as shown in Fig. (**13**) [224 - 226]. Nordmann and Petcher [225] simplified apomorphine's catechol moiety by incorporating a monohydroxy aromatic group to protect against metabolism by catecholamine o-methyl transferase (COMT) and synthesized quinagolide and CV 205-503 as analogues of CQ 32-084 and pergolide, respectively. Preliminary pharmacological evaluation showed that these two compounds retained specific and potent dopamine agonist property with longer duration of action and good oral bioavailability. Detailed stereochemical and structural studies with these compounds and the ergolines revealed that the rigid pyrrolethylamine moiety in ergolines represents the dopaminomimetic pharmacophore [225].

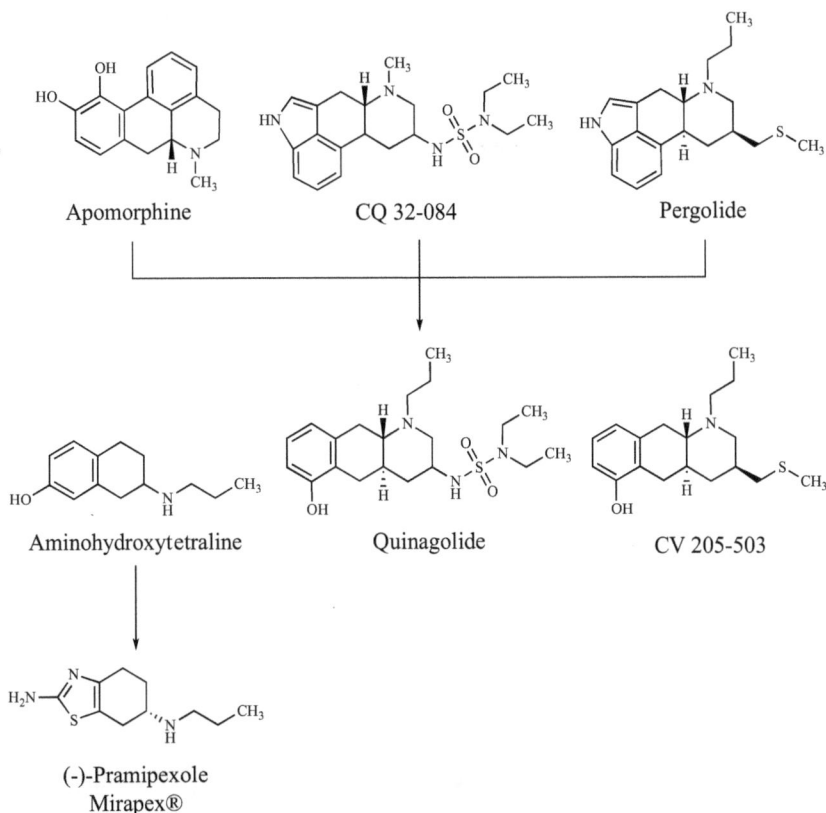

Fig. (13). Discovery of pramipexole.

During the same time period, Van Oene's group [228] investigated a number of 2-aminotetralin derivatives as centrally acting dopamine receptor agonists. While high postsynaptic effectiveness was observed with 5-hydroxyaminotetralins, aminotetralins without the 5-hydroxyl group were found to possess high dopamine autoreceptor selectivity. 2-Amino-7-hydroxytetralin (Fig. **13**) was shown to be a potent dopamine autoreceptor agonist [228].

Schneider and Mierau [227] established the absolute configurations of the enantiomers of the aminohydroxytetralin by X-ray crystallography. Based on apomorphine and aminohydroxytetralin, they discovered a series of aminothiazole derivatives as potent dopamine autoreceptor agonist. The most potent highly selective compound of this series was found to be *S*-(-)-pramipexole. The freely rotatable N-propylamino substituent in pramipexole allows an unhindered direction of the positive charge under physiological conditions that confers high potency of the compound when compared to its other congeners [227].

STUDENT SELF-STUDY GUIDE

1. What are the four cardinal motor symptoms of PD and highlight the non-motor symptoms of PD?
2. Discuss in detail the mechanisms involved in MPTP-induced neuronal cell death
3. List the enzymes involved in the biosynthesis and metabolism of dopamine and the various metabolites formed
4. Discuss dopamine receptor classification, their anatomical distribution and corresponding signal transduction mechanisms
5. Describe the four major dopaminergic pathways and corresponding dopamine actions
6. What are the neuropathological features of PD?
7. How do the *direct* and *indirect* pathways affect motor control and what is the pathophysiological basis for hypokinetic symptoms of PD?
8. Use of which medications is associated with movement disorders
9. Describe the mechanism of action and pharmacokinetics of $_L$-DOPA with particular emphasis on the rationale for use of carbidopa with $_L$-DOPA
10. Discuss adverse effects and motor complications observed with the use of $_L$-DOPA
11. What are the numerous drug interactions reported with the use of $_L$-DOPA
12. With regards to dopamine agonists, describe their mechanism of action, pharmacokinetics, FDA approved indications, and adverse effects, contraindications and precautions
13. With regards to COMT inhibitors, describe their mechanism of action, pharmacokinetics, FDA approved indications, and adverse effects, contraindications and precautions
14. With regards to selective MAO inhibitors, describe their mechanism of action, pharmacokinetics, FDA approved indications, and adverse effects, contraindications and precautions
15. Discuss the role of anticholinergics and amantadine for the management of PD symptoms

STUDENT SELF-ASSESSMENT QUESTIONS

1. A patient taking **Requip**® is most likely to experience which of the following adverse effects?

a. Sudden sleep attacks

b. Hyperglycemia

c. joint pain

d. Indigestion

e. Headache

2. Which of the following agents are contraindicated with **Azilect®**? (**Select ALL that apply**)

a. Meperidine

b. Methadone

c. Tramadol

d. Dextromethorphan

e. Levodopa

3. A patient taking _____ is most likely to experience _____ due to formation of _____ metabolites

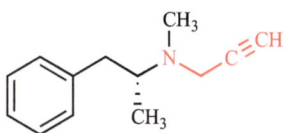

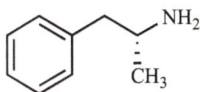

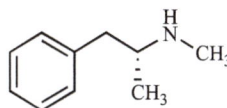

A B C

4. Which of the following is **NOT** a motor complication observed with the use of levodopa/carbidopa?

a. Wearing off

b. On/off phenomenon

c. Malignant melanoma

d. Dyskinesias

e. Dystonias

5. A patient prescribed levodopa/carbidopa should be counseled regarding (**Select ALL that apply**)

a. Occurrence of vivid dreams

b. Unusual sexual urges

c. Brown/black or dark colored urine, saliva and sweat

d. Somnolence

e. Seizures

6. Match the correct compound to the statements listed below:

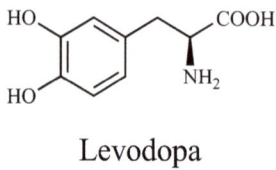

Levodopa

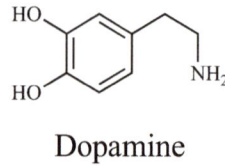

Dopamine

Statement 1 - Directly metabolized by MAO-B in the brain to DOPAC

Statement 2 - Exists predominantly in protonated form at physiologic pH

Statement 3 - Is a strongly basic compound

Statement 4 – Undergoes 3-O-methylation by COMT

Statement 5 - Penetrates BBB *via* large neutral amino acid transporter

7. Which one of the following compounds can destroy nigrostriatal dopaminergic neurons and precipitate Parkinsonism like symptoms?

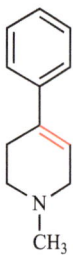

MPTP

A

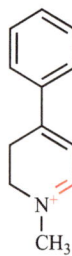

MPDP$^+$

B

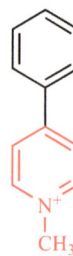

MPP$^+$

C

8. Which of the following is **NOT** a cardinal motor symptom of Parkinson Disease?

a. Resting tremor

b. Dementia

c. Bradykinesia

d. Muscular rigidity

e. Postural instability

9.Entacapone _____

a. Is a dopamine reuptake inhibitor

b. Is an anticholinergic agent

c. Blocks peripheral conversion of L-DOPA to 3-O-methyl DOPA

d. Is a direct dopamine receptor agonist

e. Is a selective irreversible inhibitor of MAO-B

10. Identify the **FALSE** statement regarding **carbidopa**

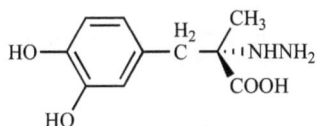

Carbidopa

a. Is a peripheral aromatic amino acid decarboxylase (AADC) inhibitor

b. Increases proportion of levodopa that crosses BBB

c. Biotransformed into dopamine in the brain

d. Does not cross blood-brain barrier (BBB)

e. Reduces nausea and vomiting associated with use of levodopa alone

CONSENT FOR PUBLICATION

Not applicable.

CONFLICT OF INTEREST

The author(s) confirms that there is no conflict of interest.

ACKNOWLEDGEMENTS

Declared none.

REFERENCES

[1]   Parkinson J. An essay on the shaking palsy. London: Sherwood, Neely, and Jone 1817; pp. 1-16.

[2]   Schapira AH, Agid Y, Barone P, *et al.* Perspectives on recent advances in the understanding and treatment of Parkinson's disease. Eur J Neurol 2009; 16(10): 1090-9.
[http://dx.doi.org/10.1111/j.1468-1331.2009.02793.x] [PMID: 19723294]

[3]   Driver JA, Logroscino G, Gaziano JM, Kurth T. Incidence and remaining lifetime risk of Parkinson disease in advanced age. Neurology 2009; 72(5): 432-8.
[http://dx.doi.org/10.1212/01.wnl.0000341769.50075.bb] [PMID: 19188574]

[4]   de Lau LM, Breteler MM. Epidemiology of Parkinson's disease. Lancet Neurol 2006; 5(6): 525-35.
[http://dx.doi.org/10.1016/S1474-4422(06)70471-9] [PMID: 16713924]

[5]   Miller IN, Cronin-Golomb A. Gender differences in Parkinson's disease: clinical characteristics and cognition. Mov Disord 2010; 25(16): 2695-703.
[http://dx.doi.org/10.1002/mds.23388] [PMID: 20925068]

[6]   Alves G, Forsaa EB, Pedersen KF, Dreetz Gjerstad M, Larsen JP. Epidemiology of Parkinson's disease. J Neurol 2008; 255(5) (Suppl. 5): 18-32.
[http://dx.doi.org/10.1007/s00415-008-5004-3] [PMID: 18787879]

[7]   Martínez-Rumayor A, Arrieta O, Sotelo J, García E. Female gender but not cigarette smoking delays the onset of Parkinson's disease. Clin Neurol Neurosurg 2009; 111(9): 738-41.
[http://dx.doi.org/10.1016/j.clineuro.2009.07.012] [PMID: 19695769]

[8]   Gómez-Esteban JC, Zarranz JJ, Lezcano E, *et al.* Influence of motor symptoms upon the quality of life of patients with Parkinson's disease. Eur Neurol 2007; 57(3): 161-5.
[http://dx.doi.org/10.1159/000098468] [PMID: 17213723]

[9]   Kapp W. The history of drugs for the treatment of Parkinson's disease. J Neural Transm Suppl 1992; 38: 1-6.
[PMID: 1491242]

[10]   McNamara P. The Pace of Innovation in Treatment of Parkinson's Disease https://www.verywellhealth.com/history-of-parkinsons-treatment-26122302019.

[11]   Kövari E, Horvath J, Bouras C. Neuropathology of Lewy body disorders. Brain Res Bull 2009; 80(4-5): 203-10.
[http://dx.doi.org/10.1016/j.brainresbull.2009.06.018] [PMID: 19576266]

[12]   Beaulieu JM, Gainetdinov RR. The physiology, signaling, and pharmacology of dopamine receptors. Pharmacol Rev 2011; 63(1): 182-217.
[http://dx.doi.org/10.1124/pr.110.002642] [PMID: 21303898]

[13]   Forno LS. Neuropathology of Parkinson's disease. J Neuropathol Exp Neurol 1996; 55(3): 259-72.
[http://dx.doi.org/10.1097/00005072-199603000-00001] [PMID: 8786384]

[14]   Pennington S, Snell K, Lee M, Walker R. The cause of death in idiopathic Parkinson's disease. Parkinsonism Relat Disord 2010; 16(7): 434-7.
[http://dx.doi.org/10.1016/j.parkreldis.2010.04.010] [PMID: 20570207]

[15]   Jankovic J, Poewe W. Therapies in Parkinson's disease. Curr Opin Neurol 2012; 25(4): 433-47.
       [http://dx.doi.org/10.1097/WCO.0b013e3283542fc2] [PMID: 22691758]

[16]   Chen JJ, Swope DM. Parkinson's disease.Pharmacotherapy A Pathophysiologic Approach. 9th ed.
       New York, NY: McGraw-Hill 2014; pp. 911-23.

[17]   Chade AR, Kasten M, Tanner CM. Nongenetic causes of Parkinson's disease. J Neural Transm Suppl
       2006; 70(70): 147-51.
       [PMID: 17017522]

[18]   Brown RC, Lockwood AH, Sonawane BR. Neurodegenerative diseases: an overview of environmental
       risk factors. Environ Health Perspect 2005; 113(9): 1250-6.
       [http://dx.doi.org/10.1289/ehp.7567] [PMID: 16140637]

[19]   Moore DJ, West AB, Dawson VL, Dawson TM. Molecular pathophysiology of Parkinson's disease.
       Annu Rev Neurosci 2005; 28: 57-87.
       [http://dx.doi.org/10.1146/annurev.neuro.28.061604.135718] [PMID: 16022590]

[20]   Boldyrev A, Bryushkova E, Mashkina A, Vladychenskaya E. Why is homocysteine toxic for the
       nervous and immune systems? Curr Aging Sci 2013; 6(1): 29-36.
       [http://dx.doi.org/10.2174/18746098112059990007] [PMID: 23237596]

[21]   Martinez TN, Greenamyre JT. Toxin models of mitochondrial dysfunction in Parkinson's disease.
       Antioxid Redox Signal 2012; 16(9): 920-34.
       [http://dx.doi.org/10.1089/ars.2011.4033] [PMID: 21554057]

[22]   Zhou C, Huang Y, Przedborski S. Oxidative stress in Parkinson's disease: a mechanism of pathogenic
       and therapeutic significance. Ann N Y Acad Sci 2008; 1147: 93-104.
       [http://dx.doi.org/10.1196/annals.1427.023] [PMID: 19076434]

[23]   Langston W. The Impact of MPTP on Parkinson's Disease Research: Past, Present, and Future. In:
       Parkinson's Disease Diagnosis and Clinical Management by Stewart A Factor and William J Weiner
       (eds). Demos Medical Publishing 2002.

[24]   Samii A, Nutt JG, Ransom BR. Parkinson's disease. Lancet 2004; 363(9423): 1783-93.
       [http://dx.doi.org/10.1016/S0140-6736(04)16305-8] [PMID: 15172778]

[25]   Doty RL, Deems DA, Stellar S. Olfactory dysfunction in parkinsonism: a general deficit unrelated to
       neurologic signs, disease stage, or disease duration. Neurology 1988; 38(8): 1237-44.
       [http://dx.doi.org/10.1212/WNL.38.8.1237] [PMID: 3399075]

[26]   Ponsen MM, Stoffers D, Booij J, van Eck-Smit BL, Wolters ECh, Berendse HW. Idiopathic hyposmia
       as a preclinical sign of Parkinson's disease. Ann Neurol 2004; 56(2): 173-81.
       [http://dx.doi.org/10.1002/ana.20160] [PMID: 15293269]

[27]   Iranzo A, Molinuevo JL, Santamaría J, *et al*. Rapid-eye-movement sleep behaviour disorder as an
       early marker for a neurodegenerative disorder: a descriptive study. Lancet Neurol 2006; 5(7): 572-7.
       [http://dx.doi.org/10.1016/S1474-4422(06)70476-8] [PMID: 16781987]

[28]   Boeve BF, Silber MH, Saper CB, *et al*. Pathophysiology of REM sleep behaviour disorder and
       relevance to neurodegenerative disease. Brain 2007; 130(Pt 11): 2770-88.
       [http://dx.doi.org/10.1093/brain/awm056] [PMID: 17412731]

[29]   Costa FH, Rosso AL, Maultasch H, Nicaretta DH, Vincent MB. Depression in Parkinson's disease:
       diagnosis and treatment. Arq Neuropsiquiatr 2012; 70(8): 617-20.
       [http://dx.doi.org/10.1590/S0004-282X2012000800011] [PMID: 22899034]

[30]   Gallagher DA, Schrag A. Psychosis, apathy, depression and anxiety in Parkinson's disease. Neurobiol
       Dis 2012; 46(3): 581-9.
       [http://dx.doi.org/10.1016/j.nbd.2011.12.041] [PMID: 22245219]

[31]   Goldman JG, Litvan I. Mild cognitive impairment in Parkinson's disease. Minerva Med 2011; 102(6):
       441-59.

[PMID: 22193376]

[32]   Seppi K, Weintraub D, Coelho M, *et al.* The Movement Disorder Society evidence-based medicine review Update: treatment for the non-motor symptoms of Parkinson's disease. Mov Disord 2011; 26 (Suppl. 3): S42-80.
[http://dx.doi.org/10.1002/mds.23884] [PMID: 22021174]

[33]   Doherty KM, van de Warrenburg BP, Peralta MC, *et al.* Postural deformities in Parkinson's disease. Lancet Neurol 2011; 10(6): 538-49.
[http://dx.doi.org/10.1016/S1474-4422(11)70067-9] [PMID: 21514890]

[34]   Mendonça DA, Jog MS. Tasks of attention augment rigidity in mild Parkinson disease. Can J Neurol Sci 2008; 35(4): 501-5.
[http://dx.doi.org/10.1017/S0317167100009197] [PMID: 18973070]

[35]   Jiménez MC, Vingerhoets FJ. Tremor revisited: treatment of PD tremor. Parkinsonism Relat Disord 2012; 18 (Suppl. 1): S93-5.
[http://dx.doi.org/10.1016/S1353-8020(11)70030-X] [PMID: 22166467]

[36]   Garcia Ruiz PJ, Catalán MJ, Fernández Carril JM. Initial motor symptoms of Parkinson disease. Neurologist 2011; 17(6) (Suppl. 1): S18-20.
[http://dx.doi.org/10.1097/NRL.0b013e31823966b4] [PMID: 22045320]

[37]   Xia R, Mao ZH. Progression of motor symptoms in Parkinson's disease. Neurosci Bull 2012; 28(1): 39-48.
[http://dx.doi.org/10.1007/s12264-012-1050-z] [PMID: 22233888]

[38]   Hallett M. Parkinson's disease tremor: pathophysiology. Parkinsonism Relat Disord 2012; 18 (Suppl. 1): S85-6.
[http://dx.doi.org/10.1016/S1353-8020(11)70027-X] [PMID: 22166464]

[39]   Grabli D, Karachi C, Welter ML, *et al.* Normal and pathological gait: what we learn from Parkinson's disease. J Neurol Neurosurg Psychiatry 2012; 83(10): 979-85.
[http://dx.doi.org/10.1136/jnnp-2012-302263] [PMID: 22752693]

[40]   Langston JW, Ballard P, Tetrud JW, Irwin I. Chronic Parkinsonism in humans due to a product of meperidine-analog synthesis. Science 1983; 219(4587): 979-80.
[http://dx.doi.org/10.1126/science.6823561] [PMID: 6823561]

[41]   Thiruchelvam M, Richfield EK, Baggs RB, Tank AW, Cory-Slechta DA. The nigrostriatal dopaminergic system as a preferential target of repeated exposures to combined paraquat and maneb: implications for Parkinson's disease. J Neurosci 2000; 20(24): 9207-14.
[http://dx.doi.org/10.1523/JNEUROSCI.20-24-09207.2000] [PMID: 11124998]

[42]   Chiba K, Trevor A, Castagnoli N Jr. Metabolism of the neurotoxic tertiary amine, MPTP, by brain monoamine oxidase. Biochem Biophys Res Commun 1984; 120(2): 574-8.
[http://dx.doi.org/10.1016/0006-291X(84)91293-2] [PMID: 6428396]

[43]   Salach JI, Singer TP, Castagnoli N Jr, Trevor A. Oxidation of the neurotoxic amine 1-methyl-4-phenyl-1,2,3,6-tetrahydropyridine (MPTP) by monoamine oxidases A and B and suicide inactivation of the enzymes by MPTP. Biochem Biophys Res Commun 1984; 125(2): 831-5.
[http://dx.doi.org/10.1016/0006-291X(84)90614-4] [PMID: 6335034]

[44]   Castagnoli N Jr, Rimoldi JM, Bloomquist J, Castagnoli KP. Potential metabolic bioactivation pathways involving cyclic tertiary amines and azaarenes. Chem Res Toxicol 1997; 10(9): 924-40.
[http://dx.doi.org/10.1021/tx970096j] [PMID: 9305573]

[45]   Watanabe H, Muramatsu Y, Kurosaki R, *et al.* Protective effects of neuronal nitric oxide synthase inhibitor in mouse brain against MPTP neurotoxicity: an immunohistological study. Eur Neuropsychopharmacol 2004; 14(2): 93-104.
[http://dx.doi.org/10.1016/S0924-977X(03)00065-8] [PMID: 15013024]

[46]   Peterson LA, Caldera PS, Trevor A, Chiba K, Castagnoli N Jr. Studies on the 1-methyl-4-phenyl-

2,3-dihydropyridinium species 2,3-MPDP+, the monoamine oxidase catalyzed oxidation product of the nigrostriatal toxin 1-methyl-4-phenyl-1,2,3,6-tetrahydropyridine (MPTP). J Med Chem 1985; 28(10): 1432-6.
[http://dx.doi.org/10.1021/jm00148a010] [PMID: 3876442]

[47]   Berry MD, Juorio AV, Paterson IA. The functional role of monoamine oxidases A and B in the mammalian central nervous system. Prog Neurobiol 1994; 42(3): 375-91.
[http://dx.doi.org/10.1016/0301-0082(94)90081-7] [PMID: 8058968]

[48]   Javitch JA, D'Amato RJ, Strittmatter SM, Snyder SH. Parkinsonism-inducing neurotoxin, N-methyl-4-phenyl-1,2,3,6 -tetrahydropyridine: uptake of the metabolite N-methyl-4-phenylpyridine by dopamine neurons explains selective toxicity. Proc Natl Acad Sci USA 1985; 82(7): 2173-7.
[http://dx.doi.org/10.1073/pnas.82.7.2173] [PMID: 3872460]

[49]   Vyas I, Heikkila RE, Nicklas WJ. Studies on the neurotoxicity of 1-methyl-4-phenyl-1,2-3,6-tetrahydropyridine: inhibition of NAD-linked substrate oxidation by its metabolite, 1-methyl-4-phenylpyridinium. J Neurochem 1986; 46(5): 1501-7.
[http://dx.doi.org/10.1111/j.1471-4159.1986.tb01768.x] [PMID: 3485701]

[50]   Soloway AH. Potential endogenous epoxides of tyrosine: causative agents in initiating idiopathic Parkinson disease. Med Hypotheses Res 2009; 5: 19-26.

[51]   aChinta SJ, Andersen JK. Redox imbalance in Parkinson's disease. Biochim Biophys Acta 2008; 1780(11): 1362-7.
[http://dx.doi.org/10.1016/j.bbagen.2008.02.005] [PMID: 18358848] Booth RG. Drugs used to treat neuromuscular disorders: Antiparkinsonian and spasmolytic agents.Foye's Principles of Medicinal Chemistry. 7th ed. Baltimore, MD: Lippincott Williams & Wilkins 2013; pp. 419-47.

[52]   Graham DG, Tiffany SM, Bell WR Jr, Gutknecht WF. Autoxidation versus covalent binding of quinones as the mechanism of toxicity of dopamine, 6-hydroxydopamine, and related compounds toward C1300 neuroblastoma cells *in vitro*. Mol Pharmacol 1978; 14(4): 644-53.
[PMID: 567274]

[53]   Graham DG. Catecholamine toxicity: a proposal for the molecular pathogenesis of manganese neurotoxicity and Parkinson's disease. Neurotoxicology 1984; 5(1): 83-95.
[PMID: 6538951]

[54]   Ramsay RR, McKeown KA, Johnson EA, Booth RG, Singer TP. Inhibition of NADH oxidation by pyridine derivatives. Biochem Biophys Res Commun 1987; 146(1): 53-60.
[http://dx.doi.org/10.1016/0006-291X(87)90689-9] [PMID: 2886124]

[55]   Soloway AH. Potential endogenous epoxides of steroid hormones: initiators of breast and other malignancies? Med Hypotheses 2007; 69(6): 1225-9.
[http://dx.doi.org/10.1016/j.mehy.2007.04.023] [PMID: 17590278]

[56]   Jenner P. Oxidative stress in Parkinson's disease. Ann Neurol 2003; 53(3) (Suppl. 3): S26-36.
[http://dx.doi.org/10.1002/ana.10483] [PMID: 12666096]

[57]   Beal MF. Mitochondria take center stage in aging and neurodegeneration. Ann Neurol 2005; 58(4): 495-505.
[http://dx.doi.org/10.1002/ana.20624] [PMID: 16178023]

[58]   Chinta SJ, Andersen JK. Redox imbalance in Parkinson's disease. Biochim Biophys Acta 2008; 1780(11): 1362-7.
[http://dx.doi.org/10.1016/j.bbagen.2008.02.005] [PMID: 18358848]

[59]   Mizuno Y, Ohta S, Tanaka M, *et al.* Deficiencies in complex I subunits of the respiratory chain in Parkinson's disease. Biochem Biophys Res Commun 1989; 163(3): 1450-5.
[http://dx.doi.org/10.1016/0006-291X(89)91141-8] [PMID: 2551290]

[60]   Mann VM, Cooper JM, Krige D, Daniel SE, Schapira AH, Marsden CD. Brain, skeletal muscle and platelet homogenate mitochondrial function in Parkinson's disease. Brain 1992; 115(Pt 2): 333-42.

[http://dx.doi.org/10.1093/brain/115.2.333] [PMID: 1606472]

[61]   Dauer W, Przedborski S. Parkinson's disease: mechanisms and models. Neuron 2003; 39(6): 889-909.
        [http://dx.doi.org/10.1016/S0896-6273(03)00568-3] [PMID: 12971891]

[62]   Haber F, Weiss J. The catalysis of hydrogen peroxide. Naturwissenschaften 1932; 20: 948-50.
        [http://dx.doi.org/10.1007/BF01504715]

[63]   Weisskopf MG, Knekt P, O'Reilly EJ, *et al.* Persistent organochlorine pesticides in serum and risk of
        Parkinson disease. Neurology 2010; 74(13): 1055-61.
        [http://dx.doi.org/10.1212/WNL.0b013e3181d76a93] [PMID: 20350979]

[64]   Betarbet R, Sherer TB, MacKenzie G, Garcia-Osuna M, Panov AV, Greenamyre JT. Chronic systemic
        pesticide exposure reproduces features of Parkinson's disease. Nat Neurosci 2000; 3(12): 1301-6.
        [http://dx.doi.org/10.1038/81834] [PMID: 11100151]

[65]   Logroscino G. The role of early life environmental risk factors in Parkinson disease: what is the
        evidence? Environ Health Perspect 2005; 113(9): 1234-8.
        [http://dx.doi.org/10.1289/ehp.7573] [PMID: 16140634]

[66]   Miller GW. Paraquat: the red herring of Parkinson's disease research. Toxicol Sci 2007; 100(1): 1-2.
        [http://dx.doi.org/10.1093/toxsci/kfm223] [PMID: 17934192]

[67]   Hatcher JM, Pennell KD, Miller GW. Parkinson's disease and pesticides: a toxicological perspective.
        Trends Pharmacol Sci 2008; 29(6): 322-9.
        [http://dx.doi.org/10.1016/j.tips.2008.03.007] [PMID: 18453001]

[68]   Coon S, Stark A, Peterson E, *et al.* Whole-body lifetime occupational lead exposure and risk of
        Parkinson's disease. Environ Health Perspect 2006; 114(12): 1872-6.
        [http://dx.doi.org/10.1289/ehp.9102] [PMID: 17185278]

[69]   Liu R, Guo X, Park Y, *et al.* Caffeine intake, smoking, and risk of Parkinson disease in men and
        women. Am J Epidemiol 2012; 175(11): 1200-7.
        [http://dx.doi.org/10.1093/aje/kwr451] [PMID: 22505763]

[70]   Kessler II, Diamond EL. Epidemiologic studies of Parkinson's disease. I. Smoking and Parkinson's
        disease: a survey and explanatory hypothesis. Am J Epidemiol 1971; 94(1): 16-25.
        [http://dx.doi.org/10.1093/oxfordjournals.aje.a121289] [PMID: 5556218]

[71]   Tanner CM, Goldman SM, Aston DA, *et al.* Smoking and Parkinson's disease in twins. Neurology
        2002; 58(4): 581-8.
        [http://dx.doi.org/10.1212/WNL.58.4.581] [PMID: 11865136]

[72]   Yu PH, Boulton AA. Irreversible inhibition of monoamine oxidase by some components of cigarette
        smoke. Life Sci 1987; 41(6): 675-82.
        [http://dx.doi.org/10.1016/0024-3205(87)90446-2] [PMID: 3613836]

[73]   Khalil AA, Davies B, Castagnoli N Jr. Isolation and characterization of a monoamine oxidase B
        selective inhibitor from tobacco smoke. Bioorg Med Chem 2006; 14(10): 3392-8.
        [http://dx.doi.org/10.1016/j.bmc.2005.12.057] [PMID: 16458520]

[74]   Nalls MA, Plagnol V, Hernandez DG, *et al.* Imputation of sequence variants for identification of
        genetic risks for Parkinson's disease: a meta-analysis of genome-wide association studies. Lancet
        2011; 377(9766): 641-9.
        [http://dx.doi.org/10.1016/S0140-6736(10)62345-8] [PMID: 21292315]

[75]   Trevitt J, Kawa K, Jalali A, Larsen C. Differential effects of adenosine antagonists in two models of
        parkinsonian tremor. Pharmacol Biochem Behav 2009; 94(1): 24-9.
        [http://dx.doi.org/10.1016/j.pbb.2009.07.001] [PMID: 19602422]

[76]   Chase TN, Bibbiani F, Bara-Jimenez W, Dimitrova T, Oh-Lee JD. Translating A2A antagonist
        KW6002 from animal models to parkinsonian patients. Neurology 2003; 61(11) (Suppl. 6): S107-11.
        [http://dx.doi.org/10.1212/01.WNL.0000095223.08711.48] [PMID: 14663022]

[77] Huang Y, Cheung L, Rowe D, Halliday G. Genetic contributions to Parkinson's disease. Brain Res Brain Res Rev 2004; 46(1): 44-70.
[http://dx.doi.org/10.1016/j.brainresrev.2004.04.007] [PMID: 15297154]

[78] Dekker MC, Bonifati V, van Duijn CM. Parkinson's disease: piecing together a genetic jigsaw. Brain 2003; 126(Pt 8): 1722-33.
[http://dx.doi.org/10.1093/brain/awg172] [PMID: 12805097]

[79] Scott WK, Nance MA, Watts RL, *et al.* Complete genomic screen in Parkinson disease: evidence for multiple genes. JAMA 2001; 286(18): 2239-44.
[http://dx.doi.org/10.1001/jama.286.18.2239] [PMID: 11710888]

[80] Hardy J, Cai H, Cookson MR, Gwinn-Hardy K, Singleton A. Genetics of Parkinson's disease and parkinsonism. Ann Neurol 2006; 60(4): 389-98.
[http://dx.doi.org/10.1002/ana.21022] [PMID: 17068789]

[81] Sidransky E, Lopez G. The link between the GBA gene and parkinsonism. Lancet Neurol 2012; 11(11): 986-98.
[http://dx.doi.org/10.1016/S1474-4422(12)70190-4] [PMID: 23079555]

[82] Ozansoy M, Başak AN. The central theme of Parkinson's disease: α-synuclein. Mol Neurobiol 2013; 47(2): 460-5.
[http://dx.doi.org/10.1007/s12035-012-8369-3] [PMID: 23180276]

[83] Polymeropoulos MH, Lavedan C, Leroy E, *et al.* Mutation in the α-synuclein gene identified in families with Parkinson's disease. Science 1997; 276(5321): 2045-7.
[http://dx.doi.org/10.1126/science.276.5321.2045] [PMID: 9197268]

[84] Krüger R, Kuhn W, Müller T, *et al.* Ala30Pro mutation in the gene encoding α-synuclein in Parkinson's disease. Nat Genet 1998; 18(2): 106-8.
[http://dx.doi.org/10.1038/ng0298-106] [PMID: 9462735]

[85] Jain S, Wood NW, Healy DG. Molecular genetic pathways in Parkinson's disease: a review. Clin Sci (Lond) 2005; 109(4): 355-64.
[http://dx.doi.org/10.1042/CS20050106] [PMID: 16171459]

[86] Maingay M, Romero-Ramos M, Kirik D. Viral vector mediated overexpression of human α-synuclein in the nigrostriatal dopaminergic neurons: a new model for Parkinson's disease. CNS Spectr 2005; 10(3): 235-44.
[http://dx.doi.org/10.1017/S1092852900010075] [PMID: 15744224]

[87] Wang G, Pan J, Chen SD. Kinases and kinase signaling pathways: potential therapeutic targets in Parkinson's disease. Prog Neurobiol 2012; 98(2): 207-21.
[http://dx.doi.org/10.1016/j.pneurobio.2012.06.003] [PMID: 22709943]

[88] Benmoyal-Segal L, Soreq H. Gene-environment interactions in sporadic Parkinson's disease. J Neurochem 2006; 97(6): 1740-55.
[http://dx.doi.org/10.1111/j.1471-4159.2006.03937.x] [PMID: 16805780]

[89] van der Merwe C, Haylett W, Harvey J, Lombard D, Bardien S, Carr J. Factors influencing the development of early- or late-onset Parkinson's disease in a cohort of South African patients. S Afr Med J 2012; 102(11 Pt 1): 848-51.
[http://dx.doi.org/10.7196/SAMJ.5879] [PMID: 23116741]

[90] Soreq L, Ben-Shaul Y, Israel Z, Bergman H, Soreq H. Meta-analysis of genetic and environmental Parkinson's disease models reveals a common role of mitochondrial protection pathways. Neurobiol Dis 2012; 45(3): 1018-30.
[http://dx.doi.org/10.1016/j.nbd.2011.12.021] [PMID: 22198569]

[91] Braak H, Del Tredici K, Rüb U, de Vos RA, Jansen Steur EN, Braak E. Staging of brain pathology related to sporadic Parkinson's disease. Neurobiol Aging 2003; 24(2): 197-211.
[http://dx.doi.org/10.1016/S0197-4580(02)00065-9] [PMID: 12498954]

[92]   Sanders-Bush E, Hazelwood L. 5-Hydroxytryptamine (Serotonin) and Dopamine.Goodman & Gilman's The Pharmacological Basis of Therapeutics. 12th ed. New York, NY: McGraw-Hill 2011; pp. 335-61.

[93]   Beaulieu JM, Gainetdinov RR. The physiology, signaling, and pharmacology of dopamine receptors. Pharmacol Rev 2011; 63(10): 182-217.
        [http://dx.doi.org/10.1124/pr.110.002642]

[94]   Kövari E, Horvath J, Bouras C. Neuropathology of Lewy body disorders. Brain Res Bull 2009; 80(4-5): 203-10.
        [http://dx.doi.org/10.1016/j.brainresbull.2009.06.018] [PMID: 19576266]

[95]   Wolters ECh, Braak H. Parkinson's disease: premotor clinico-pathological correlations. J Neural Transm Suppl 2006; 70(70) (Suppl.): 309-19.
        [PMID: 17017546]

[96]   Postuma RB, Aarsland D, Barone P, *et al.* Identifying prodromal Parkinson's disease: pre-motor disorders in Parkinson's disease. Mov Disord 2012; 27(5): 617-26.
        [http://dx.doi.org/10.1002/mds.24996] [PMID: 22508280]

[97]   Siderowf A, Lang AE. Premotor Parkinson's disease: concepts and definitions. Mov Disord 2012; 27(5): 608-16.
        [http://dx.doi.org/10.1002/mds.24954] [PMID: 22508279]

[98]   Lang AE. A critical appraisal of the premotor symptoms of Parkinson's disease: potential usefulness in early diagnosis and design of neuroprotective trials. Mov Disord 2011; 26(5): 775-83.
        [http://dx.doi.org/10.1002/mds.23609] [PMID: 21484865]

[99]   Standaert DG, Roberson ED. Treatment of central nervous system degenerative disorders.Goodman & Gilman's The Pharmacological Basis of Therapeutics. 12th ed. New York, NY: McGraw-Hill 2011; pp. 609-28.

[100]   Ehrt U, Broich K, Larsen JP, Ballard C, Aarsland D. Use of drugs with anticholinergic effect and impact on cognition in Parkinson's disease: a cohort study. J Neurol Neurosurg Psychiatry 2010; 81(2): 160-5.
        [http://dx.doi.org/10.1136/jnnp.2009.186239] [PMID: 19770163]

[101]   Yasuda T, Mochizuki H. The regulatory role of α-synuclein and parkin in neuronal cell apoptosis; possible implications for the pathogenesis of Parkinson's disease. Apoptosis 2010; 15(11): 1312-21.
        [http://dx.doi.org/10.1007/s10495-010-0486-8] [PMID: 20221696]

[102]   Olanow CW. The pathogenesis of cell death in Parkinson's disease--2007. Mov Disord 2007; 22 (Suppl. 17): S335-42.
        [http://dx.doi.org/10.1002/mds.21675] [PMID: 18175394]

[103]   Del Tredici K, Braak H. Lewy pathology and neurodegeneration in premotor Parkinson's disease. Mov Disord 2012; 27(5): 597-607.
        [http://dx.doi.org/10.1002/mds.24921] [PMID: 22508278]

[104]   Braak H, Bohl JR, Müller CM, Rüb U, de Vos RA, Del Tredici K. Stanley Fahn Lecture 2005: The staging procedure for the inclusion body pathology associated with sporadic Parkinson's disease reconsidered. Mov Disord 2006; 21(12): 2042-51.
        [http://dx.doi.org/10.1002/mds.21065] [PMID: 17078043]

[105]   Bibl M, Mollenhauer B, Esselmann H, *et al.* CSF amyloid-beta-peptides in Alzheimer's disease, dementia with Lewy bodies and Parkinson's disease dementia. Brain 2006; 129(Pt 5): 1177-87.
        [http://dx.doi.org/10.1093/brain/awl063] [PMID: 16600985]

[106]   Whitton PS. Inflammation as a causative factor in the aetiology of Parkinson's disease. Br J Pharmacol 2007; 150(8): 963-76.
        [http://dx.doi.org/10.1038/sj.bjp.0707167] [PMID: 17339843]

[107] Kim YS, Joh TH. Microglia, major player in the brain inflammation: their roles in the pathogenesis of Parkinson's disease. Exp Mol Med 2006; 38(4): 333-47.
[http://dx.doi.org/10.1038/emm.2006.40] [PMID: 16953112]

[108] Sawada M, Imamura K, Nagatsu T. Role of cytokines in inflammatory process in Parkinson's disease. J Neural Transm Suppl 2006; 70(70) (Suppl.): 373-81.
[http://dx.doi.org/10.1007/978-3-211-45295-0_57] [PMID: 17017556]

[109] Tufekci KU, Meuwissen R, Genc S, Genc K. Inflammation in Parkinson's disease. Adv Protein Chem Struct Biol 2012; 88: 69-132.
[http://dx.doi.org/10.1016/B978-0-12-398314-5.00004-0] [PMID: 22814707]

[110] Caslake R, Moore JN, Gordon JC, Harris CE, Counsell C. Changes in diagnosis with follow-up in an incident cohort of patients with parkinsonism. J Neurol Neurosurg Psychiatry 2008; 79(11): 1202-7.
[http://dx.doi.org/10.1136/jnnp.2008.144501] [PMID: 18469029]

[111] López-Sendón JL, Mena MA, de Yébenes JG. Drug-induced parkinsonism in the elderly: incidence, management and prevention. Drugs Aging 2012; 29(2): 105-18.
[http://dx.doi.org/10.2165/11598540-000000000-00000] [PMID: 22250585]

[112] Ross RT. Drug-induced parkinsonism and other movement disorders. Can J Neurol Sci 1990; 17(2): 155-62.
[http://dx.doi.org/10.1017/S0317167100030389] [PMID: 2192787]

[113] Kemp PM. Imaging the dopaminergic system in suspected parkinsonism, drug induced movement disorders, and Lewy body dementia. Nucl Med Commun 2005; 26(2): 87-96.
[http://dx.doi.org/10.1097/00006231-200502000-00002] [PMID: 15657499]

[114] Lee PE, Sykora K, Gill SS, *et al.* Antipsychotic medications and drug-induced movement disorders other than parkinsonism: a population-based cohort study in older adults. J Am Geriatr Soc 2005; 53(8): 1374-9.
[http://dx.doi.org/10.1111/j.1532-5415.2005.53418.x] [PMID: 16078964]

[115] Miller DD, Caroff SN, Davis SM, *et al.* Extrapyramidal side-effects of antipsychotics in a randomised trial. Br J Psychiatry 2008; 193(4): 279-88.
[http://dx.doi.org/10.1192/bjp.bp.108.050088] [PMID: 18827289]

[116] Chan HY, Chang CJ, Chiang SC, *et al.* A randomised controlled study of risperidone and olanzapine for schizophrenic patients with neuroleptic-induced acute dystonia or parkinsonism. J Psychopharmacol (Oxford) 2010; 24(1): 91-8.
[http://dx.doi.org/10.1177/0269881108096070] [PMID: 18801830]

[117] Cortese L, Caligiuri MP, Williams R, *et al.* Reduction in neuroleptic-induced movement disorders after a switch to quetiapine in patients with schizophrenia. J Clin Psychopharmacol 2008; 28(1): 69-73.
[http://dx.doi.org/10.1097/jcp.0b013e318160864f] [PMID: 18204344]

[118] Miletić V, Relja M. Citalopram-induced parkinsonian syndrome: case report. Clin Neuropharmacol 2011; 34(2): 92-3.
[PMID: 21407001]

[119] Grosset DG, Macphee GJA, Nairn M. Diagnosis and pharmacological management of Parkinson's disease: summary of SIGN guidelines. BMJ 2010; 340: b5614.
[http://dx.doi.org/10.1136/bmj.b5614] [PMID: 20068048]

[120] Olanow CW, Stern MB, Sethi K. The scientific and clinical basis for the treatment of Parkinson disease (2009). Neurology 2009; 72(21) (Suppl. 4): S1-S136.
[http://dx.doi.org/10.1212/WNL.0b013e3181a1d44c] [PMID: 19470958]

[121] Baumann CR. Epidemiology, diagnosis and differential diagnosis in Parkinson's disease tremor. Parkinsonism Relat Disord 2012; 18 (Suppl. 1): S90-2.
[http://dx.doi.org/10.1016/S1353-8020(11)70029-3] [PMID: 22166466]

[122] Ferreira JJ, Katzenschlager R, Bloem BR, *et al.* Summary of the recommendations of the EFNS/MDS-ES review on therapeutic management of Parkinson's disease. Eur J Neurol 2013; 20(1): 5-15.
[http://dx.doi.org/10.1111/j.1468-1331.2012.03866.x] [PMID: 23279439]

[123] Uitti RJ. Treatment of Parkinson's disease: focus on quality of life issues. Parkinsonism Relat Disord 2012; 18 (Suppl. 1): S34-6.
[http://dx.doi.org/10.1016/S1353-8020(11)70013-X] [PMID: 22166448]

[124] Politis M, Wu K, Molloy S, G Bain P, Chaudhuri KR, Piccini P. Parkinson's disease symptoms: the patient's perspective. Mov Disord 2010; 25(11): 1646-51.
[http://dx.doi.org/10.1002/mds.23135] [PMID: 20629164]

[125] Rosenthal LS, Dorsey ER. The Benefits of Exercise in Parkinson Disease. Arch Neurol 2012; 5: 1-2.

[126] Corcos DM, Comella CL, Goetz CG. Tai chi for patients with Parkinson's disease. N Engl J Med 2012; 366(18): 1737-8.
[http://dx.doi.org/10.1056/NEJMc1202921] [PMID: 22551137]

[127] Shulman LM, *et al.* Randomized Clinical Trial of 3 Types of Physical Exercise for Patients With Parkinson Disease. Arch Neurol 2012; 5: 1-8.

[128] van Nimwegen M, Speelman AD, Overeem S, *et al.* Promotion of physical activity and fitness in sedentary patients with Parkinson's disease: randomised controlled trial. BMJ 2013; 346: f576.
[http://dx.doi.org/10.1136/bmj.f576] [PMID: 23457213]

[129] París AP, Saleta HG, de la Cruz Crespo Maraver M, *et al.* Blind randomized controlled study of the efficacy of cognitive training in Parkinson's disease. Mov Disord 2011; 26(7): 1251-8.
[http://dx.doi.org/10.1002/mds.23688] [PMID: 21442659]

[130] Okun MS. Deep-brain stimulation for Parkinson's disease. N Engl J Med 2012; 367(16): 1529-38.
[http://dx.doi.org/10.1056/NEJMct1208070] [PMID: 23075179]

[131] Tawfik VL, Chang SY, Hitti FL, *et al.* Deep brain stimulation results in local glutamate and adenosine release: investigation into the role of astrocytes. Neurosurgery 2010; 67(2): 367-75.
[http://dx.doi.org/10.1227/01.NEU.0000371988.73620.4C] [PMID: 20644423]

[132] Lee KH, Hitti FL, Chang SY, *et al.* High frequency stimulation abolishes thalamic network oscillations: an electrophysiological and computational analysis. J Neural Eng 2011; 8(4)046001
[http://dx.doi.org/10.1088/1741-2560/8/4/046001] [PMID: 21623007]

[133] Poewe W, Antonini A, Zijlmans JC, Burkhard PR, Vingerhoets F. Levodopa in the treatment of Parkinson's disease: an old drug still going strong. Clin Interv Aging 2010; 5: 229-38.
[PMID: 20852670]

[134] Contin M, Martinelli P. Pharmacokinetics of levodopa. J Neurol 2010; 257 (Suppl. 2): S253-61.
[http://dx.doi.org/10.1007/s00415-010-5728-8] [PMID: 21080186]

[135] Nagatssu T. biochemistry of catecholamines. Baltimore, MD.: University Park Press 1973; pp. 289-651.

[136] Chalmers JP, Baldessarini RJ, Wurtman RJ. Effects of L-dopa on norepinephrine metabolism in the brain. Proc Natl Acad Sci USA 1971; 68(3): 662-6.
[http://dx.doi.org/10.1073/pnas.68.3.662] [PMID: 5276777]

[137] Baldessarini RJ, Fischer JE. Substitute and alternative neurotransmitters in neuropsychiatric illness. Arch Gen Psychiatry 1977; 34(8): 958-64.
[http://dx.doi.org/10.1001/archpsyc.1977.01770200096013] [PMID: 19004]

[138] Fernandez N, Garcia JJ, Diez MJ, Sahagun AM, Díez R, Sierra M. Effects of dietary factors on levodopa pharmacokinetics. Expert Opin Drug Metab Toxicol 2010; 6(5): 633-42.
[http://dx.doi.org/10.1517/17425251003674364] [PMID: 20384552]

[139] Contin M, Riva R, Martinelli P, Cortelli P, Albani F, Baruzzi A. Longitudinal monitoring of the

levodopa concentration-effect relationship in Parkinson's disease. Neurology 1994; 44(7): 1287-92.
[http://dx.doi.org/10.1212/WNL.44.7.1287] [PMID: 8035932]

[140] Bianchine JR, Shaw GM. Clinical pharmacokinetics of levodopa in parkinson's disease. Clin Pharmacokinet 1976; 1(5): 313-38.
[http://dx.doi.org/10.2165/00003088-197601050-00001] [PMID: 797502]

[141] Vogel WH. Determination and physiological disposition of p-methoxyphenylethylamine in the rat. Biochem Pharmacol 1970; 19(9): 2663-5.
[http://dx.doi.org/10.1016/0006-2952(70)90017-1] [PMID: 5478289]

[142] Tafazoli S, Spehar DD, O'Brien PJ. Oxidative stress mediated idiosyncratic drug toxicity. Drug Metab Rev 2005; 37(2): 311-25.
[http://dx.doi.org/10.1081/DMR-55227] [PMID: 15931767]

[143] Fink JS, Weaver DR, Rivkees SA, *et al.* Molecular cloning of the rat A2 adenosine receptor: selective co-expression with D2 dopamine receptors in rat striatum. Brain Res Mol Brain Res 1992; 14(3): 186-95.
[http://dx.doi.org/10.1016/0169-328X(92)90173-9] [PMID: 1279342]

[144] Durrieu G, Senard JM, Tran MA, Rascol A, Montastruc JL. Effects of levodopa and bromocriptine on blood pressure and plasma catecholamines in parkinsonians. Clin Neuropharmacol 1991; 14(1): 84-90.
[http://dx.doi.org/10.1097/00002826-199102000-00007] [PMID: 2029695]

[145] Barbeau A. The clinical physiology of side effects in long-term L-DOPA therapy. Adv Neurol 1974; 5: 347-65.
[PMID: 4155234]

[146] Barbeau A. The clinical physiology of side effects in long-term L-DOPA therapy. Adv Neurol 1974; 5: 347-65.
[PMID: 4155234]

[147] Goodwin FK. Psychiatric side effects of levodopa in man. JAMA 1971; 218(13): 1915-20.
[http://dx.doi.org/10.1001/jama.1971.03190260031009] [PMID: 5000569]

[148] Papapetropoulos S, Mash DC. Motor fluctuations and dyskinesias in advanced/end stage Parkinson's disease: a study from a population of brain donors. J Neural Transm (Vienna) 2007; 114(3): 341-5.
[http://dx.doi.org/10.1007/s00702-006-0603-6] [PMID: 17146589]

[149] Melamed E, Ziv I, Djaldetti R. Management of motor complications in advanced Parkinson's disease. Mov Disord 2007; 22(Suppl): S379-84.
[http://dx.doi.org/10.1002/mds.21680]

[150] Khor SP, Hsu A. The pharmacokinetics and pharmacodynamics of levodopa in the treatment of Parkinson's disease. Curr Clin Pharmacol 2007; 2(3): 234-43.
[http://dx.doi.org/10.2174/157488407781668802] [PMID: 18690870]

[151] Gershanik OS. Clinical problems in late-stage Parkinson's disease. J Neurol 2010; 257 (Suppl. 2): S288-91.
[http://dx.doi.org/10.1007/s00415-010-5717-y] [PMID: 21080191]

[152] Stocchi F, Jenner P, Obeso JA. When do levodopa motor fluctuations first appear in Parkinson's disease? Eur Neurol 2010; 63(5): 257-66.
[http://dx.doi.org/10.1159/000300647] [PMID: 20332641]

[153] Bouwmans AE, Weber WE. Neurologists' diagnostic accuracy of depression and cognitive problems in patients with parkinsonism. BMC Neurol 2012; 12: 37.
[http://dx.doi.org/10.1186/1471-2377-12-37] [PMID: 22702891]

[154] Stacy M. The wearing-off phenomenon and the use of questionnaires to facilitate its recognition in Parkinson's disease. J Neural Transm (Vienna) 2010; 117(7): 837-46.
[http://dx.doi.org/10.1007/s00702-010-0424-5] [PMID: 20563826]

[155] Cereda E, Barichella M, Pedrolli C, Pezzoli G. Low-protein and protein-redistribution diets for Parkinson's disease patients with motor fluctuations: a systematic review. Mov Disord 2010; 25(13): 2021-34.
[http://dx.doi.org/10.1002/mds.23226] [PMID: 20669318]

[156] Espay AJ, Fasano A, van Nuenen BF, Payne MM, Snijders AH, Bloem BR. "On" state freezing of gait in Parkinson disease: a paradoxical levodopa-induced complication. Neurology 2012; 78(7): 454-7.
[http://dx.doi.org/10.1212/WNL.0b013e3182477ec0] [PMID: 22262741]

[157] Thanvi B, Treadwell SD. Freezing of gait in older people: associated conditions, clinical aspects, assessment and treatment. Postgrad Med J 2010; 86(1018): 472-7.
[http://dx.doi.org/10.1136/pgmj.2009.090456] [PMID: 20709769]

[158] Snijders AH, Toni I, Ružička E, et al. Bicycling breaks the ice for freezers of gait. Mov Disord 2011; 15;26(3): 36-71.
[http://dx.doi.org/10.1002/mds.23530]

[159] Calabresi P, Di Filippo M, Ghiglieri V, Tambasco N, Picconi B. Levodopa-induced dyskinesias in patients with Parkinson's disease: filling the bench-to-bedside gap. Lancet Neurol 2010; 9(11): 1106-17.
[http://dx.doi.org/10.1016/S1474-4422(10)70218-0] [PMID: 20880751]

[160] Colosimo C, Martínez-Martín P, Fabbrini G, et al. Task force report on scales to assess dyskinesia in Parkinson's disease: critique and recommendations. Mov Disord 2010; 25(9): 1131-42.
[http://dx.doi.org/10.1002/mds.23072] [PMID: 20310033]

[161] Lewitt PA. Relief of parkinsonism and dyskinesia: one and the same dopaminergic mechanism? Neurology 2010; 74(15): 1169-70.
[http://dx.doi.org/10.1212/WNL.0b013e3181d90076] [PMID: 20237309]

[162] Ahmed I, Bose SK, Pavese N, et al. Glutamate NMDA receptor dysregulation in Parkinson's disease with dyskinesias. Brain 2011; 134(Pt 4): 979-86.
[http://dx.doi.org/10.1093/brain/awr028] [PMID: 21371994]

[163] Stocchi F, Tagliati M, Olanow CW. Treatment of levodopa-induced motor complications. Mov Disord 2008; 23 (Suppl. 3): S599-612.
[http://dx.doi.org/10.1002/mds.22052] [PMID: 18781681]

[164] Jankovic J, Stacy M. Medical management of levodopa-associated motor complications in patients with Parkinson's disease. CNS Drugs 2007; 21(8): 677-92.
[http://dx.doi.org/10.2165/00023210-200721080-00005] [PMID: 17630819]

[165] Sinemet [package insert] Merck & Co, Inc, Whitehouse Station, NJ; Jan 2009.

[166] Burton DA, Nicholson G, Hall GM. Anaesthesia in elderly patients with neurodegenerative disorders: special considerations. Drugs Aging 2004; 21(4): 229-42.
[http://dx.doi.org/10.2165/00002512-200421040-00002] [PMID: 15012169]

[167] Jenner P. Dopamine agonists, receptor selectivity and dyskinesia induction in Parkinson's disease. Curr Opin Neurol 2003; 16 (Suppl. 1): S3-7.
[http://dx.doi.org/10.1097/00019052-200312001-00002] [PMID: 15180131]

[168] Weiner WJ, Singer C, Sanchez-Ramos JR, Goldenberg JN. Levodopa, melanoma, and Parkinson's disease. Neurology 1993; 43(4): 674-7.
[http://dx.doi.org/10.1212/WNL.43.4.674] [PMID: 8469320]

[169] Chen JJ, Swope DM. Pharmacotherapy for Parkinson's disease. Pharmacotherapy 2007; 27(12 Pt 2): 161S-73S.
[http://dx.doi.org/10.1592/phco.27.12part2.161S] [PMID: 18041936]

[170] Hauser RA. New considerations in the medical management of early Parkinson's disease: impact of recent clinical trials on treatment strategy. Parkinsonism Relat Disord 2009; 15 (Suppl. 3): S17-21.

[http://dx.doi.org/10.1016/S1353-8020(09)70772-2] [PMID: 20082983]

[171] Tarrants ML, Denarié MF, Castelli-Haley J, Millard J, Zhang D. Drug therapies for Parkinson's disease: A database analysis of patient compliance and persistence. Am J Geriatr Pharmacother 2010; 8(4): 374-83.
[http://dx.doi.org/10.1016/j.amjopharm.2010.08.001] [PMID: 20869623]

[172] Millan MJ, Maiofiss L, Cussac D, Audinot V, Boutin JA, Newman-Tancredi A. Differential actions of antiparkinson agents at multiple classes of monoaminergic receptor. I. A multivariate analysis of the binding profiles of 14 drugs at 21 native and cloned human receptor subtypes. J Pharmacol Exp Ther 2002; 303(2): 791-804.
[http://dx.doi.org/10.1124/jpet.102.039867] [PMID: 12388666]

[173] Newman-Tancredi A, Cussac D, Audinot V, *et al.* Differential actions of antiparkinson agents at multiple classes of monoaminergic receptor. II. Agonist and antagonist properties at subtypes of dopamine D(2)-like receptor and alpha(1)/alpha(2)-adrenoceptor. J Pharmacol Exp Ther 2002; 303(2): 805-14.
[http://dx.doi.org/10.1124/jpet.102.039875] [PMID: 12388667]

[174] Elenkova A, Shabani R, Kalinov K, Zacharieva S. Increased prevalence of subclinical cardiac valve fibrosis in patients with prolactinomas on long-term bromocriptine and cabergoline treatment. Eur J Endocrinol 2012; 167(1): 17-25.
[http://dx.doi.org/10.1530/EJE-12-0121] [PMID: 22511808]

[175] Rothman RB, Baumann MH, Savage JE, *et al.* Evidence for possible involvement of 5-HT(2B) receptors in the cardiac valvulopathy associated with fenfluramine and other serotonergic medications. Circulation 2000; 102(23): 2836-41.
[http://dx.doi.org/10.1161/01.CIR.102.23.2836] [PMID: 11104741]

[176] Horvath J, Fross RD, Kleiner-Fisman G, *et al.* Severe multivalvular heart disease: a new complication of the ergot derivative dopamine agonists. Mov Disord 2004; 19(6): 656-62.
[http://dx.doi.org/10.1002/mds.20201] [PMID: 15197703]

[177] Roth BL. Drugs and valvular heart disease. N Engl J Med 2007; 356(1): 6-9.
[http://dx.doi.org/10.1056/NEJMp068265] [PMID: 17202450]

[178] Wakil A, Rigby AS, Clark AL, Kallvikbacka-Bennett A, Atkin SL. Low dose cabergoline for hyperprolactinaemia is not associated with clinically significant valvular heart disease. Eur J Endocrinol 2008; 159(4): R11-4.
[http://dx.doi.org/10.1530/EJE-08-0365] [PMID: 18625690]

[179] Vallette S, Serri K, Rivera J, *et al.* Long-term cabergoline therapy is not associated with valvular heart disease in patients with prolactinomas. Pituitary 2009; 12(3): 153-7.
[http://dx.doi.org/10.1007/s11102-008-0134-2] [PMID: 18594989]

[180] Requip [package insert]. GlaxoSmithKline Research Triangle Park: NC 2009.

[181] Morgan JC, Sethi KD. Rotigotine for the treatment of Parkinson's disease. Expert Rev Neurother 2006; 6(9): 1275-82.
[http://dx.doi.org/10.1586/14737175.6.9.1275] [PMID: 17009915]

[182] Simola N, Pinna A, Fenu S. Pharmacological therapy of Parkinson's disease: current options and new avenues. Recent Patents CNS Drug Discov 2010; 5(3): 221-38.
[http://dx.doi.org/10.2174/157488910793362421] [PMID: 20726838]

[183] Perez-Lloret S, Rey MV, Ratti L, Rascol O. Pramipexole for the treatment of early Parkinson's disease. Expert Rev Neurother 2011; 11(7): 925-35.
[http://dx.doi.org/10.1586/ern.11.75] [PMID: 21721909]

[184] Kulisevsky J, Pagonabarraga J. Tolerability and safety of ropinirole versus other dopamine agonists and levodopa in the treatment of Parkinson's disease: meta-analysis of randomized controlled trials. Drug Saf 2010; 33(2): 147-61.

[http://dx.doi.org/10.2165/11319860-000000000-00000] [PMID: 20082541]

[185] Bonuccelli U, Del Dotto P, Rascol O. Role of dopamine receptor agonists in the treatment of early Parkinson's disease. Parkinsonism Relat Disord 2009; 15 (Suppl. 4): S44-53.
[http://dx.doi.org/10.1016/S1353-8020(09)70835-1] [PMID: 20123557]

[186] Perez-Lloret S, Rascol O. Dopamine receptor agonists for the treatment of early or advanced Parkinson's disease. CNS Drugs 2010; 24(11): 941-68.
[http://dx.doi.org/10.2165/11537810-000000000-00000] [PMID: 20932066]

[187] Hayes MW, Fung VS, Kimber TE, O'Sullivan JD. Current concepts in the management of Parkinson disease. Med J Aust 2010; 192(3): 144-9.
[http://dx.doi.org/10.5694/j.1326-5377.2010.tb03453.x] [PMID: 20121682]

[188] Sprenger FS, Seppi K, Poewe W. Drug safety evaluation of rotigotine. Expert Opin Drug Saf 2012; 11(3): 503-12.
[http://dx.doi.org/10.1517/14740338.2012.678830] [PMID: 22468676]

[189] Schnitzler A, Leffers KW, Häck HJ. High compliance with rotigotine transdermal patch in the treatment of idiopathic Parkinson's disease. Parkinsonism Relat Disord 2010; 16(8): 513-6.
[http://dx.doi.org/10.1016/j.parkreldis.2010.06.009] [PMID: 20605106]

[190] Kim HJ, Jeon BS, Lee WY, et al. Overnight switch from ropinirole to transdermal rotigotine patch in patients with Parkinson disease. BMC Neurol 2011; 11: 100.
[http://dx.doi.org/10.1186/1471-2377-11-100] [PMID: 21831297]

[191] Naidu Y, Chaudhuri KR. Transdermal rotigotine: a new non-ergot dopamine agonist for the treatment of Parkinson's disease. Expert Opin Drug Deliv 2007; 4(2): 111-8.
[http://dx.doi.org/10.1517/17425247.4.2.111] [PMID: 17335409]

[192] Wüllner U, Kassubek J, Odin P, et al. Transdermal rotigotine for the perioperative management of Parkinson's disease. J Neural Transm (Vienna) 2010; 117(7): 855-9.
[http://dx.doi.org/10.1007/s00702-010-0425-4] [PMID: 20535621]

[193] Factor SA. Literature review: intermittent subcutaneous apomorphine therapy in Parkinson's disease. Neurology 2004; 62(6) (Suppl. 4): S12-7.
[http://dx.doi.org/10.1212/WNL.62.6_suppl_4.S12] [PMID: 15037666]

[194] Vaamonde J, Flores JM, Weisser R, Ibañez R, Obeso JA. The duration of the motor response to apomorphine boluses is conditioned by the length of a prior infusion in Parkinson's disease. Mov Disord 2009; 24(5): 762-5.
[http://dx.doi.org/10.1002/mds.22234] [PMID: 19224589]

[195] Apokyn[package insert] US WorldMeds, LLC, Louisville, KY; June 2012.

[196] Frucht S, Rogers JD, Greene PE, Gordon MF, Fahn S. Falling asleep at the wheel: motor vehicle mishaps in persons taking pramipexole and ropinirole. Neurology 1999; 52(9): 1908-10.
[http://dx.doi.org/10.1212/WNL.52.9.1908] [PMID: 10371546]

[197] Friedman JH, Factor SA. Atypical antipsychotics in the treatment of drug-induced psychosis in Parkinson's disease. Mov Disord 2000; 15(2): 201-11.
[http://dx.doi.org/10.1002/1531-8257(200003)15:2<201::AID-MDS1001>3.0.CO;2-D] [PMID: 10752567]

[198] Vilas D, Pont-Sunyer C, Tolosa E. Impulse control disorders in Parkinson's disease. Parkinsonism Relat Disord 2012; 18 (Suppl. 1): S80-4.
[http://dx.doi.org/10.1016/S1353-8020(11)70026-8] [PMID: 22166463]

[199] Wu K, Politis M, Piccini P. Parkinson disease and impulse control disorders: a review of clinical features, pathophysiology and management. Postgrad Med J 2009; 85(1009): 590-6.
[http://dx.doi.org/10.1136/pgmj.2008.075820] [PMID: 19892894]

[200] Calandrella D, Antonini A. Pathological gambling in Parkinson's disease: disease related or drug

related? Expert Rev Neurother 2011; 11(6): 809-14.
[http://dx.doi.org/10.1586/ern.11.70] [PMID: 21651329]

[201]   Villa C, Pascual-Sedano B, Pagonabarraga J, Kulisevsky J. Impulse control disorders and dopaminergic treatments in Parkinson's disease. Rev Neurol (Paris) 2011; 167(11): 827-32.
[http://dx.doi.org/10.1016/j.neurol.2011.01.018] [PMID: 21596410]

[202]   McKenzie GM, White HL. Evidence for the methylation of apomorphine by catechol-*O*-methy--transferase *in vivo* and *in vitro*. Biochem Pharmacol 1973; 22(18): 2329-36.
[http://dx.doi.org/10.1016/0006-2952(73)90014-2] [PMID: 4739044]

[203]   Renoux C, Dell'Aniello S, Brophy JM, Suissa S. Dopamine agonist use and the risk of heart failure. Pharmacoepidemiol Drug Saf 2012; 21(1): 34-41.
[http://dx.doi.org/10.1002/pds.2267] [PMID: 22109939]

[204]   http://www.fda.gov/Drugs/DrugSafety/ucm319779.htm

[205]   Widnell KL, Comella C. Role of COMT inhibitors and dopamine agonists in the treatment of motor fluctuations. Mov Disord 2005; 20 (Suppl. 11): S30-7.
[http://dx.doi.org/10.1002/mds.20461] [PMID: 15822107]

[206]   Bridgewater NJ. Tasmar[package insert]. Valeant Pharmaceuticals North America LLC 2014.

[207]   Stocchi F, Rascol O, Kieburtz K, *et al.* Initiating levodopa/carbidopa therapy with and without entacapone in early Parkinson disease: the STRIDE-PD study. Ann Neurol 2010; 68(1): 18-27.
[http://dx.doi.org/10.1002/ana.22060] [PMID: 20582993]

[208]   Reichmann H, Emre M. Optimizing levodopa therapy to treat wearing-off symptoms in Parkinson's disease: focus on levodopa/carbidopa/entacapone. Expert Rev Neurother 2012; 12(2): 119-31.
[http://dx.doi.org/10.1586/ern.11.203] [PMID: 22288667]

[209]   Ries V, Selzer R, Eichhorn T, Oertel WH, Eggert K. Replacing a dopamine agonist by the COMT-inhibitor tolcapone as an adjunct to L-dopa in the treatment of Parkinson's disease: a randomized, multicenter, open-label, parallel-group study. Clin Neuropharmacol 2010; 33(3): 142-50.
[http://dx.doi.org/10.1097/WNF.0b013e3181d99d6f] [PMID: 20502133]

[210]   Entacapone MT. Expert Opin Drug Metab Toxicol 2010; 6(8): 983-93.
[http://dx.doi.org/10.1517/17425255.2010.502167] [PMID: 20572781]

[211]   Elmer LW, Bertoni JM. The increasing role of monoamine oxidase type B inhibitors in Parkinson's disease therapy. Expert Opin Pharmacother 2008; 9(16): 2759-72.
[http://dx.doi.org/10.1517/14656566.9.16.2759] [PMID: 18937611]

[212]   Glezer S, Finberg JP. Pharmacological comparison between the actions of methamphetamine and 1-aminoindan stereoisomers on sympathetic nervous function in rat vas deferens. Eur J Pharmacol 2003; 472(3): 173-7.
[http://dx.doi.org/10.1016/S0014-2999(03)01906-X] [PMID: 12871751]

[213]   Hoy SM, Keating GM. Rasagiline: a review of its use in the treatment of idiopathic Parkinson's disease. Drugs 2012; 72(5): 643-69.
[http://dx.doi.org/10.2165/11207560-000000000-00000] [PMID: 22439669]

[214]   Chen JJ, Wilkinson JR. The monoamine oxidase type B inhibitor rasagiline in the treatment of Parkinson disease: is tyramine a challenge? J Clin Pharmacol 2012; 52(5): 620-8.
[http://dx.doi.org/10.1177/0091270011406279] [PMID: 21628600]

[215]   Ondo WG, Hunter C, Isaacson SH, *et al.* Tolerability and efficacy of switching from oral selegiline to Zydis selegiline in patients with Parkinson's disease. Parkinsonism Relat Disord 2011; 17(2): 117-8.
[http://dx.doi.org/10.1016/j.parkreldis.2010.10.001] [PMID: 21084213]

[216]   National Collaborating Centre for Chronic Conditions (UK). http://www.ncbi.nlm.nih.gov/pubmed/?term.

[217]   Azilect [package insert] TEVA Neuroscience, Inc, Kansas City, MO; Oct 2013.

[218] Hubsher G, Haider M, Okun MS. Amantadine: the journey from fighting flu to treating Parkinson disease. Neurology 2012; 78(14): 1096-9.
[http://dx.doi.org/10.1212/WNL.0b013e31824e8f0d] [PMID: 22474298]

[219] Schwab RS, England AC Jr, Poskanzer DC, Young RR. Amantadine in the treatment of Parkinson's disease. JAMA 1969; 208(7): 1168-70.
[http://dx.doi.org/10.1001/jama.1969.03160070046011] [PMID: 5818715]

[220] Schwab RS, England AC Jr. Amantadine HCL (Symmetrel) and its relation to Levo-Dopa in the treatment of Parkinson's disease. Trans Am Neurol Assoc 1969; 94: 85-90.
[PMID: 4907453]

[221] Blandini F, Armentero MT. New pharmacological avenues for the treatment of L-DOPA-induced dyskinesias in Parkinson's disease: targeting glutamate and adenosine receptors. Expert Opin Investig Drugs 2012; 21(2): 153-68.
[http://dx.doi.org/10.1517/13543784.2012.651457] [PMID: 22233485]

[222] Hallett PJ, Standaert DG. Rationale for and use of NMDA receptor antagonists in Parkinson's disease. Pharmacol Ther 2004; 102(2): 155-74.
[http://dx.doi.org/10.1016/j.pharmthera.2004.04.001] [PMID: 15163596]

[223] Dunkley EJ, Isbister GK, Sibbritt D, Dawson AH, Whyte IM. The Hunter Serotonin Toxicity Criteria: simple and accurate diagnostic decision rules for serotonin toxicity. QJM 2003; 96(9): 635-42.
[http://dx.doi.org/10.1093/qjmed/hcg109] [PMID: 12925718]

[224] Iqbal MM, Basil MJ, Kaplan J, Iqbal MT. Overview of serotonin syndrome. Ann Clin Psychiatry 2012; 24(4): 310-8.
[PMID: 23145389]

[225] Sneader W. Analogues of pharmacodynamics agents from fungi.Drug Discovery A History. West Sussex, England: John Wiley & Sons Ltd 2005.
[http://dx.doi.org/10.1002/0470015535]

[226] Nordmann R, Petcher TJ. Octahydrobenzo[g]quinolines: potent dopamine agonists which show the relationship between ergolines and apomorphine. J Med Chem 1985; 28(3): 367-75.
[http://dx.doi.org/10.1021/jm00381a017] [PMID: 3973904]

[227] Schneider CS, Mierau J. Dopamine autoreceptor agonists: resolution and pharmacological activity of 2,6-diaminotetrahydrobenzothiazole and an aminothiazole analogue of apomorphine. J Med Chem 1987; 30(3): 494-8.
[http://dx.doi.org/10.1021/jm00386a009] [PMID: 3820220]

[228] Van Oene JC, De Vries JB, Dijkstra D, Renkema RJW, Tepper PG, Horn AS. *In vivo* dopamine autoreceptor selectivity appears to be critically dependent upon the aromatic hydroxyl position in a series of N,N-disubstituted 2-aminotetralins. Eur J Pharmacol 1984; 102(1): 101-15.
[http://dx.doi.org/10.1016/0014-2999(84)90342-X] [PMID: 6434327]

[229] https://www.accessdata.fda.gov/drugsatfda_docs/label/2017/207145lbl.pdf

[230] https://www.accessdata.fda.gov/drugsatfda_docs/label/2019/022075s000lbl.pdf

SUBJECT INDEX

A

Abdominal 111, 268, 269, 328
　discomfort 269
　neuronal signaling 328
　pathophysiological condition 111
　thalamocortical rhythmicity 268
ACE inhibitor 91
Acetic acid 22
Acetylcholine 12, 49
　-derived cholinergic agonists 12
　receptor 49
AChE enzyme 12, 21, 22, 23, 26, 52
　regenerating 22
AChE inhibitors 24, 25, 52
　irreversible covalent 52
　phosphoric acid ester 24
　phosphorous-based covalent 25
AChEIs 37, 39, 42, 43, 49
　oral 39
Acid 11, 17, 24 47, 63, 71, 116, 249, 252, 254,
　　261, 263, 268, 274, 283, 301, 308, 311,
　　329, 330
　aminobenzoic 311
　ascorbic 63
　gamma amino butyric 249, 252
　gamma-aminobutyric 301
　homovanillic 116, 329, 330
　hypothetical carbamic 274
　inactive phenylcyclohexylglycolic 17
　isoxazolepropanoic 252
　lepropionic 283
　malonic 261
　phenylpropionic 47
　phosphoric 24
　propionic 79
　succinic 254, 268
　trifluoracetic 308
　uric 263
　vanillyl-mandelic 71
Action of local anesthetics 302
Active 18, 51, 141
　metabolites of cariprazine 141

moieties 18
　muscarinic receptor agonists 51
Adrenergic antagonists 59, 80, 86, 95, 99
Adrenergic 59, 64, 68, 78
　effect 78
　neurochemistry 59, 64
　neuron 68
Adrenergic agonist 73, 74
　and cardiac function 74
　metaproterenol 73
Adverse drug reaction (ADRs) 265, 266, 267,
　　272
Agents 10, 20, 14, 24, 25, 62, 66, 80, 81, 82,
　　87, 92, 93, 169, 170, 187, 222, 231, 258,
　　340, 342, 343, 345, 348, 349, 353
　adjunctive 343
　adrenergic 62
　antiparkinson 20
　cardioprotective 87
　cosmetic 14
　dopaminergic 340, 342, 349
　miotic 24
　oral 348
　pharmacologic 10, 25
Aggregates 324, 334
　cytoplasmic protein/lipid 324
　lipid 334
Aggregation 32, 328
　abnormal 328
Agonist activity 68, 86, 70, 73, 77, 85, 231,
　　232
　blocking orexin 232
　intrinsic 86
Agranulocytosis 110, 137, 153, 166, 269, 271
Alcohol 23, 44, 60, 191, 207, 222, 234, 238
　abuse 191
　consumption 44
　detoxification 207
Alzheimer's Disease 2, 24, 30, 31, 32, 43, 44,
　　335
　pathology 335
AMPA/Kainate receptors 258, 280
　antagonism 280
AMPA receptor 258, 295

M. O. Faruk Khan & Ashok E. Philip (Eds.)

N

allosteric (NAs) 212, 241, 242
  lipophilic state 302
Nicotine 2, 8, 9, 42, 50
  and muscarine 8, 9
  polacrilex 42
Nicotinic receptors 6, 10, 14, 27, 30, 32, 33,
    39, 301
  ganglionic 30
  neuronal 39
  stimulated presynaptic 6
  unique 10
Nigrostriatal dopaminergic neurons 361
Nigrostriatal system 338
NMDA receptor 41, 43, 122, 255, 257, 295
  activation 41
  antagonists 41, 43, 122, 257
  blockade 255, 295
Non-depolarizing muscle relaxants 16
Non-dopamine receptors 136
Non-pharmacological management 336
  of parkinson disease 336
  strategies 336
Norepinephrine 33, 59, 60, 63, 65, 99, 102,
    115, 163, 165, 166, 167, 168, 169, 171,
    172, 179, 181, 183, 202, 329, 332, 340
  infused 165
  presynaptic 169
  binding 65
  release 99, 102, 332, 340
  transferases 115
  transporter 179, 183, 202, 329
Norepinephrine reuptake 163, 164, 168, 169,
    171, 173, 179, 180, 181, 194, 197, 209
  Inhibitors (NRIs) 163, 164, 168, 169, 173,
    179, 180, 194, 197, 209
  activity 173
Norepinephrine uptake 99, 165, 166, 169, 185,
    193
  inhibiting 166, 193
Norepineprine 177
  reuptake inhibition 177
Nucleus 113, 167, 212, 213, 240, 333
  hypothalamic suprachiasmatic 213, 240
  innervates subthalamic 333
  reticular thalamic 212
Nucleus accumbens reward circuits 113

O

Obsessive-compulsive disorder (OCD) 134,
    139, 173, 181, 183, 210, 238
Oral 222, 277, 278, 347
  contraceptives 222
  formulations 278, 347
    extended-release 277
Oral bioavailability 35, 81, 135, 142, 180,
    181, 185, 189, 224, 235, 275, 277, 281,
    284
  absolute 180, 181
  relative 35
Orthostasis 142
Orthostatic 119, 120, 121, 137
  side effects 137
    ligand-binding cavity 119, 120, 121
Orthostatic hypotension 86, 130, 132, 133,
    134, 135, 139, 144, 145, 340, 346, 347,
    353
  high 144
  induced 340
  severe 86
Oxidation 76, 129, 142, 217, 218, 225, 262,
    269, 303, 310, 326
  metabolic 310
  olefinic 218
  -reduction cycle 326
Oxidative deamination reaction 188

P

Paralysis 23, 27
  peripheral muscle 27
Parasympathetic 2, 7, 9
  effects 9
  systems innervate 7
  agent 2
Parkinson Disease 322, 336, 337, 361
Parkinsonism 147, 325, 335, 336
Parkinson's Disease (PD) 20, 24, 322, 323,
    324, 325, 327, 328, 332, 333, 334, 335,
    336, 337, 356, 359
  idiopathic 20
Past medical history (PMH) 44, 191, 192, 356
Pathogenesis 122, 335
  psychotic 122
Pathways 9, 32, 39, 113, 114, 115, 137, 167,
    223, 302, 328, 331, 332, 333

U

Ubiquitin proteasome system (UPS) 335
Unconjugated plasma metabolites 40

V

Valproic acid 249, 250, 259, 260, 270, 273,
    274, 285, 286, 287, 288, 295
Vasoconstrictive effects 60, 77
Ventral tegmental area (VTA) 113, 114, 167,
    330, 331
Ventricular 85, 314
    fibrillation 314
    tachycardias 85
Ventromedial prefrontal cortex 113
Vesicular acetylcholine transporter 5
Volatile liquid vapors 306
Voltage-gated ion channels Modulation 332
Vomiting 36, 42, 132, 134, 141, 269, 274,
    275, 276, 277, 279, 339, 346

W

Weight gain 132, 133, 134, 135, 136, 139,
    140, 141, 142, 143, 145, 147, 148, 153
    antipsychotic-associated 136
Weight loss 39, 40, 280, 325, 352

Z

Zolpidem's structure 232
Zonisamide 250, 280, 281, 286, 288, 294
Zotepine 122, 147
Zyprexa 137